CONTENTS

Introduction: the management process, 1

PART 1

PLAN

Objectives, 3
Study questions, 3
Nature and purpose of planning, 4
Decision-making process, 4
  Identify problem, 4
  Explore alternatives, 5
  Choose most desirable alternative, 6
  Implement decision, 7
  Evaluate results, 7
Ethical aspects of decision making, 7
Decision-making tools, 9
  Probability theory, 9
  Simulation, models, and games, 10
  Decision trees, 11
  Program evaluation and review technique (PERT), 12
  Critical path method (CPM), 14
  Queuing theory, 14
  Linear programming, 15
  Advantages and limitations of quantitative tools for decision making, 15
    Computers, 16
Behavioral aspects of decision making, 17
  Continuum of participation, 17
Vroom and Yetton Normative Model, 19
  Types of management decision styles, 19
  Problem attributes used in the model, 21
  Individuals as decision makers, 22
    Values, 22
    Attitudes, 22
    Perceptions, 23
    Personality, 23
    Roles, 23
  Group factors in decision making, 24
    Advantages of group participation in decision making, 25
    Disadvantages of group participation in decision making, 25
  Committee aspects of decision making, 26
    Advantages of committee decision making, 27
    Disadvantages of committee decision making, 27
    Committee functioning, 27
    Techniques to facilitate group creativity, 30
    The Delphi technique, 31
Consultation, 31

Planning process, 32
   Purpose, 32
   Philosophy, 33
   Goals and objectives, 34
   Policies, 36
   Procedures, 40
   Budgets, 43
      Prerequisites to budgeting, 44
      Accounting, 44
      Operating or revenue-and-expense budgets, 45
      Capital expenditure budgets, 46
      Cash budgets, 46
      Labor or personnel budgets, 46
      Flexible budgets, 47
      Historical approach to budgeting, 47
      Standard cost, 47
      Zero-base budgeting, 48
      Periodic budgetary review, 48
      Supplementary budgets, 48
      Moving budgets, 49
      Advantages and disadvantages of flexible budgets, 49
      Advantages of budgeting, 49
      Disadvantages of budgeting, 49
   Budgeting process, 50
Cost containment, 50
Time management, 52
   Maximize managerial time, 52
   Maximize organization time, 57
      Plan, 57
      Organize, 57
      Staff, 57
      Direct, 58
      Control, 58
Marketing, 58
   Marketing concepts, 58
      Exchange, 58
      Publics, 59
      Market, 59
      Image, 59
   Marketing process, 59
      Audit, 59
      Market segmentation, 60
      Marketing mix, 61
      Implementation, 61
      Evaluation and control, 61
Learning activities, 63

PART 2

ORGANIZE

Objectives, 75
Study questions, 75

GUIDE TO NURSING MANAGEMENT

To David and Natasha

GUIDE TO
NURSING
MANAGEMENT

ANN MARRINER-TOMEY, R.N., Ph.D.

Professor, Indiana University
School of Nursing,
Nursing Management Consultant,
Indianapolis, Indiana

THIRD EDITION

with 45 illustrations

The C. V. Mosby Company

St. Louis   Washington, D.C.   Toronto   1988

MOSBY

A TRADITION OF PUBLISHING EXCELLENCE

Editor: Tom Lochhaas
Assistant editor: Laurie Sparks
Editing and production: Editing, Design & Production, Inc.
Design: Rey Umali

THIRD EDITION

Printed in the United States of America

The C. V. Mosby Company
11830 Westline Industrial Drive, St. Louis, Missouri 63146

Library of Congress Cataloging in Publication Data

Marriner-Tomey, Ann, 1943-
  Guide to nursing management.

  Includes index.
  1. Nursing services—Administration. I. Title.
[DNLM: 1. Nursing, Supervisory. WY 105 M359g]
RT89.M39 1988   362.1'73'068   87-12200
ISBN 0-8016-3207-2 (pbk.)

JS/VH/VH 9 8 7 6 5 4 3 2   05/A/606

PREFACE

Management skills are as important to nurse administrators as their clinical knowledge and skills. Unfortunately, beginning in the early 1960s, nursing education emphasized clinical skills at the expense of managerial expertise, and nurses who were interested in leadership and management had to turn to other disciplines. The bias was reflected in the dearth of writings on management in nursing literature and has been corrected only in the last decade.

Guide to Nursing Management is designed to teach nursing students the management process and to supply the practicing nurse with practical information about nursing administration. The management process—plan, organize, staff, direct, and control—is presented in detail and applied to nursing. I have drawn on hundreds of articles on such topics as staffing and quality assurance that have appeared in the nursing literature, synthesizing and organizing the content to make it readily retrievable and more meaningful. In addition I have incorporated the contributions of other disciplines' sources—notably business and the social sciences—that are superior but not readily available to most nurses. This type of approach is long overdue in nursing and should help prepare middle and top managers to deal with the tasks before them. Portions of this book have appeared as articles in the *American Journal of Nursing, Journal of Nursing Administration, Nursing Leadership, Nursing Management,* and *Supervisor Nurse.*

Since most nurses are women, female pronouns have been used in the text when referring to nurses and managers. No sexism is intended.

I wish to thank Irene Pollert for updating the blood pressure measurement procedure, Dr. Lincoln V. Lewis for reviewing the equal opportunity and affirmative action section, Valerie Brown for her consultation about computers, and Carole Owens for her typing assistance.

ANN MARRINER-TOMEY

Nature and purpose of organizing, 76
Organizational process, 76
Organizational development, 76
Organizational structure, 77
  Bureaucratic structure, 78
    Dual management, 78
    Principles of organization, 78
    Disadvantages of the bureaucratic structure, 81
  Adhocracy organizational models, 82
    Free form, 82
    Collegial management, 82
    Project management, 83
    Task forces, 86
    Matrix, 87
    Systems, 88
    Mixed model, 89
Organizational concepts, 89
  Charts, 89
  Span of management, 92
  Flat versus tall structures, 94
  Decentralization versus centralization, 95
    Delegation, 97
    Departmentalization, 101
  Line-staff relationships, 103
    Line authority, 103
    Staff authority, 103
      Assistant staff, 103
      General staff, 104
      Advisory staff, 104
      Service staff, 104
      Control staff, 104
      Functional staff, 104
    Line-staff conflict, 105
    Improving line-staff relationships, 105
Behavioral aspects of organizational change, 106
  Resistance to change, 107
  Types of change, 107
  Planning for change, 108
  Strategies for change, 110
  Job analysis, 110
  Job evaluation, 111
  Job design, 113
  Job descriptions, 115
Learning activities, 121

PART 3

STAFF

Objectives, 131
Study questions, 131
Nature and purpose of staffing, 132
Selection of personnel, 132

Recruitment and retention, 132
Screening of staff, 134
    Application forms and résumés, 134
    Letters of reference, 135
    Interview, 135
    Testing, 138
Equal opportunity and affirmative action, 139
    Orientation, 142
    Staff development, 143
        Preceptorship, 144
        Mentorship, 145
Assignment systems for staffing, 146
    Case method, 146
    Functional nursing, 146
    Team nursing, 147
    Modular nursing, 149
    Primary nursing, 149
    Leveling of staff, 150
Staffing schedules, 151
    Centralized scheduling, 152
    Decentralized staffing, 153
    Alternating or rotating work shifts, 153
    Permanent shifts, 155
    Block or cyclical scheduling, 155
    Variable staffing, 156
    Eight-hour shift, five-day workweek, 156
    Ten-hour day, four-day workweek, 156
    Ten-hour day plus five- or six-hour shift, 157
    Ten-hour shift, seven-day workweek, 157
    Twelve-hour shift, seven-day workweek, 158
    Baylor plan, 158
    Variations, 159
Variables affecting staffing, 159
    Staffing studies, 160
        Patient classification systems, 160
        Time standards, 161
        Staffing formulas, 161
    Staffing to meet fluctuating needs, 163
        Full-time staff, 163
        Part-time staff, 163
Learning activities, 166

PART 4

DIRECT

Objectives, 181
Study questions, 181
Nature and purpose of directing, 182
Theories of leadership, 182
    Great man theory, 183
    Charismatic theory, 183

Trait theory, 183
Situational theories, 184
Contingency theory, 185
Path-goal theory, 187
Life-cycle theory, 187
Integrative leadership model, 189
Development of management thought, 189
Scientific management, 189
Classic organization, 192
Human relations, 193
Behavioral science, 196
Implications for nursing administration, 204
Power and authority, 206
Sources of power, 206
Reward, 206
Coercive power, 206
Legitimate power, 206
Referent power, 206
Expert power, 206
Informal sources of power, 206
Power relations, 207
Kinds of power, 208
Authority, 208
Politics, 209
Conflict, 213
Conflict theory, 213
Sources of conflict, 213
Types of conflict, 214
Reactions to conflict, 216
Stages of conflict, 217
Conflict resolution, 218
Approaches to conflict resolution, 218
Strategies for conflict resolution, 220
Interpersonal conflict, 220
Group conflict, 221
Intergroup conflict, 229
Organizational conflict, 230
Prevention of conflict, 231
Motivation of personnel, 231
Taylor's monistic theory, 231
Maslow's hierarchy-of-needs theory, 231
Physiological needs, 232
Safety needs, 232
Love needs, 232
Esteem needs, 232
Self-actualization, 232
Alderfer's modified need hierarchy, 232
McClelland's basic needs theory, 233
Herzberg's motivation-hygiene theory or two-factor theory, 233
Argyris's psychological energy theory, 234
Vroom's expectancy theory, 234
Skinner's positive reinforcement theory, 235

Equity theory, 235
Intrinsic motivation, 236
McGregor's Theory X and Theory Y, 236
Likert's participative management theory, 237
Theory Z, 237
Historical development of motivation theory, 238
Job satisfaction, 239
Communication, 241
Communication process, 241
Communication systems, 242
Downward communication, 243
Upward communication, 243
Lateral communication, 244
Diagonal communication, 245
The grapevine, 245
Barriers to communication, 246
Improving communications, 247
Communicating with difficult people, 249
Assertiveness, 252
Barriers to assertiveness, 252
Transactional analysis, 253
Life positions, 258
Assertive techniques, 259
Learning activities, 263

PART 5

CONTROL

Objectives, 281
Study questions, 281
Nature and purpose of controlling, 282
Management of change, 282
Strategies for effecting change, 282
Empirical-rational strategies, 282
Normative re-educative strategies, 282
Power-coercive strategies, 283
Process of change, 283
Types of change, 284
Coercive change, 284
Emulative change, 284
Indoctrination, 284
Interactional change, 284
Natural change, 284
Socialization change, 284
Technocratic change, 284
Planned change, 284
Role of the manager as change agent, 285
Force-field analysis, 285
MAPS design technology, 287
Evaluation of personnel, 287
Purposes, 287

Common errors in evaluation, 288
Methods of evaluation, 289
  Anecdotal notes, 289
  Checklists, 289
  Rating scales, 289
  Ranking, 292
  Management by objectives, 293
  Peer review, 295
Appraisal interview, 296
Appraisal reports, 299
Problem employees, 300
  Substance abusers, 300
  Angry or withdrawn employees, 301
  Decreased productivity, 302
  Absenteeism, 302
  Terminating employees, 303
  Employee counseling, 304
Outplacement counseling, 305
Discipline of personnel, 307
  Need for discipline, 307
  Principles of disciplinary action, 308
    Positive attitude, 308
    Investigate carefully, 308
    Be prompt, 308
    Pocket privacy, 309
    Focus on the act, 309
    Enforce rules consistently, 309
    Be flexible, 309
    Advise the employee, 309
    Take corrective, constructive action, 309
    Follow up, 309
  Penalties, 310
    Oral reprimand, 310
    Written reprimand, 310
    Other penalties, 310
  Components of a disciplinary action program, 311
    Codes of conduct, 311
    Authorized penalties, 311
    Records of offenses and corrective measures, 311
    Right of appeal, 311
Modification of employee behavior, 311
  Reinforcement, 312
  Shaping, 312
  Extinction, 313
  Punishment, 313
  Behavior modification for the employee with a performance problem, 314
Labor relations, 316
  Why employees join unions, 316
  Labor law, 316
    Unfair labor practices by management, 317
    Unfair labor practices by unions, 317
  Unionization, 318

Organizing phase, 318
Recognition phase, 318
Contract negotiation phase, 320
Contract administration, 321
Arbitration, 322
Decertification, 323
Nurse managers' role in collective bargaining, 324
Advantages and disadvantages of collective bargaining, 324
Program evaluation, 324
Calendar of events, 325
Program evaluation model, 325
Sources of internal and external invalidity, 326
Research designs, 329
Experimental designs, 329
Pretest-posttest control group, 329
Posttest-only control group, 330
Solomon four group, 330
Factoral design, 330
Quasi-experimental designs, 330
Time series, 331
Equivalent-time-samples design, 331
Nonequivalent control group, 331
Counterbalanced designs, 331
Separate-sample pretest-posttest design, 332
Separate-sample pretest-posttest control group, 332
Multiple time-series design, 332
Recurrent institutional cycle design, 333
Regression-discontinuity analysis design, 333
Quality assurance, 333
Committee selection and functions, 334
Conceptual framework, 334
Review of the literature, 335
Instrument development, 336
Validity and reliability, 337
Methods of data collection, 338
Sampling, 339
Analysis of data, 341
Expected level of performance, 341
Tools for control, 341
Statistics, reports, and observations, 341
Audits, 341
Inventory control, 342
Break-even calculations, 344
Stress management, 345
Source of stress, 345
Stress response, 346
Symptoms of stress, 346
Stress control, 347
Values' clarification, 347
Goal setting, 348
Stress avoidance and regulation, 348
Time blocking, 348

Time management, 348
Assertiveness, 349
Feeling pauses, 349
Inner shouting, 350
Anchoring, 350
Sorting, 350
Compartmentalization, 351
Environmental changes, 351
Humor, 351
Centering, 351
Nutrition, 352
Exercise, 352
Sleep, 353
Relaxation, 353
   Abdominal breathing, 353
   Massage, 353
   Progressive relaxation, 354
   Biofeedback, 355
   Autogenic training—self-hypnosis, 355
   Meditation, 356
   Visualization and mental imagery, 356
   Poetry, 356
   Music, 357
   Baths, 357
Enhancing self-esteem, 357
Support groups, 357
Learning activities, 359

Appendix, 377

INTRODUCTION
The Management Process

The management process is universal. It is used in one's personal life as well as one's professional life. One applies it to management of oneself, a patient, a group of patients, or a group of workers. Although management process, principles, and tools can be used in a variety of situations, this presentation will focus on the process in nursing administration and the management of an agency and workers.

The management process is composed of five major functions: (1) planning, (2) organizing, (3) staffing, (4) directing, and (5) controlling. Planning is the first function, and all other functions are dependent on it. Conceptual thinking and problem solving are crucial. Data are gathered and analyzed so that alternatives can be identified and evaluated in the decision-making process. The manager must forecast what is needed for the future, set objectives for the desired results, and develop strategies for how to achieve the goals. Priorities must be set, and the strategies need to be sequenced in a time frame to accomplish the goals. Policies and procedures are developed in the planning phase. Policies are standing decisions about recurring matters, and procedures standardize methods. Budgets are used as planning and controlling tools to allocate resources. Planning is the basis for time management, which will in turn facilitate the implementation of the plans.

Organizing is the second managerial function. Having planned, the manager now organizes so that personnel can implement the plans with efficiency and effectiveness. An organizational structure is established and shown on an organizational chart. Relationships are delineated, depicted on the organizational chart, and described in position descriptions that define the scope of responsibilities, relationships, and authority. Job analysis, evaluation, and design help define qualifications for persons in each position on the organizational chart.

Staffing includes recruiting, selecting, orienting, and developing personnel to accomplish the goals of the organization. It also involves determining assignment systems, such as case method, functional, team, modular, or primary nursing, and selecting staffing schedules to meet the needs of the clients, personnel, and institution. There are many variables to be considered, and the more accurately they are assessed, the higher the probability of containing costs while providing high-quality care.

After the manager has planned, organized, and staffed, she must direct personnel and activities to accomplish the goals of the organization. Knowledge of one's leadership style, managerial philosophy, sources of power and authority, and political strategies is important. To get work done by others, the manager must resolve conflicts and motivate and discipline staff. All these tasks require good communication skills and assertive behavior.

Controlling is the last step in the management process. It ensures progress toward objectives according to plan and involves setting standards, measuring performance against those standards, reporting the results, taking corrective actions, and rewarding perfomance as appropriate. Controls should be designed for specific situations and should reveal potential or actual deviations promptly enough for corrective action to be effective.

PART 1

PLAN

OBJECTIVES

After completing this part, the reader will be able to:

Identify five steps in the decision-making process.

Describe at least three decision-making tools.

Explain the relationship between purpose, philosophy, goals, and policies.

Distinguish between different types of budgets.

Manage time effectively.

STUDY QUESTIONS

1

What are the steps in the decision-making process?

2

What tools can be used to minimize the uncertainty of decisions?

3

What are the advantages and disadvantages of group participation in decision making?

4

What is the relationship between purpose, philosophy, goals, and policies?

5

What are the advantages and disadvantages of budgets?

6

How does the reader waste time?

7

What time-saving tips could the reader use?

NATURE AND PURPOSE OF PLANNING

Planning is the first function of management. All other management functions—organizing, staffing, directing, and controlling—are dependent on planning. The nurse manager needs to be familiar with the decision-making process
and tools so that she can identify the purpose of the institution, state the philosophy, define goals and objectives, outline policies and procedures, prepare
budgets to implement her plans, and effectively manage her time and that of
the organization.

DECISION-MAKING PROCESS

Decision making, the process of selecting one course of action from alternatives, is a continuing responsibility of the nurse manager. She is confronted
by a variety of situations. Hospital or agency policies provide guidelines for
dealing with routine situations. Exceptional instances can make decisions more
difficult and may require a mature sense of judgment. Problem solving is a skill
that can be learned, and because staff nurses can learn by observing their superiors, good decision making by the supervisor may do more than solve immediate problems; more important for the long term, it can foster good decision
making by staff nurses.

Decision making is the scientific problem-solving process. It involves identifying the problem, analyzing the situation, exploring alternatives and considering their consequences, choosing the most desirable alternative, implementing
the decision, and evaluating the results.

Identify problem

The first step in the decision-making process is defining the problem. What
is wrong? Where is improvement needed? Sometimes the problem seems quite
obvious and can be dealt with routinely. If the employee repeatedly reports late
to work or abuses the privilege of sick leave, the supervisor can respond in
accordance with agency policies. However, when the supervisor is concerned
only with the infraction, she may be dealing with the effect rather than the cause
of the problem. Consequently, similar situations may continue to occur. It is
important to define the factors that are causing the problem. For instance, two
staff nurses may each complain about the intrusion of the other into her work.
Initially the problem may appear to be a personality clash or a political power
struggle. However, the cause may be the manager's failure to define the job
responsibilities of each nurse. As long as the supervisor concentrates on the
symptom instead of the problem, the difficulties will continue to arise. It is only

when the real problem has been identified that effective decision making can be initiated.

The nurse manager can identify the problem by analyzing the situation. All too frequently, decisions are made and implemented before all the facts have been gathered. To avoid this the supervisor should have a questioning attitude. What is the desirable situation? What are the presenting symptoms? What are the discrepancies? Who is involved? When? Where? How? With answers to these questions the supervisor can develop tentative hypotheses and test them against what she knows. Progressive elimination of hypotheses that fail to conform to the facts reduces the number of causes to be considered. Feasible hypotheses should be further tested for causal validity. When the manager believes she has identified the cause or causes of the problem by analyzing available information, she should begin exploring possible solutions.

Explore alternatives

There are usually a number of ways to solve a problem. Some may be quick and economical but not as effective as their alternatives. Others may be more effective but less economical. If various alternatives are not explored, the course of action is limited.

When solving a problem, the manager should determine first if the situation is covered by policy. If it is not, she must draw on her education and experience for facts and concepts that will help her determine alternatives. Drawing on one's experience is probably the most common approach to solving problems, but it may be inadequate. The more experience the manager has had, the more alternatives may be suggested that can help solve a variety of problems. However, health care is changing rapidly, and solutions to yesterday's problems may not work today. Consequently, the manager should look beyond her own experiences and learn how others are solving similar problems. This can be done through continuing education, professional meetings, review of the literature, correspondence with others, and brainstorming with staff. Inductive and deductive reasoning are both appropriate.

It is during this step that creative solutions to problems may be developed. The creative process has steps similar to the problem-solving process, but the emphasis is different. Decision making stresses choice of a solution, while the creative process emphasizes the uniqueness of the solution. Creativity is a latent quality, activated when a person becomes motivated by the need for self-expression or by the stimulation of a problem situation. Thus the first phase of the creative process is a felt need. Similarly, when a decision maker is confronted with a problem, she starts seeking a solution.

The second phase of creative problem solving is a work stage known as preparation, from which creative ideas emerge. Innovation is partially dependent on the number of options considered. By exploring relationships among potential solutions, one may identify additional solutions. Many decisions are made after slight preparation and therefore result in commonplace solutions. Superficial analysis of obvious information does not facilitate creative answers. Extensive use of libraries for data collection is useful. The creative person may take notes on readings, develop them into files with other clippings and ideas, review these materials, and combine the most appropriate aspects of old solutions into new answers.

Incubation, the third phase, is a period for pondering the situation. Repetition of the same thoughts, with no new ideas or interpretations, is a sign of fatigue and indicates that it is a good time to start the incubation period. Switching one's attention provides a necessary respite, and yet the unconscious mind continues to deal with the problem. A time should be set to reexamine the situation and review the data collected during the preparation phase.

Illumination is the discovery of a solution. It may come to mind in the middle of the night or during the performance of another task. It is recommended that the idea be written down so the details can be preserved. Having paper and pencil readily available at all times (including in the bedside stand) is helpful.

It is rare for an illumination to be ready for adoption. Verification, the fifth and final phase of creative decision making, is the period of experimentation when the idea is improved through modification and refinement. The advantages and disadvantages of each alternative must be weighed. Resources and constraints such as manpower, finances, facilities, and equipment have to be evaluated, and potential technical and human problems should be considered. Some decisions have failed at implementation because potential problems were not anticipated and dealt with. It would be unfortunate for an otherwise good alternative to be rejected for a disadvantage that could be easily overcome. By comparing the advantages and disadvantages of her options, the manager can choose the most desirable alternative.

Choose most desirable alternative

The number and quality of alternatives are largely dependent on the creativity and productivity of the manager and her staff. Leadership that prevents immediate acceptance of an apparently obvious solution and facilitates group exploration of decision-making opportunities (such as problems to solve) usually increases the number of alternatives and the quality of problem solving.

Anxiousness to reach a decision may lead to premature solutions; on the other hand, only considering a few alternatives because of haste blocks good decisions. Avoidance of the real problem, lack of clear problem definition, lack of data, early statement of attitude by a status figure, mixing idea generation and idea evaluation, lack of staff commitment because the superior who makes the decision does not implement it, or decisions made by large groups also interfere with quality solutions.

One alternative is not always clearly superior to all others. The supervisor must try to balance multiple factors such as patient safety, staff acceptance, morale, public acceptance, cost, and risk of failure. Criteria for calculating the value of decisions are useful. The following questions may be asked: Will this decision accomplish the stated objectives? If it does not, it should not be enforced and another option should be used. Does it maximize effectiveness and efficiency? One should use available resources before seeking outside assistance. Finally, can the decision be implemented? If not, it obviously will not solve the problem.

Implement decision

After a decision has been made, it needs to be implemented. A decision that is not put into action is useless. The manager will need to communicate the decision to appropriate staff in a manner that does not arouse antagonism. The decision and procedures for its implementation can be explained in an effort to win the cooperation of those responsible for its implementation. The supervisor will need to select the staff to implement the decision and provide the direction to initiate action. She may need to control the environment so staff can function as planned. Once the decision has been implemented, it should be evaluated.

Evaluate results

The final step of decision making is evaluation of the results of the implementation of the chosen alternative. Evaluative criteria may need to be developed. Audits, checklists, ratings, and rankings are tools that can be used to review and analyze the results. Because solutions to old problems sometimes create new problems, additional decisions may need to be made and evaluated.

ETHICAL ASPECTS OF DECISION MAKING

Ethics is a moral philosophy, a science of judging the relationship of means to ends, and the art of controlling means so they will serve human ends. It involves conflict, choice, and conscience. When there is a conflict, there is a choice between conflicting alternatives. The choice is influenced by values. Values are learned first from important adults and are modified by association with people of different values. Value modification and reinforcement is a lifelong process. A value is consciously prized and cherished. It is freely chosen from alternatives and is acted on in a variety of ways. Ethical choices must also consider wants, needs, and rights. People may want what they do not need. Someone may want a dessert but not need it. In fact, it may be harmful to the person. People often need what others also need. One may need food to prevent starvation. She may have a right to receive food from people who have plenty, but not from someone who would starve without it. That would infringe on the other person's rights. Duty and right are correlated. It is one's duty to protect rights. A legal obligation is legislated, but it may not be ethical. A moral dilemma occurs when a decision has equally unsatisfactory alternatives.

There are several ethical positions that do not solve dilemmas. However, they do provide ways to structure and clarify them. *Utilitarianism* is a community-oriented position that focuses on the consequences and prefers the greatest amount of good and happiness for the most people, or the least amount of harm. In contrast, *egoism* seeks solutions that are best for oneself without regard for others. One's own pleasure is the concern. *Formalism* considers the nature of the act and the related principles without thought to one's personal position or the consequences of the actions: be honest; remember the golden rule. *Rule* ethics expects obedience to laws, rules, professional codes, and authority. *Fairness* considers distribution of benefits and liabilities from the viewpoint of the least advantaged. Benefit to the least advantaged is the norm in this decision making.

There are also models for ethical relationships. With the *priestly model*, the manager is paternalistic and makes decisions without considering others' values or seeking others' input. Although nurses may have expertise that qualifies them to make some decisions, they have no right to make moral decisions affecting other people. Autocratic leadership may use the priestly model. The *engineering model* suggests that one person presents facts to another and sets aside her own code of ethics to do what the other wants. Staff working for line authority may be an example of this model. The *contractual model* provides a contract that identifies general obligations and benefits for two or more people. It deals with the morals of both parties and is appropriate for superior-subordinate relationships. Under the *collegial model*, individuals share mutual goals and reach decisions through discussion and consensus. When there are shared values, this model helps build teams and minimize conflict.*

To make an ethical decision, one must first consider what is intended to be a means and an end and then determine what good or evil is found in the means and the end. If a major evil is intended either as a means or an end, it is an unethical decision.

If the ramifications of the decision are probable, but not willed as a means or an end, there are several factors to consider. The good or evil of each alter-

---

*Robert Veatch's models for ethical medicine are discussed in Aroskar, M.A.: Ethics of nurse-patient relationships, Nurse Educ. **5**:18-20, March-April 1980.

native should be evaluated. A necessary good outweighs a useful good. Paying workers wages outweighs paying for profit sharing. Urgency increases the necessity; Therefore, physical needs must be met before self-actualizing needs. An agency should provide adequate wages for food and shelter before providing continuing education. The probability of an outcome should be considered. A possible negative outcome is out-weighed by a probable good. One will work to earn a living even though there is a slight risk of back strain. The intensity of one's influence is considered because her impact on someone else may have undesirable consequences. For instance, if someone is fired for incompetence, it may cause a hardship for her family. If the supervisor did not tell her what was expected or how to do the job, the supervisor would have been a considerable factor in that employee's poor job performance. Firing the employee would seem evil. If, however, the worker is frequently tardy or absent through no fault of the supervisor, the consequences of firing the worker seem justified. If there is no proportionate reason for permitting an evil, the act is unethical. If there is an alternative that provides more good and less risk of evil, it should be chosen. If there is not, there is proportionate reason for risking an evil.

DECISION-MAKING TOOLS

Most decisions involve varying degrees of uncertainty. Managers use research of various kinds to minimize the uncertainty of their decisions.

Probability theory

Probability theory can be applied when risk or uncertainty is present in a decision. It operates on the assumption that factors occur in accordance with a predictable pattern. For example, if a person tosses a coin 200 times, we can predict that it will show heads 100 times and tails 100 times. Deviations can be set within a predictable margin. Inferences based on statistical analysis of existing data can be used to predict results.

Sometimes a sample of the population may be analyzed. Measures of probable error become increasingly important when one is dealing with a sample because the smaller the probable error, the greater the amount of confidence that can be put in the findings. One must consider the reliability of sampling and the additional time and expense involved in collecting more information. Probability can become a substitute for otherwise unknown information. When probabilities can be substituted for unknowns, the margin of error for the solution may be limited but not completely removed.

There are three criteria that assume that previous experience is necessary to work with probability. In the "maximax" criterion the manager maximizes the maximum possible gain. The manager is very optimistic about the factors influencing her decision and selects the option from which she can achieve the best results. This is a dangerous criterion in that it does not consider possible complications. When applying the "maximin" criterion, the supervisor is very pessimistic and expects the worst possible results. She selects the option that allows her to maximize the least favorable results. She considers what complications can occur for each option, assumes that everything that can go wrong will go wrong, and selects the alternative that offers the best results when everything possible goes wrong. The "minimax" criterion can be applied when the supervisor has made a decision she regrets. Something unexpected prevented her from achieving the most favorable results. The supervisor then subtracts the complication from the most favorable results and tries to minimize her regrets.

Uncertainty arises when the supervisor has to make a decision for which there is no historical data on which to calculate probabilities. Under uncertain conditions there is no best criterion to apply. The supervisor considers objective and subjective options according to her own optimistic or pessimistic philosophy and guesses which alternative will render the most desirable results.

Simulation, models, and games

Simulation is a way of using models and games to simplify problems by identifying the basic components and using trial and error to determine a solution. Through simulation, the manager may compare alternatives and their consequences. The computer may be used to help solve simulations. These methods may be used to study organizational changes, scheduling, assembly line management, and time sequences.

A model represents something else, most commonly objects, events, processes, or systems. It is a technique of abstraction and simplification for studying something under varying conditions. Manipulation is used to test the impact of proposed changes on the system without disturbing the subject of the model. Almost all quantitative methods used to guide decision making are models. They are particularly useful because of their convenience and low cost as compared to manipulating real occurrences. Although models vary considerably in the accuracy with which they represent real situations, they increase predictive capabilities over such methods as guesswork and intuition.

Models are developed to describe, explain, and predict phenomena. The critical element of model building is conceptualization. Consequently, models can provide abstractions that facilitate communication. Models vary in the degree of abstraction used. A life-size mannequin is a realistic model that nursing students use to learn to make occupied beds. A model of a building or a piece of equipment built to scale is quite concrete, whereas blueprints or photographs, organizational charts, and mathematical models are abstract.

The more variables added to the model, the more realistic but cumbersome it becomes. The objective of modeling is to provide a simplified, abstract version of reality. The manager must strive for the appropriate level of abstractness. She may base her decision on an oversimplified model if she does not attempt to expand her knowledge of the situation. Simplified models may be useful for quantitative analysis and prediction. But one must be cautious, because a person with the least knowledge about a situation may be the most certain about how to solve the problem. If description and understanding are important, then more comprehensive models should be developed. Continuing to research a problem may contribute to a more realistic model, but it may also delay the decision too long. The cost of gathering additional information may be prohibitive. Therefore, the cost of model refinement needs to be balanced against the benefits obtained.

Game theory is a simulation of system operations. The player tries to develop a strategy that will maximize gains and minimize losses, regardless of what the competitor does. War games are commonly used to train personnel and to test plans and equipment under field conditions. Management games are used primarily to train personnel rather than to solve competitive problems. They are particularly useful for training in decision making by simulating real-life operations in a laboratory setting.

Decision trees

A decision tree is a graphic method that can help the supervisor visualize the alternatives available, outcomes, risks, and information needs for a specific problem over a period of time. It helps her to see the possible directions that actions may take from each decision point and to evaluate the consequences of a series of decisions. The process begins with a primary decision having at least two alternatives. Then the predicted outcome for each decision is considered, and the need for further decisions is contemplated. The matrix resembles a tree as the decision points are diagramed (Fig. 1-1).

The results diagramed on the tree are founded on the manager's experience and judgment but may be supported by computational data. For complex problems, probability statistics may be used to explore further factors that favor or oppose expected events. Although the decision tree does not depict an obviously correct decision, it allows the supervisor to base her decision on a consideration of various alternatives and their probable consequences. It helps her realize that subsequent decisions may be dependent on future events. Decision trees are useful for short- and medium-range planning as well as for decision making. Unfortunately, decision trees for more than 2 or 3 years become cumbersome and speculative.

In Fig. 1-2 the nursing staff decides to have a ward picnic for the psychiatric patients. The alternatives are to have the picnic indoors or outdoors, and the chance events are rain or no rain. If the picnic is scheduled indoors and it rains,

Fig. 1-1. Decision tree.

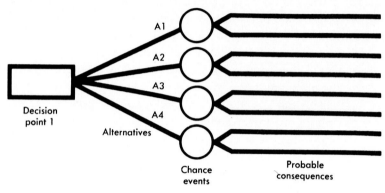

Fig. 1-2. Decision tree for psychiatric ward picnic.

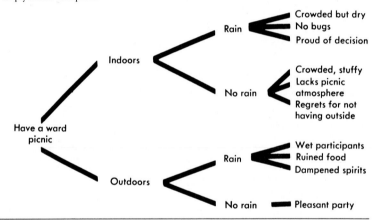

the patients may be crowded but dry; there would be no bugs; and the staff would feel proud of their decision. If the picnic is scheduled indoors and it does not rain, the patients may feel crowded; the room may seem stuffy; the party will lack a picnic atmosphere; and the staff may have regrets for not scheduling the picnic outside. On the other hand, if the picnic is scheduled outdoors and it rains, the participants will get wet; the food will be ruined; and spirits will be dampened. If the picnic is scheduled outdoors and it does not rain, it will be a pleasant experience.

Program evaluation and review technique (PERT)

PERT is a network system model for planning and control under uncertain conditions. It involves identifying the key activities in a project, sequencing the

Fig. 1-3. PERT model. This PERT model indicates that subtask *1* must be completed before *2, 3,* and *4* can be done; *2, 3,* and *4* before *5, 5* before *6* and *7, 6* before *9; 6* and *7* before *8, 8* and *9* before *10*. A coding system can be used to determine what the numbers mean. For example, 1 = program planned, 2 = staff informed. Arrows show direction of work flow. Optimistic, most likely, pessimistic, and expected times are recorded for each activity.

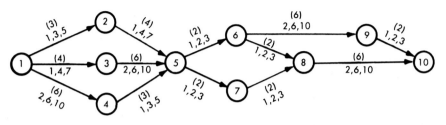

activities in a flow diagram, and assigning the duration time for each phase of the work. It is particularly appropriate for one-of-a-kind projects that involve extensive research and development.

PERT recognizes that certain tasks must be completed before the total project can be completed and, furthermore, that subtasks must be completed before others can be started. The key events are identified. They may be numbered, labeled, or numbered and labeled on the flow chart. The activities that cause the progress from one event to another are indicated by arrows with the direction of the arrow showing the direction of the work flow.

PERT also deals with the problem of uncertainty with respect to time by estimating the time variances associated with the expected time of completion of the sub-tasks. Three projected times are determined: (1) the optimistic time (t_o), which estimates the completion time without complications; (2) the most likely time (t_m), which estimates the completion time with normal problems; and (3) the pessimistic time (t_p), which estimates the completion time given numerous problems. Thus the shortest, average, and longest times needed to complete an activity are calculated. The expected time (t_e) is calculated from these figures using the following formula:

$$t_e = \frac{t_o + 4(t_m) + t_p}{6}$$

If the optimistic time is 2 weeks, the most likely time 4 weeks, and the pessimistic time 6 weeks, the expected time would be 4 weeks:

$$t_e = \frac{2 \text{ weeks} + 4(4 \text{ weeks}) + 6 \text{ weeks}}{6} = \frac{24 \text{ weeks}}{6} = 4 \text{ weeks}$$

The PERT model helps the manager determine priorities (Fig. 1-3). Use of resources can be considered when setting priorities. Assignments may be changed temporarily, overtime may be allowed, or temporary help hired to facilitate the activity flow and to manipulate the time required to move from one event to another.

Critical path method (CPM)

CPM, closely related to PERT, calculates a single time estimate for each activity, the longest possible time. A cost estimate is figured for both normal and crash operating conditions. Normal means the least-cost method, and crash refers to conditions in less than normal time. Simple sequences can be worked out manually and more complex ones by computer. CPM is particularly useful where cost is a significant factor and experience provides a basis for estimating time and cost. Managers can observe the critical path and compare the progress to the projected dates.

Network analysis techniques facilitate planning and result in objective plans. They make it possible to identify the critical path and show interrelationships between parts, thus facilitating improvements in structure and communications. They are particularly useful for task force or project forms of organization and for projects.

Queuing theory

Queuing theory deals with waiting lines or intermittent servicing problems. It is a mathematical technique for determining the most efficient balance of factors related to intermittent service. It is particularly applicable when units to receive service arrive in a random fashion, but the time required for service is predictable. It balances the cost of waiting versus the prevention of waiting by increasing service. It acknowledges that although delays are costly, eliminating them may be even more costly. By decreasing or eliminating the waiting line to reduce waiting line costs, there is an increase in cost of labor and physical facilities. The time of arrival is an important factor to consider in determining the optimal size of facilities and staffing. Sometimes actual observations may be made and tallies kept of how many units or clients require service each hour of the workday or during certain seasons. For example, through observation one may determine that many junior and senior high school students attend VD or family planning clinics during after-school hours. The VD or family planning clinics in a small college community may have fewer demands for service during holiday seasons and summer vacation because many students have returned to their hometown communities. The supervisor may adjust staffing accordingly. In the hospital setting, the supervisor may choose to use part-time people or split shifts to help compensate for an increased work load during the morning when most patients are bathed and once-a-day treatments are given, and again during late afternoon or early evening when most patients are admitted.

When observations cannot be made for an extended period to determine a stable pattern of work load, the Monte Carlo technique may be applied. It provides a large sample of random numbers that may be generated by a computer to determine rather precise predictions of servicing load per hour.

Linear programming

Linear programming uses matrix algebra or linear mathematical equations to determine the best way to use limited resources to achieve maximal results. The technique is based on the assumption that a linear relationship exists between the variables and that the limits of the variations can be calculated. Three conditions must exist before linear programming can be utilized: (1) Either a maximal or minimal value is sought to optimize the objective. The value may be expressed as cost, time, or quantity. The manager may wish to minimize time and expense while maximizing quantity and quality of production. She may wish to reduce the time lost through inefficient allocation of resources or minimize the number of people required to do a job. (2) The variables affecting the goal must have a linear relationship. The ratio of change in one variable to the change in another variable must be constant. If it takes 3 minutes to do a task, it should take 15 minutes to do the task 5 times. (3) Constraints or obstacles to the relationships of the variables exist. Linear programming would not be needed if there were no restrictions.

Simple allocations can often be made by observation and experience, but in large operations the problems may be complex and involve thousands of possible choices. Linear programming is a sophisticated, shortcut technique in which a computer can be used to determine solutions. It could be used to determine a minimal-cost diet for meeting certain nutritional standards or for assigning community health nurses to territories. A school of nursing might use this technique to determine class sizes, class hours, and instructors by feeding into a computer equations containing such variables as student's desire or requirement to enroll in particular classes, number of students, number of professors qualified to teach the course, and the hours available to conduct the course. Because linear programming is dependent on linear relationships and many decisions do not involve them, the manager may need to apply nonlinear programming.

Advantages and limitations of quantitative tools for decision making

Quantitative tools lend themselves to a rational, systematic approach to problem solving for decisions that can be expressed mathematically. They encourage disciplined thinking. They are not limited to the six or seven variables the human mind can consider at one time, and they may evaluate thousands of interrelationships simultaneously. Decisions made with the use of quantitative tools are likely to be superior to decisions that rely heavily on judgment. Unfortunately, many managerial problems involve intangible, nonmeasurable factors that reduce the effectiveness of the tools. The mathematical expressions are based on assumptions. If those assumptions are not true for a given situation, the tool becomes useless.

Computers. Computers provide several advantages over paper-based record systems. Information can be stored in smaller areas, search and analytical tasks can be done, and information can be obtained faster and more efficiently. Unfortunately, if used improperly, computers can magnify weaknesses in an organization.

Computers can be applied in nursing in three major categories: (1) Clinical systems, (2) management information systems, and (3) educational systems. In clinical systems, computers help with patient histories, medical records, and patient monitoring. Computerized record systems can improve the usability of patient information because data from the chart can be rearranged to be useful to various health care professionals. Physicians can enter their diagnoses, protocols, and notes directly into the computer, saving nurses transcribing time. The instructions can be printed out at the appropriate auxiliary department. Nurses can also record their notes directly into the computer and no longer need to spend so much time and energy accumulating and summarizing data to develop care plans. Standard screens with standard choices increase efficiency for recording observations and doing care plans. Nurses are made aware of changes that require their intervention quickly because information from ancillary departments can be sent automatically to the nursing station terminal. The computer can sort and analyze data and facilitate communication about the patients among health care providers.

Patient monitoring systems record patient responses and can alert nurses to changes. Computers can record the patient's progress on paper or on the monitor, sound an alarm, and often transmit information from the patient's bedside to monitors at the nursing station. In addition to monitoring patients continuously and detecting changes, computers can analyze and interpret the data. Through computer monitoring, nurses can respond quickly to changes in patients' conditions.

Computers have many applications in management information systems. They can be used for patient classification systems, supplies and material management, staff scheduling, policy and procedure changes and announcements, patient charges, budget information and management, personnel records, statistical reports, administrative reports, and memos.

In educational systems, computer-assisted instruction allows students to proceed at their own speed, provides immediate feedback, and can allow dissemination of information to remote areas.

When using computers as decision-making tools, nurses should take advantage of good commercial software that is available and should investigate the possibility of using existing systems. Securing the confidentiality of patient and personnel records by carefully locking up diskettes or by constructing a pass-words system is very important.*

BEHAVIORAL ASPECTS OF DECISION MAKING
Continuum of participation

Participation in decision making is based on the principle that all members of a group or organization should be encouraged to contribute to decisions. The extent of participation allowed is dependent on such factors as organizational philosophy, managerial style, and organizational climate. Agencies that discourage participation have an authoritarian climate. Directions and control are located at the top of the hierarchy, where decisions primarily are made by top management. They are communicated down to staff, and unquestioned obedience is expected. Agencies that allow greater participation at lower echelons are democratic in nature. Tannenbaun and Schmidt developed the continuum of leadership behavior and participation related to the degree of authority used by the leader and the amount of freedom granted subordinates in reaching decisions (Fig. 1-4). The actions on the extreme left characterize the manager who maintains a high degree of control, whereas the actions on the right characterize the leader who releases a high degree of control. Neither extreme is without limitations.

Manager makes the decision and announces it. In this situation the manager identifies the problem, explores alternative solutions, chooses one of them, and then reports her decision. She provides no opportunity for others to participate, may or may not give consideration to others' thoughts and feelings, and may or may not imply coercion.

Manager "sells" decision. Here the manager identifies the problem and makes a decision. However, instead of merely announcing the decision, she tries to persuade subordinates to accept it. This procedure recognizes the possibility of some resistance and seeks to reduce it by such acts as explaining to employees what they gain from the decision.

Manager presents ideas and invites questions. Now the manager, who has made a decision and has tried to persuade subordinates to accept it, provides an opportunity for others to ask questions to get a fuller explanation of her thinking and intentions. This discussion allows exploration of the implications of the decision.

Manager presents tentative decision subject to change. In this situation the

---

*For more information, see Zielstorff, R.D., editor: Computers in nursing. Rockville, Md., Aspen Systems Corp.

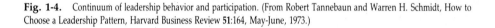

Fig. 1-4. Continuum of leadership behavior and participation. (From Robert Tannebaun and Warren H. Schmidt, How to Choose a Leadership Pattern, Harvard Business Review 51:164, May-June, 1973.)

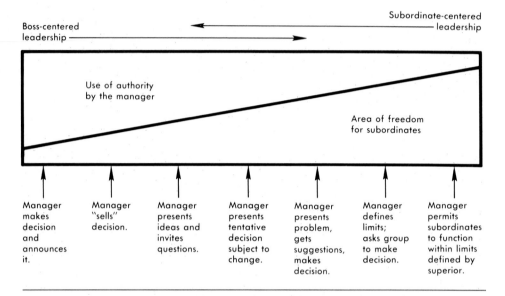

Boss-centered leadership

Subordinate-centered leadership

Use of authority by the manager

Area of freedom for subordinates

| Manager makes decision and announces it. | Manager "sells" decision. | Manager presents ideas and invites questions. | Manager presents tentative decision subject to change. | Manager presents problem, gets suggestions, makes decision. | Manager defines limits; asks group to make decision. | Manager permits subordinates to function within limits defined by superior. |

manager presents her tentative decision for reaction by the people who will be affected by it. She reserves the power to make the final decision but takes others' thoughts and feelings into account when making the decision.

Manager presents problem, gets suggestions, makes decision. Now the manager identifies the problem but gets suggestions from subordinates before making a decision. This approach uses the knowledge and experiences of others. The manager selects what she considers the best solution from the expanded list of alternatives developed by herself and others.

The manager defines the limits and requests the group to make a decision. The manager identifies the problem, sets the boundaries within which the decision must be made, and gives the group, including herself, the power to make the decision.

The manager permits the group to make decisions within prescribed limits. This represents the extreme degree of group freedom where the group identifies the problem, explores alternatives, and makes the decision. The only limits imposed on the group's decision are from top-level administration. The manager commits herself in advance of the decision making to help implement the decision of the group. She may or may not be a part of the group decision making. If so, she acts with no more authority than any other member of the group.

Whether the manager chooses a more autocratic or democratic approach depends on several factors. The following questions should be asked: How important is the quality of the decision? Does the manager have sufficient information to make a good decision? If not, others should be involved in the decision. If so, have prior autocratic decisions been accepted by the subordinates? If not, others should be involved. Is acceptance of the decision critical for its implementation? If so, the implementers should be involved with the decision making. Subordinates should be included in decision making if they share organizational goals and are not in conflict with preferred solutions.

VROOM AND YETTON NORMATIVE MODEL

Vroom and Yetton address decision making as a social process and emphasize how managers do rather than should behave in their normative model. They identify the following alternative decision processes: A = autocratic, C = consultative, G = group, I = first variant, and II = second variant.

Types of management decision styles*

AI   You solve the problem or make the decision yourself, using information available to you at that time.

AII You obtain the necessary information from your subordinate(s), then decide on the solution to the problem yourself. You may or may not tell your subordinates what the problem is in getting the information from them. The role played by your subordinates in making the decision is clearly one of providing the necessary information to you, rather than generating or evaluating alternative solutions.

CI   You share the problem with relevant subordinates individually, getting their ideas and suggestions without bringing them together as a group. Then you make the decision that may or may not reflect your subordinates' influence.

CII You share the problem with your subordinates as a group, collectively obtaining their ideas and suggestions. Then you make the decision that may or may not reflect your subordinates' influence.

GII You share a problem with your subordinates as a group. Together you generate and evaluate alternatives and attempt to reach agreement (consensus) on a solution. Your role is much like that of chairman. You do not try to influence the group to adopt "your" solution and you are willing to accept and implement any solution that has the support of the entire group.

(GI is omitted because it applies only to more comprehensive models outside the scope of the article.)

Vroom identifies seven rules that do most of the work of the model. Three rules protect decision quality and four protect acceptance.†

---

*Reprinted by permission of the publisher: Vroom, V.: A new look at managerial decision making, Organization Dynamics 1(4):67, Spring 1973. Copyright © 1971 by AMACOM, a division of American Management Associations.
†Reprinted by permission of the publisher: Vroom, V.: A new look at managerial decision making, Organizational Dynamics 1(4):69-71, Spring 1973. © 1971 by AMACOM, a division of American Management Associations.

1. *The Information Rule.* If the quality of the decision is important and if the leader does not possess enough information or expertise to solve the problem by himself, AI is eliminated from the feasible set. (Its use risks a low-quality decision.)
2. *The Goal Congruence Rule.* If the quality of the decision is important and if the subordinates do not share the organizational goals to be obtained in solving the problem, GII is eliminated from the feasible set. (Alternatives that eliminate the leader's final control over the decision reached may jeopardize the quality of the decision.)
3. *The Unstructured Problem Rule.* In decisions in which the quality of the decision is important, if the leader lacks the necessary information or expertise to solve the problem by himself, and if the problem is unstructured, i.e., he does not know exactly what information is needed and where it is located, the method used must provide not only for him to collect the information but to do so in an efficient and effective manner. Methods that involve interaction among all subordinates with full knowledge of the problem are likely to be both more efficient and more likely to generate a high-quality solution to the problem. Under these conditions, AI, AII, and CI are eliminated from the feasible set. (AI does not provide for him to collect the necessary information, and AII and CI represent more cumbersome, less effective, and less efficient means of bringing the necessary information to bear on the solution of the problem than methods that do permit those with the necessary information to interact.)
4. *The Acceptance Rule.* If the acceptance of the decision by subordinates is critical to effective implementation, and if it is not certain that an autocratic decision made by the leader would receive that acceptance, AI and AII are eliminated from the feasible set. (Neither provides an opportunity for subordinates to participate in the decision, and both risk the necessary acceptance.)
5. *The Conflict Rule.* If the acceptance of the decision is critical, and an autocratic decision is not certain to be accepted, and subordinates are likely to be in conflict or disagreement over the appropriate solution, AI, AII, and CI are eliminated from the feasible set. (The method used in solving the problem should enable those in disagreement to resolve their differences with full knowledge of the problem. Accordingly, under these conditions, AI, AII, and CI, which involve no interaction or only "one-on-one" relationships and therefore provide no opportunity for those in conflict to resolve their differences, are eliminated from the feasible set. Their use runs the risk of leaving some of the subordinates with less than the necessary commitment to the final decision.)
6. *The Fairness Rule.* If the quality of decision is unimportant and if acceptance is critical and not certain to result from an autocratic decision, AI, AII, CI, and CII are eliminated from the feasible set. (The method used should maxi-

mize the probability of acceptance as this is the only relevant consideration in determining the effectiveness of the decision. Under these circumstances, AI, AII, CI, and CII, which create less acceptance or commitment than GII, are eliminated from the feasible set. To use them is to run the risk of getting less than the needed acceptance of the decision.)

7. *The Acceptance Priority Rule.* If acceptance is critical, not assured by an autocratic decision, and if subordinates can be trusted, AI, AII, CI, and CII are eliminated from the feasible set. (Methods that provide equal partnership in the decision-making process can provide greater acceptance without risking decision quality. Use of any method other than GII results in an unnecessary risk that the decision will not be fully accepted or receive the necessary commitment on the part of subordinates.)

As one asks the diagnostic questions and applies the rules to specific situations, one may eliminate all but one decision style from the feasibility set. However, it is more likely that several decision styles could be used and still protect both the decision quality and acceptance requirements. Then the time factor is used to determine which of the feasible options will require the least time.

Vroom and Yetton focus on three classes of outcomes that influence the ultimate effectiveness of decisions: (1) the quality of the decision, (2) acceptance of the decision by the subordinates, and (3) available time needed to make the decision. The authors found that managers can diagnose a situation quickly and accurately by answering seven questions.*

Problem attributes used in the model

Problem Attributes	Diagnostic Questions
A. The importance of the quality of the decision.	Is there a quality requirement such that one solution is likely to be more rational than another?
B. The extent to which the leader possesses sufficient information/expertise to make a high-quality decision by himself.	Do I have sufficient information to make a high-quality decision?
C. The extent to which the problem is structured.	Is the problem structured?
D. The extent to which acceptance or commitment on the part of subordinates is critical to the effective implementation of the decision.	Is acceptance of decision by subordinates critical to effective implementation?
E. The prior probability that the leader's autocratic decision will receive acceptance by subordinates.	If you were to make the decision by yourself, is it reasonably certain that it would be accepted by your subordinates?

*Reprinted by permission of the publisher: Vroom, V.: A new look at managerial decision making, Organizational Dynamics 1(4):69, Spring 1973. Copyright © 1971 by AMACOM, a division of American Management Associations.

F. The extent to which subordinates are motivated to attain the organizational goals as represented in the objectives explicit in the statement of the problem.	Do subordinates share the organizational goals to be obtained in solving this problem?
G. The extent to which subordinates are likely to be in conflict over preferred solutions.	Is conflict among subordinates likely in preferred solutions?

Individuals as decision makers

The underlying belief of an autocratic manager is that others are not as competent as she. The autocrat fears that decisions made by others may be more costly, less effective, and represent a threat to her power. Sometimes, when a decision involves highly technical consideration, it may best be made by technicians or specialists. Others argue, however, that specialists are not always effective decisions makers, do not see the total picture, and do not appreciate the human factors.

Three major behavioral characteristics influence decision making: (1) perception of the problem, (2) a personal value system, and (3) the ability to process data. Perception is a psychological process that makes sense out of what one sees, hears, smells, tastes, or feels. It is affected by one's previous experiences and personal value system; thus, people may perceive the same situation differently. There are also differences in ability to process data, to remember facts, and to explore alternatives.

Values. Values represent basic convictions about what is right, good, or desirable; as a result, they help an individual to decide which mode of conduct is preferable to the others. Value systems list an individual's values in order of their relative importance and provide the foundation of attitudes, perceptions, personality, and roles. These values cloud objectivity and rationality by containing interpretations of what is right and wrong and implications that certain behaviors or outcomes are preferred over others. They are relatively stable and enduring and generally influence decisions and behaviors.

Attitudes. Attitudes are mental states of readiness that are organized through experience and exert specific influences upon a person's response to the people, objects, and situations to which they are related. Attitudes, like values, are learned from parents, teachers, and peers, but attitudes are less stable than values. They influence decisions and behavior and are close to the core of personality.

In the late 1950s, Leon Festinger proposed the theory of cognitive dissonance to explain the linkage between attitudes and behavior. *Cognitive dissonance* means a perceived inconsistency or incompatibility between attitudes and behavior. Festinger maintained that this inconsistency is uncomfortable and that people will try to reduce the dissonance and consequently the discomfort. People seek a stable state with a minimum of dissonance. For example, if someone thinks he is getting paid more than he is worth, he is likely to work harder, but if he thinks he is underpaid, he may slow down and do less.

Perceptions. Perception involves receiving, organizing, and interpreting stimuli. The perceptions then influence behavior and form attitudes. People select various cues that influence their perceptions and consequently often mis-perceive another person, group, or object. *Selective perception* means that people select information that supports their viewpoints. Knowing oneself increases the accuracy of perception of others. People tend to identify their own charac-teristics in others. Consequently, people who accept themselves are more likely to view others favorably. A *stereotype* is a judgment made about people on the basis of their ethnic background that can contribute to selective perception. A *self-fulfilling prophecy* occurs when people expect certain behavior, use selective perception to see it, and treat others as if it were so. For example, if a supervisor thinks blacks are lazy and irresponsible, he may not assign them challenging assignments. That could lead to boredom and demotivation, which reinforces the stereotype and becomes a self-fulfilling prophecy.

Personality. Personality is a relatively stable set of characteristics, tempera-ments, and tendencies that are significantly formed by inheritance and by social, cultural, and environmental factors.

Roles. *Role theory* is a collection of concepts, definitions, and hypotheses that predict how actors will perform in certain roles and under what circumstances given behaviors can be expected. *Roles* are acts or behaviors expected of a person who occupies a given social position. *Positions* are locations in social systems, such as nurse or teacher. People who occupy positions collectively share common behaviors. Specific behaviors associated with positions constitute roles. Positions and roles have counterparts or counterroles such as nurse-client, teacher-student, or leader-follower.

Positions may be *ascribed* or *achieved*. A person has little or no control over ascribed positions such as age, sex, or birth order in the family. Some degree of control is possible for achieved positions such as marital status, occupation, and social status.

Role structure involves individuals, behaviors, and positions. The *individual* or actor, ego, referent, or self has a set of attributes that can be described from a variety of viewpoints. An interactionist would look at the interaction of roles, the psychiatrist at personality, and the structuralist at position tasks. *Behaviors* are actions taken by the role enactor. These acts are learned and influenced by norms. They are often voluntary and goal-directed. *Prescription* refers to what should be done by a person in a certain position. *Positions* often require specific skills, intelligence, or temperament and may be held based on one's age, sex, and education. Positions often imply titles such as nurse or teacher. People in positions are exchangable but the positions are not.

Role socialization is a process of acquiring specific roles and involves role expectations, role learning, and role enactment. *Role expectations* are beliefs held by others about the specific behaviors inherent in specific positions. Role expectations may be general or specific, formal or informal, and extensive or narrow in scope. Some expectations are very clear, whereas others are not. General expectations allow more latitude in the implementation of the role than do specific ones. For example, nurses should be kind and gentle in general. More specifically, nurses use two-way communications skills. Some formal expectations are written, such as codes of ethics and behavioral objectives, whereas informal expectations are communicated indirectly. Expectations for age and sex are extensive in scope in that they transcend other roles. Expectations that apply in only a few positions are narrow in scope. Thus, only nurses working in cardiac intensive care units are expected to read and interpret electrocardiograms, and only the nurse managers are expected to write a budget.

Role learning involves locating oneself accurately in the social structure. It begins at infancy and early childhood as one prepares to assume adult responsibilities. It involves the development of basic skills such as language, interpersonal competence, and role taking. *Role taking* is the ability of the person to act out perceptions of how she and others would behave in certain positions. Playing nurse is an example of learning role taking.

Role enactment refers to behaviors and is related to the number of positions held, the intensity of involvement in those positions, and the preemptiveness of them. People hold multiple positions at any one time, a situation that sometimes causes conflict and difficulty with role enactment. One may not have enough time to implement each role effectively and there can be conflicts among various role expectations. A professional nurse who takes a course will have less time for child care. Intensity of involvement is the degree of effort exerted to enact a role. It may vary from noninvolvement to engrossing involvement. For example, a nurse may merely pay for membership in an organization, or the nurse may become an officer and serve on several committees. Preemptiveness is the amount of time a person spends enacting one role as compared with others.

Role stress or role dissonance is the difference between role enactment and role expectations. The greater the difference, the greater the stress. *Role ambiguity* results from a lack of clear role expectations. *Role shock* arises from discrepancies between anticipated and encountered roles. *Role conflict* is a consequence of contradictory or mutually exclusive roles.

Group factors in decision making

A group comprises two or more people who perceive themselves to share common interests and come together to accomplish an activity through face-to-face interaction. People join groups to satisfy security, fulfill social and esteem needs, enhance their personal status and careers, sustain friendships, and accomplish goals. In organizations, formal groups are deliberately created to perform specific tasks. These may be command groups formed of a supervisor and subordinates or temporary task groups composed of people who do not necessarily report to the same supervisor. The informal group evolves naturally.

Within an agency it is unusual for an individual to complete the decision-making process by herself. Even if she makes the decision, others will probably be involved in the implementation. Commitment to the decision is important to its implementation and may be increased by participation in the decision-making process. One should be aware, however, that there are disadvantages as well as advantages to group participation in decision making.

Advantages of group participation in decision making. Because of their broader experiences, groups have a wider range of knowledge to draw on than does the individual. Participation allows the nurse to express her views and attempt to persuade others, thereby increasing her self-expression, innovation, and development. One is more apt to be committed to implementation if she has had the opportunity to share in the decision-making process. Group decisions, however, are time consuming and expensive. Still, because of the members' diverse backgrounds, it may be less time consuming for a group to make a decision than for an individual to gather information and analyze it. In the end this may be no more expensive than having a higher-paid manager make the decision.

Disadvantages of group participation in decision making. Group decisions may result from social pressures. The subordinate may be influenced by her desire for group acceptance or by an attempt to appease her superior. Hierarchical pressures can reduce the subordinate's participation to acquiescence to the manager's desires. Formal status is likely to inhibit interaction when the supervisor has less expertise than the staff. A competent superior is more likely to possess self-confidence and allow interaction. It is not always easy to determine another's competence, and one cannot expect the level of expertise to match the degree of participation.

Group participants change and so do the problems. A minority may rule if an individual or a few people dominate the group. Members may become more interested in winning an argument than in determining the best alternative. Choosing the most acceptable solution may produce consensus, which is not necessarily the optimal alternative and may simply foster the status quo.

Groupthink. When a group becomes too cohesive and demands too much conformity, the group is likely to develop patterns of behavior that interfere with good decision making. Symptoms of groupthink include a highly cohesive group, the illusion of invulnerability, collective rationalization, a tendency to

25

moralize, self-righteousness, a feeling of unanimity, stereotypes of other groups, pressure to conform, and self-censorship to keep quiet. Opposing ideas are discouraged and dismissed.

Group norms form gradually and informally in a variety of ways. People bring expectations with them from past situations. The first pattern that emerges in a group often sets group expectations, and important incidents establish precedents. Explicit statements by group members and conscious decisions by the group also help determine norms. Norms apply to behavior, not to thoughts and feelings. They are generally developed only for behavior that is considered important by most group members and usually allow for a range of acceptable behaviors. Group norms are enforced because they make predictable what behavior is expected of group members, reinforce specific roles, and help avoid embarrassing interpersonal problems. They probably reflect the preferences of powerful group members and help ensure group success.

Group cohesiveness occurs when members of the group like each other and want to be members of the group. A charismatic leader, good reputation of the group, shared goals, similarity of attitudes and values, and small enough size to allow interaction increase group cohesiveness. There is a direct correlation between cohesiveness and conformity to group norms. However, group norms may not be consistent with those of the organization.

There are several steps a manager can take to discourage groupthink. When assigning a policy-planning mission to a group, the leader should be impartial instead of stating preferences and expectations. At least one member of the committee can be assigned the role of devil's advocate. One or more outside consultants or qualified internal colleagues who are not core members of the group can be invited to each meeting on a staggered basis to challenge the views of the core members. Members of the core group can discuss the group's deliberations with trusted colleagues periodically and report their reactions back to the group. The group may be divided into subgroups to meet separately under different leadership, report back to the larger group, and discuss differences. Two or more independent groups may be assigned to explore the same policy question. Results can then be compared. The leader should encourage each committee member to be a critical evaluator and to air objections and doubts diplomatically. This can be reinforced by the leader's acceptance of criticism of her own suggestions.

Committee aspects of decision making

A committee is a group of people chosen to deal with a particular topic or problem. The authority delegated to committees varies widely. A staff committee serves merely in an advisory capacity. A line committee is a plural executive responsible for making decisions affecting subordinates. Formal committees are part of the organizational structure and have specific duties and authority. Informal committees have not been delegated authority and are often primarily for discussion. Formal committees tend to be permanent; informal committees are more likely to be temporary. Committees are usually most useful when appointed for a specific purpose. A committee appointed to collect data, analyze findings, and make recommendations is an ad hoc committee. There are advantages and disadvantages to decision making by committees.

Advantages of committee decision making. Although the ultimate responsibility for a decision is the top administrator's, that burden can be shared through the use of committees. Group deliberation and judgment can be advantageous for decision making. Complex problems may be more manageable when department heads and specialists participate. Sharing in the decision-making process increases the department head's understanding of the situation and commitment to the decision. Most decisions based on consensus after deliberation are widely satisfactory. The unanimity of committee decisions helps increase the support and confidence of subordinates.

Disadvantages of committee decision making. Although the top administrator's burden for decision making can be shared by committees, it requires more leadership ability to conduct business in that manner. Committee decisions may make the manager appear to be a figurehead and decrease her prestige in the community. A weak administrator may in fact be controlled by her staff instead of being in control herself. She may use committees to avoid responsibilities or to delay decisions. A committee may have a fixed responsibility, but it is the group rather than the individual that is held accountable because it is difficult to identify who is responsible for a poor decision. A committee decision is a slow, ponderous process that is consequently expensive. Pressures for unanimity may discourage input from more aggressive and creative members. Consensus through compromise may decrease the quality of the decision. Indecisiveness can result in adjournment without action taken and contribute to a minority tyranny of the strongest members.

Committee functioning. Despite the obvious disadvantages and misuses of committees, there is an increasing emphasis on group participation. Committee decisions are particularly useful for policy formulation and planning. Consequently, the manager should consider how to maximize the use of committees.

There are several kinds of committees, including (1) interdepartmental committees involving nursing with nonnursing departments, (2) committees based on organizational position and job function, (3) standing committees, and (4) task forces. Interdepartmental committees help coordinate goals and activities among departments and help solve interdepartmental problems. The situational problems between departments can best be solved by people with first-hand experience, rather than by committees. Consequently, alternatives to committee meetings should be considered for problem solving. Dual leadership is sometimes used to give equal consideration to each department. That tends to result in a lack of leadership. Alternating chairpersons may serve the same purpose as having cochairpersons.

Committees based on organizational position and job function provide a vehicle for group cohesion and power. Supervisor and head nurse committees are common. Standing committees represent focal points of action in the institution. In hospitals, standing committees may be formed to make recommendations about patient care evaluation, continuity of care, patient education, and staff development. Schools of nursing often have standing committees for by-laws, curricula, admissions, progression, and graduation. A task force is a time-limited committee that assesses a situation, makes recommendations, and is dissolved. People with the most knowledge and skills related to the problem should serve on the task force.

Defining the scope and authority of the committee helps members know what their responsibilities are. Members should know if they are simply to discuss an issue, provide the supervisor with ideas, make recommendations, or be responsible for the decision. With their job clearly defined, there is less chance that committee members will waste their time dealing with issues beyond the scope of their responsibility. An awareness of the limits placed on them also allows committee members to evaluate their work better. It may be advisable to review committees periodically to dissolve those no longer needed, consolidate those duplicating responsibilities, and create new ones.

The size of the committee is important. It should be large enough to facilitate deliberation and have a membership with a breadth of knowledge and expertise. If it is too large, it encourages indecision and inefficiency, because the larger the group, the more time it takes to allow each member to participate and for the group to reach a consensus. Effective committee size may range from five to fifteen. Five is considered an ideal size if the five members have adequate knowledge and skills. Appropriate membership is critical for effective committee functioning. Members need the necessary knowledge and skills, should possess authority, must be suitably representative, and should be able to work well within a group.

Feedback to and from nonmembers and administration enhances committee effectiveness. Developing input channels helps foster group acceptance for committee recommendations. For example, staff nurses may give input to their head nurse who represents them at administrative team meetings. Periodic status reports to administration and nonmembers are not only a means of communication; they help committee members focus on goals and evaluate progress.

Good leadership can increase the effectiveness of a committee. The chairperson can facilitate committee work by preparing agendas, circulating reports before meetings, making research results available to members, collecting necessary facts before the meeting, defining the proposal for action, and conducting the meeting efficiently. Agendas circulated to members well in advance of meetings allow committee members to know what to expect and to come to the meeting prepared to deal with the subject. The circulation of reports and other information before the meeting helps prevent the waste of meeting time while members review studies or think aloud. It reduces the chances of a decision being railroaded, a report being meekly accepted, or postponement of a decision until after members have more opportunity to study the proposal.

Committees go through stages of team development. They typically form, organize, solve problems, implement solutions, and disband. During the forming stage, individuals are likely to feel anxious, fearful, doubtful, and self-protective. The leader concentrates on putting the members at ease, explaining the purpose, developing a workable climate, and exerting leadership. Tension tends to be high, suspiciousness is common, and disagreement emerges with the power struggles that occur during the organizing phase. The leader needs to clarify goals, policies and procedures, code of conduct, and communication patterns. Loyalty, trust, confidence, dignity, and pride develop during problem solving. The leader seeks to approve recommendations by consensus through a systematic and logical approach. Self-interest, excitement, recognition, and rewards are common during implementation. The leader tends to the plan of action, the acceptance of decisions, and the generation of feedback. Members may have positive or negative feelings about disbanding. The leader should express appreciation and give positive reinforcement.

The committee chairperson needs to handle various problems during the meeting, such as the overly talkative, the inarticulate, and the ramblers. In general, the chairperson lets the group take care of the overly talkative as much as possible. Embarrassing or sarcastic remarks are not appropriate. The overly talkative may be slowed down with some difficult questions or interrupted with a comment like, "That's an interesting point. Let's see what the group thinks of it." Input can be invited from all committee members, starting with the others first. The rambler is likely to talk about everything except the subject. When the member stops for a breath, the chairperson thanks the member, refocuses attention by restating the relevant points, and moves on. Some members may come up with comments that are obviously incorrect. The chairperson can say something like, "That's one way of looking at it," or "I see your point, but can we reconcile that with (the true situation)?" Side conversations can be distracting. The chairperson tries not to embarrass the people involved. One can be called by name and asked an easy question, or the last opinion can be restated and one asked her opinion of it. When two or more members clash or the committee is divided into factions, the chairperson should emphasize points of agreement, minimize points of disagreement if possible, and draw attention to objectives. The inarticulate may lack the ability to put thoughts into proper words; the silent person may feel timid, insecure, bored, indifferent, or superior. Interest can be aroused by asking people for their opinions. That technique can also be used to encourage people to talk. The action of the chairperson depends on what is motivating the committee member.

The chairperson should keep the discussion on the subject and help integrate committee deliberation. Thus, rather than resorting to compromise, members may develop a point of view that differs from the preconceived notions that they brought to the meeting. The chairperson should not force members to take a position until after the subject has been fully considered. Members who take a premature stand may feel the need to defend that position for the sake of winning an argument rather than for the quality of the decision. The chairperson can encourage each member to be a critical evaluator and to consider the consequences of an action. Outside experts may be invited in, or task forces can be selected to study issues and report back to the committee. It may be useful to have a follow-up meeting after a consensus has been reached to allow for, and to deal with, second thoughts.

Committees permit simultaneous participation, and yet people may still leave the meeting with varying interpretations of what happened. Consequently, it is advisable to have a secretary take minutes and for the chairperson to circulate the draft for modification before having the minutes approved by the committee. The chairperson should also follow up on the decisions made and report her findings to the committee. Was the recommendation implemented? If so, what were the results? If not, why not?

Techniques to facilitate group creativity. Under favorable circumstances a group working together can identify more ideas than an individual or that group of individuals working separately. Brainstorming is a technique a supervisor can use to get a free flow of ideas. She should encourage the members to contribute a large number of freewheeling ideas without fear of criticism or ridicule. This can improve the quality of ideas offered and result in new combinations through rearrangement, reversal, substitution, and other modifications.

Brainstorming seems to work best for simple and specific problems. Complex problems can be divided into parts and handled separately. If the problem is too complex, the discussion may lack focus and be very time consuming. Brainstorming may be most useful when group members understand at least part of the problem. Although the brainstorming session may not produce a viable solution, its stimulation may continue beyond the meeting and cause employees to take another look at their routinized activities.

Creativity is probably fostered best in a permissive atmosphere where mutual respect prevails and people are encouraged to express their views and ideas even if they are at variance with current policies and practices. A free interchange of ideas with considerable borrowing and adaptation fosters the production of creative ideas.

The Delphi Technique. The Delphi Technique allows members who are dispersed over a geographic area to participate in decision making without meeting face to face. A problem is identified, and members are asked to suggest potential solutions through the use of a questionnaire. Members anonymously return the first questionnaire. Results of the first questionnaire are centrally compiled. Each member is sent a copy of the results. After viewing the results of the first questionnaire, members are asked for their suggestions again. Review of the results of the first questionnaire typically triggers new solutions or stimulates changes in original positions. This process continues until consensus is reached. Little change usually occurs after the second round.

The Delphi Technique insulates group members from one another's influence and does not require physical presence, so it is particularly appropriate for scattered groups. Unfortunately, it is time consuming and may not develop alternatives as more interaction might.

CONSULTATION

Consultation is a helping relationship. It is a process of interaction between the consultant, who has the specialized knowledge and skills, and the consultee, who asks for assistance with problem solving. It has a beginning and an end and is a temporary, voluntary, educational relationship. The consultee identifies a problem and seeks help from an expert. Because the consultant is usually not a part of the hierarchical structure of the organization, the consultant is an outsider who advises. Implementation of the recommendations is dependent on the consultee, thus giving the process a take-it-or-leave-it quality. The consultation process usually involves problem solving, but the consultant may serve several roles. The consultant may help identify problems, educate staff about related issues, identify obstacles to problem solving, offer advice about how to solve problems, serve as a change agent, develop interpersonal relationships, mediate conflicts, or do tasks that organizational members do not have the skill to do. The consultant typically collects and analyzes data, recommends or intervenes, and then terminates the relationship.

Consultants become known by doing something and telling others about it, volunteering to present workshops and speeches, publishing books and articles, being active in professional organizations, circulating flyers and announcements, and getting their names on lists of consultants.

An internal consultant knows the system, history, political realities, norms, and language better than an outside consultant and will probably devote more time to the problem. An internal consultant is viewed as less costly because she is usually not compensated extra for consultative services. Unfortunately, there are disadvantages to hiring an internal consultant. She may be part of the problem; lack perspective to see the whole; not have independence of movement; not have an adequate power base; encounter resistance because of her relationship with the hierarchy, vested interest, or organizational politics; or not have a diverse background.

An external consultant has a more diverse background, brings new ideas and a different perspective to the situation, is independent of the power structure, and is consequently high powered. Unfortunately, the external consultant does not know the history and politics of the institution and may not care.

Once it has been determined that there is a need for consultation, what the purpose is, and who the consultant should be, a contractual agreement is necessary. The agreement may be verbal or written, but it should determine the fee, hours of the consultant's time, expected outcome, and criteria for termination. The fee may be negotiated as a flat fee, a fee based on hours spent at the agency that includes travel and preparation time, or an hourly rate for all the time the consultant spends on the project, including research and report writing. The hours are largely controlled by the compensation structure. The consultant may have a regular schedule or be "on call." In most cases the outcome is accepted whether it is judged acceptable or not. Common outcomes are a written analysis with recommendations, decisions reached, systems devised or revised, and projects completed. Usually the termination occurs at a natural closure point such as the resolution of the problem or completion of the project. However, contingency plans should be made in case there are personality conflicts or the project takes too long and exceeds the budget.

PLANNING PROCESS

The planning process is a critical element of management. The process must be learned by nurse administrators, because it will not happen by accident. Planning is largely conceptual, but the results of planning are clearly visible. The statement of the purpose or mission, philosophy, goals, objectives, policies, and procedures are all consequences of planning. They set the stage for smooth operations.

Purpose

Organizations exist for a reason. Clarification of the purpose is the first priority for planning. Most nursing services exist to provide quality nursing care to clients. Some also encourage teaching and research. Each specialty area, with its own specific purposes, contributes to the overall purpose of the institution: The purpose of the in-service education department is to orient staff to the job and to provide educational programs to improve the quality of the staff work. The burn unit exists to provide quality nursing service to patients with burns.

Purpose influences philosophy, goals, objectives, policies, and procedures. For example, if a progressive care unit exists to help patients adjust to their diseases, it should be staffed with professional nurses particularly skilled in teaching and counseling. If, however, the unit exists to cut hospital and patient expenses, it may be a minimal care unit with reduced services given by non-professional workers. The relationships among the purpose, philosophy, goals, objectives, policies, and procedures should be examined periodically for consistency.

SAMPLE PURPOSE

The purpose of General Hospital is to combine scientific knowledge with unselfish service for healing the body, mind, and spirit. Related instruction, public service programs, and research will be facilitated in the interest of high-quality health care.

Philosophy

The philosophy is a statement of beliefs and values that direct one's practice. It should be written, placed in appropriate documents, and reviewed periodically. If the philosophy is stated in vague, abstract terms that are not easily understood, it is useless. Conflicting philosophies between overlapping units cause confusion and should be avoided. Workers are most likely to interpret the philosophy from the pronouncements and actions of the leaders in the institution. Therefore, conformity of action to belief is important.

SAMPLE PHILOSOPHY
DEPARTMENT OF NURSING SERVICE*

Nursing has a significant role in a society that values the maintenance and improvement of health along a positive continuum for individuals and groups. Nursing functions dependently, interdependently, and independently in its relationship with other health care providers—all of whom share goals of prevention of disease and disability, care of the ill, promotion and maintenance of optimal health for individuals and groups, and achievement of a dignified death.

The worth, dignity, and autonomy of individuals (employees, patients, and others) are recognized, as is each individual's right to self-direction and responsibility for his or her own life. Although each individual varies in ability to adapt to stressors in a dynamic environment, each possesses the ability and potential to learn to adapt more constructively. Additionally, each individual has basic physical, social, emotional, and spiritual needs that are expressed in the environment in which the individual lives and must be responded to on the basis of the uniqueness of the individual and his or her environment, needs, and previous experiences.

The function of the department of nursing service is to provide an organizational structure conducive to provision of high-quality nursing care, the most effective utilization

---

*Adapted from Department of Nursing Service Philosophy, University of Colorado Medical Center.

of resources, and support and participation in education and research programs. It must manage the activities for which it is directly responsible and provide for the professional growth of its employees.

In addition the department of nursing service encourages the utilization of the most up-to-date knowledge available, constantly adding to that body of knowledge, teaching others to utilize the knowledge constructively to improve health care and its delivery system, and providing a milieu in which these activities can take place. In fulfilling this responsibility the department of nursing service encourages knowledge expansion by providing assistance with, and participation in, the educational and research activities of the medical center. Opportunities for knowledge acquisition are provided by workshops, classes, seminars, conferences, clinical experiences, and so on for all nursing personnel and by encouraging personnel to continue in their own developmental and educational pursuits.

The primary emphasis of the department of nursing service is the provision of patient care; therefore, all nursing personnel (including the administrative staff) must maintain a clinical component and excellence in nursing practice.

Research and educational pursuits are directed toward the improvement of the provision of health care to all individuals and groups in our society, the improvement of health care delivery system, and the effective utilization of nursing personnel (inclusive of role expansion and innovative uses of nursing personnel) based on competence, education, skill, knowledge, ability, and training.

To achieve the level of nursing care desired, the nursing care provider must develop respectful, understanding relationships and utilize systematic problem-solving and decision-making processes based on accurate assessments, appropriate knowledge, and sound judgment. The nursing care provider must be able to have effective interaction with individuals and groups under stress and to terminate those interactions when they are no longer needed or can no longer be utilized by the recipient.

The department of nursing service recognizes the need to strive toward the achievement of shared goals for nursing with the school of nursing and to provide opportunities for nursing service involvement in the educational process and nursing education involvement in the nursing care process. The department of nursing service collaborates with medical and hospital administration in the management of the hospitals, determines and manages its own practice, and works with other departments in the hospitals to improve care provision, resource utilization, and educational and research endeavors. Additionally, the department of nursing service shares responsibility with other major departments and divisions in the medical center aimed at excellence of care provision, effective resource utilization, and support of educational and research endeavors.

Goals and objectives

Goals and objectives state actions for achieving the purpose and philosophy. In fact, if the purpose and philosophy are to be more than good intentions, they must be translated into explicit goals. The more quantitative the goal, the more likely it is to receive attention toward its accomplishment and the less likely it is to be distorted. Goals are central to the whole management process—planning, organizing, staffing, directing, and controlling. Planning defines the goals. The institution is organized and staffed to accomplish the goals. Direction stimulates personnel toward accomplishment of the objectives, and control compares the results with the objectives to evaluate accomplishments.

Goals and objectives may address services rendered, economics, use of resources—people, funds, and facilities—innovations, and social responsibilities. Objectives are selective rather than global, are multiple, and cover a wide range of activities. The immediate, short-, and long-term goals need to be balanced, interdependent, and put in order of importance. It is common to have more short-term than long-term goals.

Classic theory contends that the board of directors and top administration should determine institutional goals. Behavioral scientists are interested in having workers involved in setting goals and identifying real versus stated goals. The real goals can be identified by observing the day-by-day decisions and actions. Service interest, profit motives, governmental regulations, union representation, and personal goals all influence decision making.

It is appropriate for the board of directors and top administrators to set institutional goals and objectives; for the director of nurses, her assistant and associate directors, supervisors, and head nurses to set the goals and objectives for the nursing service; for the head nurse, her team leaders, primary nurses, and staff nurses to determine the unit goals and objectives; and for each nurse to determine her goals and objectives with her immediate supervisor. The overlap created by the director of nursing's working on institutional and nursing service goals and the head nurse contributing to nursing service and her unit's goals helps facilitate continuity and compatibility of goals. Participation in the determination of goals and objectives increases commitment to them, transforming them from stated to real goals. Because goals are dynamic, they will change over time. They should be reviewed periodically so they will be changed in an evolutionary rather than a radical manner. Goals should be specific rather than vague and challenging yet reachable. Necessary support elements should be available.

SAMPLE GOALS AND OBJECTIVES
DEPARTMENT OF NURSING SERVICE*

I. *Goal:* Staff development programs continue to increase in importance as a result of technological advances and increased specialization. Programs designed to meet this increased need for knowledge must he promoted, as must leadership development programs.

Objective: To increase effectiveness and efficiency of staff development programs with emphasis on clinically specialized knowledge and leadership development programs.

A. To continue the development, implementation, and evaluation of programs for nursing service personnel in the pediatric area.

---

*Adapted from Department of Nursing Service Goals, University of Colorado Medical Center.

    B. To evaluate and revise as appropriate the head nurse orientation and ongoing staff development program.

    C. To develop an orientation and ongoing staff development program for team leaders.

    D. To evaluate the efficiency and effectiveness of the nursing assistant program and role and recommend appropriate alternatives.

II. *Goal:* Personnel utilization must be efficient and effective with responsibility and tasks performed correlated with education, knowledge, and competence.
   Objective: To evaluate and increase efficiency and effectiveness of nursing service personnel.

    A. To increase the utilization of interunit consultation among nursing service personnel.

    B. To coordinate and evaluate the preoperative teaching program with the surgical patient care units and the preoperative patient assessment performed by operating room personnel.

    C. To evaluate the cost-effectiveness of primary nursing.

    D. To initiate the development of standards of performance for selected nursing service job classifications.

    E. To evaluate various staffing methodologies by considering flexibility in addition to efficiency and effectiveness.

III. *Goal:* Health care costs continue to be of significant concern with increasing external controls being implemented. All nursing service positions most be justifiable with specific, validated tools.
   Objective: To evaluate and justify staffing patterns in each patient care area.

    A. To complete the implementation of the patient classification tool in all inpatient clinical areas.

    B. To identify a tool to measure patient complexity in the ambulatory care setting and test the validity of the tool.

    C. To utilize data comparing hours of patient care provided with hours of patient care needed to adjust staffing patterns.

IV. *Goal:* Accountability of the health care provider and regulation of health care quality continue to receive increased emphasis by external agencies; therefore, concurrent and retrospective audit of nursing care must be ongoing with data collected utilized for quality of care improvements and maintenance.
   Objective: To establish and implement a concurrent audit system while continuing retrospective audits for the purpose of quality of care improvements.

    A. To complete one new retrospective audit in each clinical area.

    B. To continue combined medical and nursing audits in each clinical area.

    C. To reaudit all diagnoses that required corrective actions to determine the effectiveness of the actions.

    D. To delineate the type of concurrent audit system to be utilized and initiate its implementation.

Policies

Policies and procedures are means for accomplishing goals and objectives. Policies explain how goals will be achieved and serve as guides that define the general course and scope of activities permissible for goal accomplishment. They serve as a basis for future decisions and actions, help coordinate plans, control performance, and increase consistency of action by increasing the probability that different managers will make similar decisions when independently facing similar situations. Consequently, morale is increased when personnel perceive that they are being treated equally. Policies also serve as a means by which authority can be delegated.

Policies should be comprehensive in scope, stable, and flexible so they can be applied to different conditions that are not so diverse that they require separate sets of policies. Consistency is important, since inconsistency introduces uncertainty and contributes to feelings of bias, preferential treatment, and unfairness. Fairness is an important characteristic that is attributed to the application of the policy. Policies should be written and understandable.

Policies can be implied or expressed. Implied policies are not directly voiced or written but are established by patterns of decisions. They may have either favorable or unfavorable effects and represent an interpretation of observed behavior. Courteous treatment of clients may be implied versus expressed. The presence or absence of workers who are over 50 or 55 years of age, minority members, women, or pregnant women may lead to an interpretation of implied policies. Sometimes policies are implied simply because no one has ever bothered to state them. At other times they may deliberately be only implied because they are illegal or reflect questionable ethics. Sometimes implied policy conflicts with expressed policy. These double standards should be avoided.

Expressed policies may be oral or written. Oral policies are more flexible than written ones and can be easily adjusted to changing circumstances. However, they are less desirable than written ones because they may not be known.

The process of writing policies reveals discrepancies and omissions and causes the manager to think critically about the policy, thus contributing to clarity. Once written, they are readily available to all in the same form; their meaning cannot be changed by word of mouth; misunderstandings can be referred to the written words; the chance of misinterpretation is decreased; policy statements can be sent to all affected by them; they can be referred to whoever wishes to check the policy; and they can be used for orientation purposes. Written policies indicate the integrity of the organization's intention and generate confidence in management.

A disadvantage of written policies is the reluctance to revise them when they become outdated. However, even oral policies become obsolete. Managers should review policies periodically, and if that fails, personnel can appeal for a revision.

Policies can emerge in several ways—originated, appealed, or imposed. The originated, or internal, policies are usually developed by top management to guide subordinates in their functions. Strategy for originated policy flows from the objectives of the organization as defined by top management and may be broad in scope, allowing subordinates to develop supplemental policies, or well defined with little room for interpretation. All of the lower managerial decisions should implement the broader policy defined by top management.

Sometimes policies are generated at the operating and first-line supervisory levels and imposed upward. The extent to which this happens is influenced by the organizational atmosphere and adequacy of policies generated by top management. At times policies may be formulated simultaneously from both directions.

When a manager does not know how to solve a problem, disagrees with a previous decision, or otherwise wants a question reviewed, she appeals to her superior for a decision. As appeals are taken up the hierarchy and decisions are made, precedents known as appealed policy develop and guide future managerial actions.

Policies developed from appeals are likely to be incomplete, uncoordinated, and unclear. Unintended precedents can be set when decisions are made for a given situation without consideration for possible effects on other dimensions of the organization. This aimless formation of policy makes it difficult to know what policies exist. Sometimes managers dislike facing issues until forced to do so and consequently delay policy making until precedents have been set. Appeals policies can be foresighted and consistent, especially when the manager knows that her decision constitutes policy. Nevertheless, when a number of policies are being appealed, it is time to assess policies for gaps and needs for updating and clarification so originated policies can dominate. One can expect health agencies to need policies about patient care assignments, noting physicians' orders, administration of medications, patient safety, charting, and infection control.

Imposed, or external, policies are thrust on an organization by external forces such as government or labor unions. Policies of the organization must conform to local, state, and federal laws. Collective bargaining and union contracts direct labor policies. Professional and social groups—such as the American Nurses' Association, National League for Nursing, church, school, and charitable organizations—mold policy.

The planning process involves defining, communicating, applying, and maintaining policies. The development of a policy can originate anywhere in an organization and should involve personnel who will be affected by the policy. They have valuable information for sound policy formation and can ensure that the policy will be implemented. Before writing a policy one must consider if there are specific, recurring problems, how frequently they occur, whether they are temporary or permanent in nature, and if a policy statement would clarify thinking and promote efficiency.

When policies are written, the purpose, philosophy, goals, and objectives should serve as guides. Policies should be consistent and help solve or prevent specific problems. Clear, concise statements that establish areas of authority and perhaps include reference to supporting policies minimize exceptions. Managers need sufficient guidance with accompanying freedom for action. It is advisable to have the policy statement reviewed and approved by superiors and the affected managers before the policy is formalized.

Policies are of no use if no one knows of their existence. Oral communication is appropriate to introduce and explain new policies. It is appropriate to send a letter of purpose and a copy of policies to personnel affected by them. The written policies can then be referred to later. Policies should be written in a specific, concise, and complete manner and stored in a policy manual that is easily accessible to all personnel to whom the policies apply. The manual will be well organized if policies are classified, noted in the table of contents, and indexed by topic. Policies should be easily replaceable with revised ones.

Once a policy has been stated and approved, it is applied. Policy formation is a continuous process so the policy is continually reappraised and restated as necessary. Continuing surveillance to determine that the policy is understood and applied is important. Periodic analysis and evaluation of existing policies can suggest the need for revision. Personnel should be encouraged to help formulate, review, and revise policies.

SAMPLE POLICIES

Annual leave

Annual leave is accrued at the rate of 1 ¼ working days per month up to 15 days per year. Accrued leave is credited to the employee's record at the end of each month providing the employee worked more than half of the working days in that month. Any leave taken may be used in any portion of ¼ days. At least half of the leave accrued each year must be used. Annual leave may be accumulated up to 30 days. No annual leave is allowed for employees until 6 months' service is completed. In the event an employee's services are terminated during this 6-month period, any leave accrued will be lost.

Sick leave

Sick leave is accrued at the rate of 1 ¼ working days per month up to 15 days per year. Any sick leave accrued by the employee may be used at any time by illness of the employee or the illness of the employee's immediate family requiring her presence. If the employee does not have sufficient accrued sick leave for a period of illness, any available annual leave may be used after all available sick leave has been used. If there is no accrued leave available to use, the employee may be granted leave without pay.

Leave without pay

No leave without pay can be granted until all annual leave accrued has been used. Leaves in this category are certain types of educational leaves or any leave in which annual leave or sick leave is not available or not allowed. Leave without pay is granted on an individual basis.

Procedures

Procedures supply a more specific guide to action than policy does. They help achieve a high degree of regularity by enumerating the chronological sequence of steps. Procedures are intradepartmental or interdepartmental and consequently do not affect the entire organization to the extent that policy statements do.

Procedure manuals provide a basis for orientation and staff development and are a ready reference for all personnel. They standardize procedures and equipment and can provide a basis for evaluation. Good procedures can result in time and labor savings.

Improvement in operating procedures increases productivity and reduces cost. Waste in performing work can be decreased by applying work simplification that strives to make each part of a procedure productive. First one decides what work needs simplification by identifying problem areas. Next the work selected is analyzed carefully and in detail. Charts that depict the components of the work and the work flow are useful for motion or procedural analysis.

A questioning attitude helps determine why work is done, by whom, when, where, and how. What is the purpose of the procedure? Does it need to be done? Can it be eliminated? For example, are "closed" and "surgical" beds really necessary or could "open" beds be used for all purposes? Who does the work? Can someone else do it better, or can it be assigned to someone with less skill? Is there duplication of efforts? Can two or more activities be combined? Will changing the time sequence improve the procedure? Can transportation be reduced by changing the location? Once these questions have been answered, work should be simplified by rearranging, combining, or eliminating components. Then the improved methods must be communicated so they can be implemented.

Writing procedures demands a consistent format that considers the definition; purpose; materials needed and how to locate, requisition, and dispose of them; steps in the procedure; expected results; precautions; legal implications; nurse, patient, and physician responsibilities; and appropriate charting. Each step in the procedure leading to the accomplishment of a goal should be necessary and in proper relationship to the other steps. Balance between flexibility and stability should be maintained. As with the policy manual, the procedure manual should be easily accessible, well organized with a table of contents, and indexed. Each procedure should be easily replaceable with a revised one. Because there is a tendency to add new procedures instead of revising existing ones, it is important to review and revise the procedure manual periodically.

In reviewing, check the effectiveness and workability with personnel to determine if the procedure has been followed. Procedures should be realistic and written in simple language that is easy to understand. Changes should be dated and provided to all appropriate personnel.

Before spending valuable time writing procedures, one must consider if a procedure is actually needed. With preservice and on-the-job preparation, is there really a need to have on each unit procedures on how to feed a patient and how to make a bed? Goals can be reached in a variety of ways, and consequently nursing students are taught principles rather than procedures. There are textbooks with bedside nursing procedures, and many disposable products with directions are available. It seems most important for the procedure manual to contain information that may vary from institution to institution. Not all parts of the procedure format may be necessary for each procedure. New personnel and float nurses can serve as valuable resources for the nursing manager to consult when she is determining what content is important for the procedure manual.

SAMPLE PROCEDURE

Blood pressure measurement

A. Definition: Amount of pressure exerted against the arterial wall as the blood is forced by the pumping action of the heart
B. Purpose: To determine the changes in the arterial walls, the condition of the heart, and the volume of the blood
C. Materials needed
  1. Stethoscope
  2. Mercury sphygmomanometer
  3. Cuffs (12 to 14 cm for adults; 18 to 20 cm for large adults; 2.5 to 9.5 cm for children)
D. Location of materials
  1. Stethoscope, sphygmomanometer, and cuffs are located at the nursing stations.
  2. Materials do not need to be requisitioned.
E. Steps in procedure

Steps in procedure	Key points
1. Collect equipment and check to see that it is in working order.	Be sure that all connections are right. Examine rubber bladder and pressure bulbs for leaks. Check that the edge of the meniscus of the mercury manometer is at the zero mark.
2. Cleanse earpieces of stethoscope with a Zephiran or alcohol sponge.	
3. Wash your hands.	
4. Enter patient's room and verify name.	Assess environmental conditions that may influence pressure.
5. Explain procedure to patient.	It is very important to gain the cooperation

E. Steps in procedure—cont'd

Key points

of the patient because distress will alter the reading of the blood pressure.

Identify other factors that may affect the blood pressure reading (such as exercise, eating, weight, changes in posture, full bladder).

6. Position patient in a relaxed, reclining, or sitting position with the arm flexed, palm up, and with the whole forearm supported at heart level (fourth intercostal space) on a smooth surface.

If arm is placed above the level of the heart, the reading will be falsely low; if placed below the level of the heart, the reading will be falsely high.

Quiet must be maintained to allow hearing the blood pressure sounds.

7. Position yourself no more than 3 ft away from the sphygmomanometer with the meniscus of the mercury model at eye level.

8. Select correct cuff size.

Average adult size is 12 to 14 cm; large adult, 18 to 20 cm; child, 2.5 to 9.5 cm.

9. Measure length of bladder to fit two-thirds distance between shoulder and elbow. It should be 20% wider than the diameter of the arm, or 40% wider than its circumference.

If cuff is too narrow, pressure reading will be abnormally high; if too wide, the reading will be falsely low.

10. Palpate brachial artery in the medial surface of the arm and place the center of the bladder directly over the brachial artery 2.5 cm above the antecubital space.

11. Apply cuff snugly and smoothly.

If cuff is wrapped too loosely, the results will be falsely high.

12. Palpate radial pulse by placing index and middle finger on radial pulse. Inflate cuff rapidly until radial pulsation disappears. Identify this reading as the palpatory systolic reading.

13. Wait 30 to 60 sec before reinflation of cuff to 30 cm above the palpatory systolic reading.

This waiting period is necessary to allow time for the release of blood trapped in the veins.

Failure to do so may prevent recognition of auscultatory gap (sound initially appears at a high level, fades completely, and reappears 10 to 40 mm later), accounting for falsely low systolic pressure.

14. Position stethoscope with ear tips forward.

15. Place diaphragm or bell of stethoscope over brachial artery in antecubital fossa with as little pressure as possible and with no space between skin and stethoscope.

Heavy pressure distorts the artery, and sounds are heard below the diastolic pressure.

E. Steps in procedure—cont'd

Key points

16. Tighten screw on bulb and inflate cuff rapidly to 30 mm above palpatory systolic pressure.

Column of mercury (Hg) must be in a vertical position. If it is tilted, results will be falsely high. The edge of the mercury meniscus should be exactly at zero.

17. Deflate cuff 2 to 4 mm Hg per heart beat to zero level.

Deflating too slowly will cause a falsely high reading.

18. Note reading at the meniscus on the mercury column at which the first two regular tapping sounds (Korotkoff phase I) are heard. This is the systolic pressure.

If sounds are difficult to hear, raise the arm a few seconds to drain venous blood before inflating cuff; inflate cuff, then lower the arm, deflate, and listen for sounds; or have patient open and close fist ten times after the systolic level has been obtained.

19. Deflate cuff at an even rate of 2 to 4 mm while the sounds change from faint and clear tapping sounds (Korotkoff phase I), to a swishing quality (Korotkoff phase II), to crisper and louder sounds (Korotkoff phase III), to abrupt muffling of sound (Korotkoff phase IV), to the point at which sounds disappear (Korotkoff phase V).

The best index of diastolic pressure in adults is the point at which the sounds disappear. The onset of muffling (fourth phase) is the best index of diastolic pressure in children.

20. Expel any air in cuff and remove from patient's arm.

21. Return equipment to nursing station.

F. Charting
   1. Chart systolic pressure over diastolic pressure on graphic sheet at foot of patient's bed.
   2. Chart systolic pressure over diastolic pressure on flow chart in patient's chart. If sounds were heard to zero, chart systolic, fourth phase (muffling sound), and disappearance of sound (for example, 148/72/0 or 100/60/50).
   3. Specify position of patient: "L" (lying), "ST" (standing), "SIT" (sitting), "RA" (right arm), or "LA" (left arm).

Budgets

A budget is a plan for the allocation of resources and a control for ensuring that results comply with the plans. Results are expressed in quantitative terms. Although budgets are usually associated with financial statements, such as revenues and expenses, they also may be nonfinancial statements covering output, materials, and equipment. Budgets help coordinate the efforts of the agency by determining what resources will be used by whom, when, and for what purpose. They are frequently prepared for each organizational unit and for each function within the unit.

Planning is done for a specific time period, usually a fiscal year, but may be subdivided into monthly, quarterly, or semiannual periods. The budgeting period is determined by the desired frequency of checks and should complete a normal cycle of activity. Budget periods that coincide with other control devices—such as managerial reports, balance sheets, and profit-and-loss statements—are helpful.

The extent to which accurate forecasts can be predicted must be considered. If the budget forecasts too far in advance, its usefulness is diminished. On the other hand, factors such as seasonal fluctuations make it impossible to predict long-range needs from short-budget periods. Managers, therefore, necessarily revise budgets as more information becomes available. Top management and the board of directors also may prepare long-term budgets of 3, 5, 10, or more years, but these are not used as direct operating budgets.

Prerequisites to budgeting. Some conditions are necessary for the development and implementation of a budgetary program. First there is need for a sound organizational structure with clear lines of authority and responsibility. Each employee knows her responsibilities and to whom she is responsible. Each person has the authority to do what she is responsible for and is held accountable for her actions. Organization charts and job descriptions are available. Goals and objectives are set for areas of responsibilities. Then budgets are developed to conform to the pattern of authority and responsibility.

Nonmonetary statistical data—such as number of admissions, average length of stay, percentage of occupancy, and number of patient days—are used for planning and control of the budgetary process. Someone must be responsible for collecting and reporting statistical data.

Charts of accounts are designed to be consistent with the organizational plan. Revenues and expenses are reported by responsibility areas, thus providing historical data that are valuable for planning and providing budgetary control for evaluation as performance can be compared to plans. The nurse manager focuses her attention on the principle of management by exception by noting what is not going as planned so she can take necessary action.

Managerial support is essential for a budgetary program. Although budgeting is done at the departmental level, it must be valued by top administration. Managers must be willing to devote their time and energy to the budgeting process. They are most likely to do that when they are familiar with the principles of budgeting and its usefulness for planning and controlling. Budget education is necessary.

Formal budgeting policies and procedures should be available in a budget manual. Objectives of the budgetary program are defined. Authority and responsibility for budgeting are clarified. Instructions for budget development are discussed in detail. Samples of standardized forms are available. A calendar of the budgeting activities with the schedule for each stage of the program is presented. Procedures for review, revision, and approval of budgets are discussed in detail.

Accounting. *Accounting* is a system that accumulates bookkeeping entries into summaries that tell the financial situation of an enterprise. Several terms must be understood to interpret financial accounting reports. *Entity* is a definable organizational unit. The accountant considers only transactions between one entity and another. Transactions that occur within the entity or do not involve it are not considered. If each department is an entity, performance can be compared between departments. However, if the agency as a whole is the entity, the transfer of resources from one department to another would not be taken into account. Accounts deal only with *transactions*, definable changes in the financial situation of an entity—income, expenditure, depreciation. *Cost valuation* values goods at their cost minus any depreciation. *Double entry* compares the assets, what is owed to or owned by the entity, with the liabilities, what is owed by the entity to others. Accountants are to balance total assets with the total liabilities and net worth. The double entry makes it possible to know where the entity stands financially at any given time. *Accrual* allows one to know the overall assets and liabilities by entering transactions on the accounting records at the time a commitment is made rather than waiting until it is billed or paid. *Matching* is the principle of matching revenues with expenses during a budget period.

There are several standard accounting practices. *Consistency* means that categories of transactions may not be changed during or between reporting periods without noting the changes and providing comparable figures. *Materiality* means that transactions can be combined for accounting purposes unless one transaction has a significant impact by itself. *Conservatism* is the act of understating revenue and overstating expenses to provide a margin of safety. *Industry practices* are specific to industries. Special fund accounts designated by donors and a separate account for charitable care provided are examples of industry practices.

Operating or revenue-and-expense budgets. The operating budget provides an overview of an agency's functions by projecting the planned operations, usually for the upcoming year. The operating table reveals an input-output analysis of expected revenues and expenses. Among the factors that the nurse manager might include in her operating budget are personnel salaries, employee benefits, insurance, medical-surgical supplies, office supplies, rent, heat, light, housekeeping, laundry service, drugs and pharmaceuticals, repairs and maintenance, depreciation, in-service education, travel to professional meetings, educational leaves, books, periodicals, subscriptions, dues and membership fees, legal fees, and recreation such as Christmas parties and retirement teas.

Both controllable and noncontrollable expenses are projected. The manager determines the number of personnel needed and the level of skills required of each. Wage levels and quality of materials used are other controllable expenses. Indirect expenses, such as rent, lighting, and depreciation of equipment, are noncontrollable. The noncontrollable expenses and the probability of rises in material prices or labor costs during the budgetary period demand that an operating budget include some cushion funds to provide for changes beyond the agency's control.

The operating budget deals primarily with salaries, supplies, and contractual services. Nonfinancial factors, such as time, materials, and space, may be translated into dollar values. Work hours, nurse-patient interaction hours, units of materials, equipment hours, and floor space also can be assigned dollar values.

Capital expenditure budgets. Capital expenditure budgets are related to long-range planning. Capital expenditures include physical changes such as replacement or expansion of the plant, major equipment, and inventories. These items are usually major investments and reduce the flexibility in budgeting because it takes a long time to recover the costs. For instance, a patient may be charged per treatment or per day for use of equipment, but it may take many months or even years to recover the cost of the equipment.

The hospital administrator usually establishes the ceiling for capital expenses. Under this budget, the nurse manager must establish priorities if requests exceed availability of funds. When filling out request forms for capital items, it is advisable to include names of manufacturers and suppliers, trade-in credits, and estimates of purchase, delivery, installation, and maintenance costs. Written justification for each item should be stated.

Inventories are helpful in budgeting. If supplies are checked routinely, utilization and replacement figures are available for projection of future needs. Central supply services enhance budgetary control, and storage space facilitates inventory maintenance. Stocked supply shelves on each unit with replacement service twice a day can provide a simplified recording system. Disposable equipment and supplies need careful evaluation to determine if they are more economical than nondisposables.

Cash budgets. Cash budgets are planned to make adequate funds available as needed and to use profitably any extra funds. They ensure that the agency has enough, but not too much, cash on hand during the budgetary period. This is necessary because income does not always coincide with expenditures. The manager must anticipate fluctuations in resource needs caused by such factors as seasonal variations. If the manager has insufficient cash on hand, she will not be able to purchase needed resources. At the other extreme, if too much cash is available, interest or other earnings that money could generate are lost. Budgeting cash requirements may not significantly affect profits, but it does ensure a liquid position and is a sign of prudent management. Using a cash budget, the nurse manager estimates the amount of money to be collected from clients and other sources and allocates that cash to expenditures. If the budget is well planned, it will provide cash as needed and produce interest on excess funds.

Labor or personnel budgets. Personnel budgets estimate the cost of direct labor necessary to meet the agency's objectives. They determine the recruitment, hiring, assignment, layoff, and discharge of personnel. The nurse manager decides on the type of nursing care necessary to meet the nursing needs of the estimated patient population. How many aides, orderlies, LPNs, and RNs are needed during what shifts, what months, and in what areas? The current staffing patterns, number of unfilled positions, and last year's reports can provide a base for examination and proposals. Patient occupancy and the general complexity of cases affect staffing patterns. Seasonal fluctuations must be considered. Personnel budgets also are affected by personnel policies, such as salary related to position and number of days allowed for educational and personal leave. Overtime costs should be compared with the cost of new positions. Employee turnover, recruitment, and orientation cost must be considered.

Flexible budgets. Some costs are fixed and do not change with the volume of business. Other costs vary proportionately with changes in volume. Some variable expenses are unpredictable and can be determined only after change has begun. Thus the need for flexible budgets. They show the effects of changes in volume of business on expense items, and periodic budget reviews help managers compensate for changes. Relationships between the volume of business and variable costs may be predicted by a historical analysis of costs and development of standard costs.

Historical approach to budgeting. The historical approach is most effective for calculating the relationship between volume of business and variable costs when a company manufactures a few products and each product contributes a relatively stable percentage to the total sales volume. Using the historical approach, the nurse manager may observe that there are more fractures during skiing season. Consequently, more casting materials are used at that time, and there is a need for increased staffing on the orthopedic ward. A supervising community health nurse in a small college town may note that there is less use of family planning services during the summer months and again during December when students leave for vacations. Consequently, there is less need for contraceptive devices and staffing during those months. There may be an increased demand for immunizations just before elementary schools start in the fall. By plotting on a graph the high and low volumes, the nurse manager can predict the expected costs for each level between the extreme volumes. This historical perspective helps determine the amount of supplies to stock and staffing patterns.

Standard cost. Standard cost may be developed to predict what labor and supplies should cost. Multiplying the standard cost by the volume predicts the variable cost. The supervising community health nurse can predict the standard number of clinic visits and the number of birth control pills that will be required by each family-planning client who has chosen birth control pills as a method of contraception. Multiplying the number of pills needed by each client by the number of clients using birth control pills, the nurse manager can predict the inventory needed and the cost. She also can project the number of clinic visits needed and plan staffing.

Zero-base budgeting. Many budgeting procedures allocate funds to departments based on their previous year's expenditures. Then the department managers decide how the funds will be used. This procedure usually allows for enrichment and enlargement of programs but seldom for decreases in or deletion of programs. Obsolescence is seldom examined, and this leads to increased costs.

With zero-base budgeting, no program is taken for granted. Each program or service must be justified each time funds are requested. Managers decide what will be done, what will not be done, and how much of an activity will be implemented. A decision package is prepared. The package includes a list of the activities that make up a program, the total cost, a description of what level of service can be performed at various levels of funding, and the ramifications of including them in or excluding them from the budget. The manager may identify the activity, state the purpose, list related activities, outline alternative ways of performing activities, and give the cost of the resources needed.

After decision packages are developed, they are ranked in order of decreasing benefits to the agency. They can be divided into high-, medium-, and low-priority categories and reviewed in order of rank for funding. Resources are allocated based on the priority of the decision package. The cost of each package is added to the cost of approved packages until the agreed-on spending level is reached. Lower ranked packages are then excluded.

A major advantage to zero-base budgeting is that it forces managers to set priorities and justify resources. Unfortunately, the process is time consuming.

Periodic budgetary review. Managers should review the budget at periodic intervals, compare actual with projected performances, and make necessary changes. However, if changes are made too frequently or are of considerable magnitude, the original budget becomes useless. One way to minimize variance between the annual budget and the revised budget is to anticipate such factors as increased labor costs and the inflationary cost of materials. When discrepancies are found between actual performance and the budget, management must determine the cause of variation to make appropriate adjustments for future plans. A variance may not be reason for changing the budget. It may be a symptom that alerts management to the need for further investigation and explanation. What may demand change is not the budget but the situation.

Supplementary budgets. Some budgetary flexibility may be obtained through a supplemental monthly budget. A basic or minimal budget is planned, usually for a year's time, to outline the framework for the agency's plans, establish

48

department objectives, and coordinate departments. Then a monthly supplementary budget is prepared on the basis of the volume of business forecast for that month.

Moving budgets. The moving budget may be used when forecasting is difficult. The moving budget plans for a certain length of time, such as a year. At the end of each month, another month is added to replace the one just completed. Thus the budgetary period remains constant. The projections progress a month at a time but always for a fixed period such as one year. It is an annual budget revised monthly. As January is completed, the January budget for the forthcoming year is added to the moving budget.

Advantages and disadvantages of flexible budgets. The major advantage of flexible budgets is the study and analysis necessary to prepare one. Fixed and variable costs and their effect on the total cost are analyzed. Unfortunately, flexible budgets are very costly to prepare. Their construction takes considerable time. It is difficult to predict short-term variations in volume, and it is unlikely that the information can result in savings of variable expenses.

Advantages of budgeting. Budgets plan for detailed program activities in advance. They help fix accountability by assignment of responsibility and authority. They state goals for all units, offer a standard of performance, and stress the continuous nature of planning and control process. Budgets encourage managers to make a careful analysis of operations and to base a decision on careful consideration. Consequently, hasty judgments are minimized. Weaknesses in the organization can be revealed and corrective measures taken. Staffing, equipment, and supply needs can be projected and waste minimized. Financial matters can be handled in an orderly fashion, and agency activities can be coordinated and balanced.

Disadvantages of budgeting. Budgets convert all aspects of organizational performance into monetary values for a single comparable unit of measurement. Consequently, only those aspects that are easy to measure may be considered, and equally important factors, such as organizational development and research efforts, may be ignored. Symptoms may be treated as causes. Reasons for the symptoms should be explored, because a decrease in revenue from the family planning clinic may be related to the way people are treated at the clinic, a new competitive service in the neighborhood, or other factors. The budget may become an end in itself instead of the means to an end. Budgetary goals may supersede agency goals and gain autocratic control of the organization. There is a danger of overbudgeting; the budget becomes cumbersome, meaningless, and expensive. Forecasting is required but uncertain because budgetary control is subject to human judgment, interpretation, and evaluation. Skill and experience are required for successful budgetary control. Budget planning is time consuming and expensive.

Budgeting process

Financial planning responsibilities need to be identified before budget preparation begins. The governing board, administrator, budget director, steering committee, and department heads are often involved in the budgetary process. The *governing board* is responsible for the general planning function. It selects the budget steering committee, determines the budgetary objectives, and reviews and approves the master budget. The *administrator* is responsible for the formulation and execution of the budget. She correlates the governing board's goals with the guidelines for budget preparation and supervises the budget preparation. The *budget director* is responsible for the budgeting procedures and reporting. She establishes a completion timetable, has forms prepared, and supervises data collection and budget preparation. The budget director serves as the chairperson of the *steering committee*. The committee approves of the budget before it is submitted to the governing board. *Department heads* prepare and review goals and objectives and prepare the budgets for their departments.

The first step in the budget process is the establishment of operational goals and policies for the entire agency. The governing board should approve a long-range plan of 5 to 10 years that reflects the community's future health needs and other community health care providers' activities. Because the situation changes over time, flexibility is built into the plan. Then operational goals must be translated into quantifiable management objectives for the organizational units. The department heads use the organizational goals as a framework for the development of departmental goals. A formal plan for budget preparation and review including assignment of responsibilities and timetables must be prepared. Historical, financial, and statistical data need to be collected on a monthly basis so that seasonal fluctuation can be observed. Departmental budgets need to be prepared and coordinated. During this phase, units of service, staffing patterns, salary and nonsalary expenses, and revenues are forecasted so that preliminary rate setting can be done. Next, departmental budgets are revised, and the master budget is prepared. At this point, operating, payroll, nonsalary, capital, and cash budgets can be incorporated into the master budget. Then the financial feasibility of the master budget is tested, and the final document is approved and distributed to all parties involved.

During the budget period, there should be periodic performance reporting by responsibility centers.

COST CONTAINMENT

The goal of cost containment is to keep costs within acceptable limits for volume, inflation, and other acceptable parameters. It involves cost awareness, monitoring, management, and incentives to avoid, reduce, and control costs.

The Tax Equity Fiscal Responsibility Act of 1982 added case-mix into Medicare based on diagnostic-related groups (DRGs). This is a case-based, prospective reimbursement system whereby rates are set before care is given. This system encourages the implementation of cost-effective health care services. The results of DRGs include fewer patients in acute care settings caused by early discharge, an increase in the acuteness of hospitalized patients, an increase in the use of ambulatory and home care facilities, and a focus on cost effectiveness.

Cost awareness focuses the employee's attention on costs. It increases organizational awareness of what costs are, the process available for containing them, how they can be managed, and by whom. Delegating budget planning and control to the unit level increases awareness. The managers should be provided a course about budgeting and be oriented to the agency budgeting process before being assigned the responsibility. They should be provided with a budget manual that contains budget forms, budget calendar, and budget periods.

Cost fairs in frequented areas like the cafeteria increase awareness by displaying frequently disappearing items that are labeled with the cost per unit and by posting lists of estimated costs of inventory losses. Staff development programs, unit conferences, and poster contests help increase awareness. Tagging supply items and posting a computer printout of unit charges for supplies and services are revealing. Reviewing a patient's itemized bill during a conference can also be effective.

Cost monitoring focuses on how much will be spent where, when, and why. It identifies, reports, and monitors costs. Staffing costs should be identified. Recruitment, turnover, absenteeism, and sick time are analyzed. Inventories are controlled. A central supply exchange chart prevents hoarding of supplies and allows identification of lost items.

Cost management focuses on what can be done by whom to contain costs. Programs, plans, objectives, and strategies are important. Responsibility and accountability for the control should be established. A committee can identify long- and short-range plans and strategies. A suggestion box can be used. Contests for the idea that saves the most money are useful.

Money has been saved by means such as forming a staff pool to maximize flexibility in staffing for census fluctuations, closing units for cleaning or remodeling and encouraging staff vacations when census is low, balancing the work load among shifts to minimize peaks and valleys in assigned tasks, reducing shift overlap, tape-recording shift reports, revising forms, improving drug ordering and delivery systems, modifying food services, allowing volunteers to discharge and transport patients, and reducing the amount of time nurses spend doing nonnursing functions.

Cost incentives motivate cost containment and reward desired behavior. Contests for the best money-saving ideas, perfect attendance, and nurse of the month help recognize personnel efforts.

Cost avoidance means not buying supplies, technology, or services. Supply and equipment costs should be carefully analyzed. Costs and effectiveness between disposable and reusable items are compared. The receipt, storage, and delivery of disposables and labor and processing costs of reusable items are part of the analysis. The least expensive and most effective supplies, equipment, and services should be identified. Expensive and less effective items should be avoided.

Cost reduction means spending less for goods and services. The amount of reduction is dependent on the size of the agency, previous efficiency, skill of managers, and cooperation of employees. Safety programs that reduce the costs of worker's compensation, and absenteeism programs that reduce sick time, absenteeism, and turnover reduce costs.

Cost control is effective use of available resources through careful forecasting, planning, budget preparation, reporting, and monitoring. Cost-effectiveness compares costs and identifies the most beneficial outcomes to costs. This is done by specifying programs, identifying the goals, analyzing alternatives, comparing the costs per program unit of service and the amount of service needed, assessing the effect of the outcome, and determining cost outcome and cost-effectiveness.

TIME MANAGEMENT

If productivity were only a function of time, one would expect all to produce equally. And yet, although everyone has the same number of hours in a day and the same number of days per week, some people accomplish more than others. Granted, some people work longer and harder than others to accomplish more, but some just make better use of their time. Because nurses work long hours, they should work smarter—not harder—to get more done in less time.

Maximize managerial time

The nurse manager may start a plan for maximizing use of her time by conducting an inventory of her activities. After recording what she did every 15 minutes for a typical week, she assesses how she spent her time. How much time was spent in which activities? Was the way the time was spent determined by conscious decisions, habit, work demands, default, or spontaneity? What does she like to do? What activities does she want to increase? What does she want to decrease? How can she reduce the time wasters?

Next the nurse determines her short-, medium-, and long-range goals. What does she want to accomplish? What does she want to do soon? Which goals need to be completed before others? Which ones will take the longest to achieve? Setting priorities helps resolve goal conflicts and directs how she will spend her time.

Once she has determined and ranked her goals, she plans strategies for how to accomplish them. What activities must she do? What are low-priority activities that can be eliminated? Next the nurse manager schedules activities. A tickler box with divider cards for months and weeks can be used by filing task cards behind the appropriate month and week card. As she looks at her major responsibilities for a whole year, she may have some flexibility in determining when certain jobs are done and can use those to help balance the work load around tasks that have to be done at certain times, such as preparing the budget. Various calendar systems can also be used. One may do major project planning on a year-at-a-glance calendar. Desk ink blotters that depict a month at a time can help regulate that month's work. A week-at-a-glance or a day-at-a-glance calendar is convenient for carrying in one's purse. Daily work sheets depicting what work should be done during which hour may also be useful.

The nurse manager needs to assess her peak and low times to plan a detailed schedule more effectively. Is she most alert and creative in the early morning or late at night? Is she a slow starter in the morning? Does she reach a low energy point in the middle of the afternoon? The nurse's prime internal time— her most creative time for working alone—is a good time to schedule work that should not be interrupted. When is her prime external time, her best time to work with others? If she reaches a low point in the afternoon, that may be a good time to schedule office visits. She may offer her guest a cup of coffee or tea, which tends to facilitate communication, sip on her own drink, and listen.

Time should be set aside for certain activities each day. Scheduled activities are recorded. Scheduled and unscheduled times are noted, and contact and thinking times are identified. The secretary may be given available hours for scheduling office visits.

A few minutes at the beginning of each day should be allowed for planning. A running list of what needs to be done in order of importance can be written down each morning to plan what will be done that day. Desk-organizing files— which are merely folders with such labels as urgent, return calls, dictate, read, file, and low priority—can help determine what to do each day. Scheduled free time can be used to deal with these activities. A few minutes at the end of the day are used to evaluate what happened.

Learning how to say no graciously saves time. It is advisable for the nurse manager to acknowledge the request, state and explain her position, check back for understanding with the other person, and avoid defensiveness. For example, when asked to speak at a meeting she might respond, ''I would love to discuss our institutional goals with your committee. However, I have another commitment at that time. Barbara Jones and Sue Smith are both very familiar with the institutional goals. Perhaps you could ask one of them to speak. Does that sound agreeable to you?"

Delegation also saves time and can help develop others. The manager needs to evaluate the risk involved in delegating by assessing the criticality of the expected results and the confidence in resources. The planning strategy ascertains specifications including the expected results, rationale, requirements, and constraints. The delegated authority should be specified, and support needed should be anticipated. When communicating the delegated assignment, the manager should ensure understanding, give and receive feedback, and address concerns. To monitor the delegated assignment, the manager should set up a milestone-tracking system, review scheduled status reports, and give feedback on the interim reports. Support is provided by responding to the delegatee's needs, acknowledging the status reports, and being available for guidance and problem solving. The supervisor should intervene only when the action seems warranted and, even then, by avoiding interference and explaining one's actions. Reverse delegation can be avoided by clarifying specifications, transferring authority, and expressing confidence in the delegatee. The results should be evaluated by examining the specifications, evaluating the monitoring results, and giving feedback on the final results.*

Managers can get much done during transition times. Incoming mail may be read while one is on "hold" when returning phone calls. Reports can be read while commuting to and from work. Isometric exercises can be done at most any time. Lunch and coffee breaks may be used for personal business. Because many women are watching their weight, lunch breaks may be better used for exercise, such as walking and jogging, or meditation than for eating a large lunch.

Much time can be saved by streamlining paperwork. Scheduling a block of time to answer mail prevents interruptions. If the situation warrants, a standard reply can be used. Some responses can be made on the query memo if no file copy is needed. Typing carbon responses to letters onto the back of the query letter saves filing time and space. Color coding is useful, and the recording of destruction dates on files reduces the need to review the materials later. Dictation usually takes less time than writing by hand, and calls can be used when a record is not necessary. Selective reading by scanning tables of contents and reading summaries at the end of long responses and reports saves time. Managers should not concentrate on details unless necessary as they are quickly forgotten. Scanning for major points is often adequate.

Learning speed-reading techniques such as tapping, L pattern, S swirl, area

---

*Delegation is discussed more fully in Executive delegation: achieving results through people, Stamford, Conn., 1985, Learning International.

reading, and reading for meaning can help overcome common reading problems of single-word fixation, involuntary regression by rereading, subvocalization of words as one reads, and inability to concentrate.

Listening and memory techniques also save time ultimately. When listening for understanding, one should assume value in what the speaker is saying by being attentive, delaying judgment, maintaining eye contact, and using attentive body language. One then needs to assess the content of the information by focusing on central ideas, looking for relationships between ideas, and selecting an organizing structure such as main and supporting ideas, advantages and disadvantages, or putting information into chronological order. One should analyze the information by listening to what is being said, identifying how it is being said by inferring emotions from body language and tone of voice, and considering speaker's motivation for saying it. Distractions may need to be reduced so the listener can concentrate. Verbal, mental, and physical techniques can be used to stimulate memory. *Repeating, clarifying,* and *summarizing* are effective verbal techniques. Focusing, imaging, linking, locating, and chunking are mental techniques. *Focusing* by putting attention on one thing at a time helps block out distractions. *Imaging* creates a vivid mental image that helps one remember something. When introduced to Leona Dean, the nurse might picture her leaning on a dean of a specific school to help remember her name. *Linking* makes associations between things that make them easier to remember later. Associations may be cause and effect, parts of a whole, or things that are near each other, logically go together, contrast with each other, or happen concurrently. Creating an association that leads from point one to point two to point three and creating an image of those associations will help one remember a speech. *Locating* is a memory technique that uses a known structure, often one's home, to arrange and remember information by putting it in specific locations. One might progress through an orientation program by visualizing the hallway in the office and thinking of who is in each office as one walks through the hall and what service that person provides new staff. *Chunking* helps one remember by dividing large amounts of information into smaller, more manageable pieces. One could chunk information needed into separate sections of a report, or the nurse could locate what items are needed in specific separate offices. Physical techniques for stimulating memory are *note taking, filing,* and *follow-up memos.**

Telephone calls instead of office visits or correspondence save time. Secretaries can screen calls so that other activities are not interrupted and, in fact, may be able to handle much of the business. A call-back system can be used to complete the business the secretary cannot handle. If late morning and late

---

*These skills can be developed more fully by studying Stimulating memory, Stamford, Conn., 1986, Learning International, Inc.

afternoon are chosen for returning calls, calls are likely to be kept short, because people are anxious to eat lunch or to go home.

Forms for telephone messages are less likely to get lost than scraps of paper. It helps if phone messages are collected in one place. One should keep a list of commonly called phone numbers handy. If major topics for conversation are outlined before making a call, it is less likely that one will forget something and need to call back. One can set the tone of the call. A businesslike call started by "What can I do for you?" will get more accomplished in less time than a friendly call started with, "How are you?" Conference calls also save time by focusing more on business than socializing. The purpose for the conversation helps determine whether a meeting or a conference call is necessary.

The secretary may also screen office visits. Once again she may be able to handle much of the business herself. When the manager schedules reception hours, the secretary can schedule appointments for the appropriate length of time and inform the manager of the purpose of the meeting so that she can be adequately prepared. One may need to close the office door to get a task completed without interruptions. Sitting with one's back to the door may decrease interruptions because people will notice that the manager is busy.

The length of a meeting can be better controlled if it is not in the manager's office. The manager may go to the subordinates' work area or meet visitors in a reception area where she is free to leave whenever she desires. By standing up when someone drops into the office, the manager prevents the visitor from sitting down. Thus she controls the situation. She can assess the priority, make an appointment for another time, keep the visit short, or invite the visitor to sit down for a longer discussion. Many drop-in visits can be prevented by scheduling lunch with subordinates on a regular basis. This allows the manager opportunity to keep informed, discuss matters of common interest, and eat lunch at the same time.

Managers spend considerable time in meetings, much of which is wasted. Meetings are used for participative problem solving, decision making, coordination, information sharing, and morale building. The manager first considers the purpose of the meeting and if it is not necessary, she does not conduct it. Key participants are identified, and if they cannot attend, the meeting is not held. People who do not need to attend are not invited. The manager should consider alternatives to a meeting, such as a memo, telephone call, or conference. Subordinates can represent her at some meetings both to save managerial time and to develop the subordinate. The manager may limit her time in meetings by attending only that segment when she is to make a contribution. Scheduling meetings before lunch and quitting time facilitates ending meetings on time. A centrally located meeting place saves travel time. The purpose of the meeting should be clearly defined, and an agenda should be circulated before the meeting.

Meetings should start on time, because time is expensive. Starting a meeting 15 minutes late for twenty people who earn $10 an hour costs $50 in down time. Stating the purpose of the meeting and following the agenda are the manager's responsibilities. She should start with high-priority items so that only low-priority items will be left over. The manager should control interruptions, restate conclusions, make assignments and deadlines clear, and end the meeting on time. If the business is completed early, the manager dismisses the meeting. Minutes are circulated preferably within a day after the meeting; this allows people to be informed without having to attend the meeting unless their input is specifically needed. Minutes also remind participants of their assigned tasks.

Maximize organization time

Plan. Much time can be saved through appropriate organizational planning. The purpose for the existence of the agency should be determined, and the goals and objectives should be defined and ranked in order of importance. The nurse manager determines who is responsible for coordinating activities, who makes what decisions, and who needs to be informed about certain decisions. She also determines what decisions need to be made before others, what action needs to be taken first, and what deadlines must be set. The determining and ranking of goals focuses activities and prevents people from spending time doing inappropriate or unimportant tasks. People who are adequately informed of what is expected of them will not waste time wondering what they are supposed to do. Making time estimates and setting time limits help regulate work flow. Through appropriate planning, problems can be prevented. The decreased amount of time spent in crisis management increases the time available for creative work.

Organize. The manager structures the agency to accomplish the tasks necessary to meet the agency's goals. Organizational charts help clarify who is responsible to whom and for what. Job descriptions further clarify these matters. Multiple bosses, confusion over who is responsible and who has authority for what, and duplication of tasks can be prevented with planning. Autonomy and independence reduce the amount of time otherwise spent in conflict management.

Staff. Selection of well-qualified staff is critical for time saving, because they require less supervisory time for development and corrective action. Staff development further reduces time lost by better preparing staff to do their jobs. Appropriate use of manpower through assessment of work to be done, careful planning of the number and mix of personnel, and matching the staff member's interest and abilities to her job further reduce waste. When the nurse's interests are matched to the organizational goals and she feels appreciated, she is likely to have increased job satisfaction. Consequently there is little absenteeism and less turnover. The nurse manager should watch for chronic absenteeism, try to determine the reason, and correct it. She also expects punctuality, because tardiness is a loss of time. If the nurse manager finds that employees' personal problems are affecting their work, she should refer personnel for appropriate assistance so that they will have more energy to do their jobs.

Direct. It is the nurse manager's responsibility to delegate what a less qualified, lower-paid person can handle. She is the one who identifies the task to be delegated, determines the best person to do the job, and communicates the assignment clearly. She allows the subordinate to help determine how the task will be accomplished and keeps authority commensurate with the responsibility. She sets controls, monitors results, and provides support as needed. It is essential that the manager teach others how to do the work instead of doing it herself. She can save considerable time by streamlining communication systems and by not holding any more meetings than necessary. The nurse manager should also facilitate open communications and assertive behavior and handle conflict immediately before it drains time and energy.

Control. The nurse manager sets standards, monitors results, and gives feedback. She adjusts closeness of supervision to the needs of the employee, takes disciplinary action as soon as it is justified, and fires personnel who are not meeting minimum standards. Good management conserves time and energy.

MARKETING

"Marketing is the analysis, planning, implementation, and control of carefully formulated programs designed to bring about voluntary exchanges of values with target markets for the purpose of achieving organizational objectives. It relies heavily on designing the organization's offering in terms of the target markets' needs and desires and on using effective pricing, communication, and distribution to inform, motivate, and service the markets."*

Marketing concepts

Exchange. Marketing is based on resource dependency or exchange. Organizations offer satisfactions such as goods, services, or benefits to markets that in return provide needed resources such as goods, services, time, money, or energy. Exchange involves four conditions: (1) There are at least two parties. (2)

---

*P. Kotler, Marketing for nonprofit organizations, Englewood Cliffs, N.J., 1982, Prentice-Hall, Inc., p. 6.

Each party offers something that the other believes to be of value. (3) Each party is capable of communication and delivery. (4) Each party is free to accept or reject the offer (Kotler, 1982, p. 37).

Publics. "A public is a distinct group of people and/or organizations that has an actual or a potential interest and/or impact on an organization" (Kotler, 1982, p. 47). Input publics supply resources and constraints and consist of suppliers, donors, and regulatory publics. Those inputs are then managed by the organization's internal publics such as the board of directors, management, staff, and volunteers to accomplish the organization's mission. Intermediary publics are used to promote and distribute goods and services to consumers. The consuming publics, such as patients, clients, and students, consume the output of the organization.

Market. "A market is a potential arena for the trading of resources." It is "a distinct group of people and/or organizations that have resources which they want to exchange, or might conceivably be willing to exchange, for distinct benefits" (Kotler, 1982, p. 50).

Image. "An image is the sum of beliefs, ideas, and impressions that a person has of an object" (Kotler, 1982, p. 57). Publics with a positive image of an organization will be drawn to it, whereas publics with a negative image will avoid or disparage the organization.

There are two opposite theories about image formation. *Object-determined* maintains that people perceive the reality of the object. They experience the object and process the sensory data in a similar way despite different backgrounds. Therefore, when people see a building in a beautiful setting they perceive it as a beautiful hospital. *Person-determined* theory maintains that people have different degrees of contact with an object; they selectively perceive different aspects of the object, and through individual ways of processing the sensory data, they experience selective distortion. In this case, some people may perceive the hospital as beautiful while others do not.

Image is a function of deeds and communications. Good deeds without telling others or talking without actions is not enough. A strong, favorable image develops from satisfied publics who tell others their opinions.

Marketing process

Marketing involves informing the market of services provided and fitting services to market needs. It is a complex process that generally includes the audit, market segmentation, marketing mix, implementation, and evaluation and control.

Audit. The marketing audit involves identification, collection, and evaluation of information that needs to be examined to evaluate market relations. The *market and market segments* need to be identified. How large is the area to be served? Is it rural, urban, or both? How many potential customers are there? What are their ages, occupations, income levels, and interests? How many are aware of your services? Are there seasonal differences?

The *organization* should be assessed. What are the organization's philosophy, goals, objectives, and priorities? What are the services provided, strengths, and weaknesses? How do your services compare with those of others? What conditions of the industry affect you? What internal and external controls affect you?

As *services* are further analyzed, note distinctive superiorities. What services are heavily used? Why? What services are underutilized? Why? Are there voids? If so, can they be filled? How can needed materials, supplies, and manpower be obtained? Who pays for the services?

Who are the *competitors*? How many are there? Are their numbers increasing or decreasing? Who are the principal competitors? What areas do they serve? How do their size and strength compare? How do their charges compare?

What is the profile of present and future *clients* for your services? Are client profiles different among services? What is the frequency of client usage of your services?

What is the organization's pricing philosophy? How are *prices* determined? How are prices viewed by the staff, clients, and competitors?

In what *location* is your service provided? How accessible is it to clients? How far will clients have to travel to obtain the service? Will you travel to provide a service? If so, how far? Will you charge for travel expenses?

What is the purpose of *promotion*? Is it reaching the intended publics? Is it effective? What media are being used? What media reach whom?

Many *assessment tools* can be used to collect data for the audit. Questionnaires administered by mail, telephone, or interview, in-depth interviews, and observations are common. A consumer panel can be used to discuss relevant issues. A mediator helps keep a representative group of consumers discussing a specific topic in focus groups. Nominal groups aim at generating consensus about a particular issue. Records can be reviewed, and scientific research designs can be planned and implemented to collect data.

A *sampling plan* is important. Who will be surveyed? What will the sample size be? Large size samples are more reliable than small samples. How will the sample be chosen? A random sample is the most reliable.

Statistical techniques such as frequency distributions, means, standard deviations, regression analysis, correlation analysis, factor analysis, discriminant analysis, and cluster analysis can be useful. Statistical techniques are technical, and therefore, statistical consultation is often advisable.

Market segmentation. Segmentation identifies subsets of the total market that have similar characteristics. Segmentation is based on the assumptions that consumers are different, these differences affect market behavior, and one can isolate segments within the total market. The criteria most often used to describe segments are (1) geography—rural or urban; (2) demography—age, sex, race; (3) psychography—values, habits, lifestyles; (4) behavior—repeated use of services; and (5) buying process—awareness of services, benefits sought.

There are three major marketing strategies related to segments. Differentiated marketing aims directly and differentially at several specific segments. Concentrated marketing aims at a specific segment. Undifferentiated marketing ignores segments and deals with all as one market.

Marketing mix. The marketing mix makes use of the audit's results related to the needs of targeted segments. It involves the four *p*'s: product, price, place, and promotions.

Product is something provided for consumption to satisfy a need or want. The inventory of services, analysis of costs, benefits, and target markets indicate which products are overused, underused, and cost-effective and which are perceived as strong or weak. This information should be used to determine the appropriate product mix.

Price is another major consideration. Because physicians rather than patients usually determine the services used, and health care bills are usually paid by third-party payers, nondollar costs such as time and convenience must be considered. Minimization of nondollar costs should benefit the health care agency and the consumer.

Place involves the physical location, appearance of the location, its accessibility and availability, resource utilization, the expertise and courtesy of staff, referral mechanisms, and distribution. The goal is to the the service to the consumer with efficient distribution and as little inconvenience as possible.

Marketing promotion informs potential consumers of the existence and availability of products and services and persuades them of the benefits to the consumers. Tailoring services to consumer desires is important. Marketing promotion leads to awareness, understanding, interest, decision, utilization, satisfaction, reutilization, and recommendation.

Implementation. Implementation can be done incrementally or as an entire package. Designing and implementing a marketing program are expensive projects and require personnel with expertise in marketing. Outside consultants can be hired when qualified people are not available within the organization. Dealing with local political conflicts, reaching communities that are out of touch with their own real demands, and sorting real demands from surface expectations are challenging tasks.

Evaluation and control. The last phase of the marketing process is evaluation and control. It involves identifying goals and objectives, measuring planned and actual results, determining reason for variance between planned and actual results, correcting actions based on causal analysis, and revising goals. Evaluation can be done more or less often—daily through weekly, monthly, yearly to a more extended basis to determine if implementation is accomplishing desired results.

LEARNING ACTIVITIES

1

After referring to the case study in the appendix, use your imagination to identify a problem, explore alternatives, decide what unit to add, and plan to implement your decision. To determine what units to add, consider societal trends, such as increased life expectancy and a decreased fertility rate; health care delivery trends, such as regional planning, movement from hospital to community base, and more emphasis on preventive care; trends in the nation's health, such as high incidences of heart disease, cancer, and accidents; and community trends. If the community has a high incidence of heart attacks, a cardiac care unit may be added. If the incidence of cancer is high, an oncology unit may be added. If there has been an increase in the number of burn victims because of new industry, a burn unit might be added. With a focus on health and prevention of illness, the community may need an ambulatory pediatric outpatient unit.

2

Draw a PERT chart for the activities involved with the new addition. Consider completion of the building; ordering equipment and supplies; recruitment, selection, and orientation of staff; development of goals; development of budget; and admission of the first patients.

3

Using the case study in the appendix:

Write the purpose for Lake View Hospital.

Write the philosophy for Lake View Hospital.

Develop the goals and objectives for one of the new units.

Write a policy for Lake View Hospital.

Develop a budget for one of the new units.

4

To practice time management, record what you do every 15 minutes for a typical week and assess how you spent your time. Identify time wasters. Determine your short-, medium-, and long-range goals and list them in order of priority. Plan strategies to accomplish your goals. Assess your peak and low times. Plan your schedule. Prepare a daily "to do" list.

BIBLIOGRAPHY

Books

Adams, J.L.: Conceptual blockbusting: a guide to better ideas, ed. 2, New York, 1979, W.W. Norton & Co.

Albers, H.H.: Principles of management: a modern approach, New York, 1974, John Wiley & Sons, Inc.

Albers, H.H., and Schoer, L.: Programmed organization and management principles, New York, 1966, John Wiley & Sons, Inc.

Alexander, E.L.: Nursing administration in the hospital health care system, St. Louis, 1978, The C. V. Mosby Co.

Arndt, C., and Daderian Huckabay, L.M.: Nursing administration: theory for practice with a systems approach, St. Louis, 1975, The C. V. Mosby Co.

Bagwell, M., and Clements, S.: A political handbook for health professionals, Boston, 1985, Little, Brown & Co.

Bailey, J.T., and Claus, K.E.: Decision making in nursing, St. Louis, 1975, The C. V. Mosby Co.

Barrett, J.: The head nurse: her changing role, New York, 1962, Appleton-Century-Crofts.

Belcher, D.W.: Compensation administration, Englewood Cliffs, N.J., 1974, Prentice-Hall, Inc.

Berger, M.S., et al., editors: Management for nurses, ed. 2, St. Louis, 1980, The C. V. Mosby Co.

Berman, H.J., and Weeks, L.E.: The financial management of hospitals, ed. 6, Ann Arbor, Mich., 1986, Health Administration Press.

Brooten, D.A.: Managerial leadership in nursing, Philadelphia, 1984, J.B. Lippincott Co.

Buchholz, R.A.: Essentials of public policy for management, Englewood Cliffs, N.J., 1985, Prentice-Hall, Inc.

Charns, M.P., and Schaefer, M.J.: Health care organizations: a model for management, Englewood Cliffs, N.J., 1983, Prentice-Hall, Inc.

Christian, W.P., and Hannah, G.T.: Effective management in human services, Englewood Cliffs, N.J., 1983, Prentice-Hall, Inc.

Clark, C.C., and Shea, C.A.: Management in nursing: a vital link in the health care system, New York, 1979, McGraw-Hill Book Co.

Cleverley, W.O.: Essentials of health care finance, ed. 2, Rockville, Md., 1986, Aspen Publications.

Connor, P.E.: Dimensions in modern management, ed. 3, Boston, 1982, Houghton Mifflin Co.

Cowart, M., and Allen, R.F.: Changing conceptions of health care, Grove Road, 1981, Charles B. Black, Inc.

Curtin, L., and Flaherty, M.J.: Nursing ethics: theories and pragmatics, Bowie, Md., 1982, Robert J. Brady Co.

Dale, E.: Management: theory and practice, ed. 4, New York, 1978, McGraw-Hill Book Co.

Di Vincenti, M.: Administering nursing service, ed. 2, Boston, 1977, Little, Brown & Co.

Donnelly, J.H., Jr., Gibson, J.L., and Ivancevich, J.M.: Fundamentals of management: functions, behavior, models, Austin, Tex., 1971, Business Publications, Inc.

Donovan, H.M.: Nursing service administration: managing the enterprise, St. Louis, 1975, The C. V. Mosby Co.

Eckles, R.W., Carmichael, R.L., and Sarchet, B.R.: Essentials of management for first-line supervision, New York, 1974, John Wiley & Sons, Inc.

Feldman, D.C., and Arnold, H.J.: Managing individual and group behavior in organizations, New York, 1983, McGraw-Hill Book Co.

Filley, A.C.: Interpersonal conflict resolution, Glenview, Ill., 1975, Scott, Foresman & Co.

Flippo, E.B.: Management: a behavioral approach, Boston, 1970, Allyn & Bacon, Inc.

Ford, J.G., Trygstad-Durland, L.N., and Nelms, B.G.: Applied decision making for nurses, St. Louis, 1979, The C. V. Mosby Co.

French, W.L.: The personnel management process, ed. 5, Boston, 1982, Houghton Mifflin Co.

Ganong, J.M., and Ganong, W.L.: Cases in nursing management, Germantown, Md., 1979, Aspen Systems Corp.

Ganong, J.M., and Ganong, W.L.: HELP . . . with annual budgetary planning, Chapel Hill, N.C., 1976, W.L. Ganong Co.

Ganong J.M. and Ganong W.L.: Nursing management, ed. 2, Germantown, Md., 1986, Aspen Systems Corp.

Garrett, T.M.: Business ethics, ed. 2, Englewood Cliffs, N.J., 1986, Prentice-Hall, Inc.

Gibson, J.L., Ivancevich, J.M., and Donnelly, J.H.: Organizations: behavior, structure, processes, Plano, Tex., 1985, Business Publications, Inc.

Gillies, D.A: Nursing management: a systems approach, Philadelphia, 1982, W.B. Saunders Co.

Haimann, T., and Scott, W.G.: Management in the modern organization, Boston, 1974, Houghton Mifflin Co.

Hampton, D.R.: Contemporary management, ed. 2, New York, 1981, McGraw-Hill Book Co.

Hampton, D.R., Summer, C.E., and Webber, R.A.: Organizational behavior and the practice of management, ed. 5, Glenview, Ill., 1986, Scott, Foresman & Co.

Haynes, W.W, and Massie, J.L.: Management: analysis, concepts and cases, Englewood Cliffs, N.J., 1969, Prentice-Hall, Inc.

Hein, E.C., and Nicholson, M.J., editors: Contemporary leadership behavior: selected readings, Boston, 1986, Little, Brown & Co.

Hicks, H.G.: The management of organizations: a systems and human resources approach, New York, 1972, McGraw-Hill Book Co.

Hoffman, F.M.: Financial management for nurse managers, Norwalk, Conn., 1984, Appleton-Century-Crofts.

Holle, M.L., and Blatchley, M.E.: Introduction to leadership and management in nursing, ed. 2, Monterey, Calif., 1987, Wadsworth Health Sciences Division.

Jacobs, P.: The economics of health and medical care, ed. 2, Rockville, Md., 1987, Aspen Publications.

Kaluzny, A.D., et al.: Management of health services, Englewood Cliffs, N.J., 1982, Prentice-Hall, Inc.

Kast, F.E., and Rosenzweig, J.E.: Organization and management: a systems and contingency approach, ed. 4, New York, 1985, McGraw-Hill Book Co.

Katz, D., and Kahn, R.L.: The social psychology of organizations, ed. 2, New York, 1978, John Wiley & Sons, Inc.

Kaufman, R.: Identifying and solving problems: a systems approach, ed. 3, La Jolla, Calif., 1982, University Associates, Inc.

Kazmier, L.J.: Management: a programmed approach, with cases and applications, ed. 4, New York, 1980, McGraw-Hill Book Co.

Keane, C.B.: Management essentials in nursing, Reston, Va., 1980, Appleton & Lange, Inc.

Kirk, R.K.: Nursing management tools, Boston, 1981, Little, Brown & Co.

Koontz, H., and O'Donnell, C.: Principles of management: an analysis of managerial functions, New York, 1972, McGraw-Hill Book Co.

Lakein, A.: How to get control of your time and your life, New York, 1974, The New American Library, Inc.

Lancaster, J., and Lancaster, W.: Concepts for advanced nursing practice: the nurse as a change agent, St. Louis, 1981, The C. V. Mosby Co.

Langford, T.L.: Managing and being managed, Englewood Cliffs, N.J., 1981, Appleton & Lange, Inc.

LeBoeuf, M.: Working smart, New York, 1979, Warner Books.

Lipson, S.H., and Hensel, M.D.: Hospital manpower budget preparation manual, Ann Arbor, Mich., 1975, Health Administration Press.

Longest, B.B.: Management practices for health professionals, ed. 3, Reston, Va., 1984, Appleton & Lange, Inc.

MacKenzie, R.A.: The time trap: how to get more done in less time, New York, 1975, McGraw-Hill Book Co.

Marriner, A., editor: Contemporary nursing management: issues and practice, St. Louis, 1982, The C. V. Mosby Co.

McConnel, C.R.: The effective health care supervisor, Rockville, Md., 1982, Aspen Systems Corp.

McFarland, D.: Management principles and practices, New York, 1974, Macmillan, Inc.

McQuillan, F.: Realities of nursing management: how to cope, Bowie, Md., 1978, Robert J. Brady Co.

National Center for Health Services Research and Development: Administrative cost determination manual for hospital inpatient-accounting, Rockville, Md., July, 1972, U.S. Department of Health, Education and Welfare, Public Health Service, Health Services and Mental Health Administration [DHEW publication no. (HSM) 73-3020].

National Center for Health Services Research and Development: Financial planning in ambulatory health programs, Rockville, Md., July, 1973, U.S. Department of Health, Education and Welfare, Public Health Service, Health Services and Mental Health Administration [DHEW publication no. (HRA) 74-3027].

Neal, M.C.: Nurses in business, Baltimore, 1985, Williams & Wilkins, Inc.

Newman, W.H., Summer, C.E., and Warren, E.K.: The process of management, ed. 5, Englewood Cliffs, N.J., 1981, Prentice-Hall, Inc.

Osburn, H.G., and Manese, W.R.: How to install and validate employee selection techniques, Washington, D.C., 1971, American Petroleum Institute.

Price, M., Franck, P., and Veith, S.: Nursing management: a programmed text, ed. 2, New York, 1980, Springer Publishing Co.

Rinehart, E.L.: Management of nursing care, New York, 1969, Macmillan, Inc.

Robbins, S.P.: Organizational behavior: concepts, controversies, and applications, ed. 3, Englewood Cliffs, N.J., 1986, Prentice-Hall, Inc.

Rowland, H.S., and Rowland, B.L.: Nursing administration handbook, ed. 2, Germantown, Md., 1985, Aspen Systems Corp.

Rubin, I.M., Fry, R.E., and Plomick, M.S.: Managing human resources in health care organizations: an applied approach, Reston, Va., 1978, Reston Publishing Co., Inc.

Scanlan, B.K.: Principles of management and organizational behavior, New York, 1973, John Wiley & Sons, Inc.

Schweiger, J.L.: The nurse as manager, New York, 1980, John Wiley & Sons, Inc.

Seawell, L.V.: Hospital financial accounting theory and practice, Chicago, 1975, Hospital Financial Management Association.

Shaffer, F.A.: Costing out nursing: pricing our product, New York, 1985, National League for Nursing.

Shanks, M.D., and Kennedy, D.A.: Administration in nursing, New York, 1970, McGraw-Hill Book Co.

Sheridan, R.S., Bronstein, J.E., and Walker, D.D.: The new nurse manager: a guide to management development, Rockville, Md., 1984, Aspen Systems Corp.

Simms, L.M., Price, S.A., and Ervin, N.E.: The professional practice of nursing administration, New York, 1985, John Wiley & Sons, Inc.

Sisk, H.L.: Management and organization, Cincinnati, 1973, South-Western Publishing Co.

Stevens, B.J.: The nurse as executive, ed. 2, Wakefield, Mass., 1982, Aspen Publishing Co.

Stevens, B.J.: First-line patient care management, ed. 2, Wakefield, Mass., 1983, Aspen Publishing Co.

Stevens, W.F.: Management and leadership in nursing, New York, 1978, McGraw-Hill Book Co.

Stone S., et al., editors: Management for nurses: a multidisciplinary approach, ed. 2, St. Louis, 1986, The C. V. Mosby Co.

Sullivan, E.J., and Decker, P.J.: Effective management in nursing, Reading, Mass., 1985, Addison-Wesley Publishing Co.

Terry, G.R.: Principles of management, Homewood, Ill., 1972, Richard D. Irwin, Inc.

Terry, G.R., editor: Management: selected readings, ed. 8, Homewood, Ill., 1982, Richard D. Irwin, Inc.

Veninga, R.L.: The human side of health administration, Englewood Cliffs, N.J., 1982, Prentice-Hill, Inc.

Voich, D., and Wren, D.A.: Principles of management: resources and systems, New York, 1968, Ronald Press Co.

Winston, S.: Getting organized, New York, 1978, W.W. Norton and Co.

Journals
Planning

Fox, D.H., and Fox, R.T.: Strategic planning for nursing, J. Nurs. Adm. **8**:11-17, May 1983.

Frey, M.: Planning for nursing service, Hosp. Prog. **57**:78-81, October 1976.

Kirk, R.: Professional development: nurse executives can mean business, J. Nurs. Adm. **16**:7-10, October 1986.

Lukacs, J.L.: Strategic planning in hospitals: applications for nurse executives, J. Nurs. Adm. **14**:11-17, September 1984.

McLemore, M.M.: Nurses as health planners, J. Nurs. Adm. **10**:13-17, September 1980.

Nagy, E.J., and Galimore, D.: The nursing administrator's role in health planning, J. Nurs. Adm. **9**:31-35, December 1979.

Rue, L.W: The how and who of long-range planning, Business Horizons **16**:23-30, December 1973.

Stybel, L.J.: Organic research as a planning tool for the nurse administrator, J. Nurs. Adm. **7**:28-31, March 1977.

Swansburg, R.C.: Planning: a function of nursing administration. I. Supervisor Nurse **9**:25-28, April 1978.

Swansburg, R.C: Planning: a function of nursing administration. II. Supervisor Nurse **9**:76-80, May 1978.

Zilm, F. (Consultant: Thier, N.): The planning process and development of a time line, J. Nurs. Adm. **9**:40-44, September 1979.

Decision making

Archer, S.E.: PERT: a tool for nurse administration, J. Nurs. Adm. **4**:26-32, September-October 1974.

Barnard, C.: The environment of decision, J. Nurs. Adm. **12**:25-29, March 1982.

Brown, R.V.: Do managers find decision theory useful? Harvard Business Rev. **48**:78-89, May-June 1970.

Corcoran, S.: Decision analysis: a step-by-step guide for making clinical decisions, Nurs. Health Care **7**:149-154, March 1986.

Daniel, W.W., and Terrell, S.A.: An introduction to decision analysis, J. Nurs. Adm. **8**:20-28, May 1978.

Fair E.W.: Short cuts to problem solving, Supervisor Nurse **12**:62, April 1981.

Frederiksen, N.: Implications of cognitive theory for instruction in problem solving, Rev. Educational Research **54**(3):363-407, Fall 1984.

Harper, R.W., and Rhodes, M.A.: Development and application of flow-charting techniques in nursing practice, J. Nurs. Adm. **7**:11-19, May-June 1977.

Hayes, R.H.: Qualitative insight from quantitative methods, Harvard Business Rev. **47**:108-117, August 1969.

Hibbert, J., Craven, R., and Balinski, J.: Instant problem solving, Nurs. Management **12**:37-38, December 1981.

Hill, B.S.: A pedagogue's prescription to improve nursing practice, RN **39**:37-40, November 1976.

Kuenstler, D.W.: Problem solving in nursing management, Supervisor Nurse **10**:34-42, September 1979.

La Monica, E., and Finch, F.E.: Managerial decision making, J. Nurs. Adm. **7**:20-28, May-June 1977.

Lancaster, W., and Lancaster, J.: Rational decision making: managing uncertainty, J. Nurs. Adm. **12**:23-28, September 1982.

LeClear, B.M.: The liaison nurse: centralizing problem-solving, Supervisor Nurse **7**:42-43, March 1980.

Magee, J.F.: Decision trees for decision making, Harvard Business Rev. **42**:131, July-August 1964.

Maier, N.R.F.: Specific leadership behaviors that affect problem solving, Personnel Psychol. **24**:35-44, 1971.

Maier N.R.F., and Hoffman, L.R.: Quality of first and second solutions in group problem solving, J. Appl. Psychol. **44**:278-283, 1960.

Maier, N.R.F., and Solem, A.R.: Improving solutions by turning choice situations into problems, Personnel Psychol. **15**:151-157, 1962.

Markert, R.J.: Identifying problems in a hospital nursing staff, Supervisor Nurse **12**:21-22, January 1981.

Marriner, A.: The decision-making process, Supervisor Nurse **8**:58-67, February 1977.

Marriner, A.: Behavioral aspects of decision making, Supervisor Nurse **8**:40-47, May 1977.

McKenzie, M.E.: Decisions: how you reach them makes the difference, Nurs. Management **16**:48-49, June 1985.

McWilliams, C.A.: Systems analysis can solve nursing management problems, Supervisor Nurse **11**:17-26, May 1980.

Schaefer, J.: The interrelatedness of decision making and the nursing process, Am. J. Nurs. **74**:1852-1855, October 1974.

Taylor, A.G.: Decision making in nursing: an analytical approach, J. Nurs. Adm. **8**:22-30, November 1978.

Taylor, A.G.: Decision making in nursing: an analytical approach, J. Nurs. Adm. **8**:39-42, December 1978.

Thomson, W.: Management for nurses: the problem of priorities, Nurs. Mirror **134**:50-51, May 19, 1971.

Tregoe, B.: Management problem solving and decision making, Training Dev. J. **20**:20-22, August 1966.

Von Bergen, C.W., and Kirk, R.J.: Groupthink: when too many heads spoil the decision, Management Rev. 44-49, March 1978.

Vroom, V.: A new look at managerial decision making, Organizational Dynamics **1**:67-70, 1973.

Weisman, C.S., Alexander, C.S., and Morlock, L.L.: Hospital decision making: what is nursing's role? J. Nurs. Adm. **11**:31-36, September 1981.

Wong, P., Doyle, M., and Straus, D.: Problem solving through "process management," J. Nurs. Adm. **5**:37-39, January 1975.

Zilm, F.: The planning process and development of time line, J. Nurs. Adm. **9**:40-44, September 1979.

Ethical aspects of decision making

Aroskar, M.A.: Anatomy of an ethical dilemma: the theory, Am. J. Nurs. **80**:658-663, April 1980.

Aroskar, M.A.: Ethics of nurse-patient relationships, Nurse Educ. **5**:18-20, March-April 1980.

Aroskar, M.A.: Institutional ethics committees and nursing administration, Nurs. Econ. **2**:130-136, March-April 1984.

Benoliel, J.Q.: Ethics in nursing practice and education, Nurs. Outlook **31**:210-215, July-August 1983.

Binder, J.: Organizational responsibility in health care, Nurs. Econ. **1**:193-198, November-December 1983.

Christman, L.: Moral dilemmas for practitioners in a changing society, J. Nurs. Adm. **3**:15-17, March-April 1973.

Churchill, L.: Ethical issues of a profession in transition, Am. J. Nurs. **77**:873-874, May 1977.

Curtin, L.: Nursing ethics: theories and pragmatics, Nurs. Forum **17**:4-11, January 1978.

Curtin, L.: A proposed model for critical ethical analysis, Nurs. Forum **17**:12-17, January 1978.

Curtin, L.: Should we feed Baby Doe? Nurs. Management **15**:22-28, August 1984.

Davis, A.J.: Dilemmas in practice: to tell or not, Am. J. Nurs. **81**:156-158, January 1981.

Davis, A.J.: Helping your staff address ethical dilemmas, J. Nurs. Adm. **12**:9-13, February 1982.

Flaherty, M.J.: Perspectives in nursing: guilt by association? Nurs. Management **12**:32-33, November 1981.

French, D.G.: Ethics: Nurse, am I going to live? Nurs. Management **15**:43-46, November 1984.

Kaserman, I.: A nursing committee and the code for nurses, Am. J. Nurs. **77**:875-876, May 1977.

Levenstein, A.: The art and science of supervision: a new beginning, Supervisor Nurse **11**:10-11, December 1980.

Levine, M.E.: Nursing ethics and the ethical nurse, Am. J. Nurs. **77**:845-847, May 1977.

McNally, J.M.: Values. I. Supervisor Nurse **11**:27-30, May 1980.

McNally, J.M.: Values. II. Supervisor Nurse **11**:52-53, June 1980.

McNally, J.M.: Values. III. Supervisor Nurse **11**:17-18, July 1980.

McNally, J.M.: Values. IV. Supervisor Nurse **11**:38-39, August 1980.

Prato, S.A.: Ethical decisions in daily practice, Supervisor Nurse **12**:18-20, July 1981.

Rabb, J.D.: Implications of moral and ethical issues for nurses, Nurs. Forum **15**:168-179, February 1976.

Romanell, P.: Ethics, moral conflicts, and choice, Am. J. Nurs. **77**:850-855, May 1977.

Silva, M.C.: Science, ethics, and nursing, Am. J. Nurs. **74**:2004-2007, November 1974.

Smith, S.J., and Davis, A.J.: Ethical dilemmas: conflicts among rights, duties, and obligations, Am. J. Nurs. **80**:1463-1466, August 1980.

Sredl, D.R.: The head nurse as ethical and legal leader, Nurs. Management **14**:55-58, November 1983.

Committees

Beachy, P., and Biester, D.J.: Restructuring group meetings for effectiveness, J. Nurs. Adm. **16**:30-33, December 1986.

Chopra, A.: Motivation in task-oriented groups, J. Nurs. Adm. **3**:55-62, January-February 1973.

Cooper, S.S.: Committees that work, J. Nurs. Adm. **3**:30-35, January-February 1973.

Culbertson, R.A.: The governing body and the nursing administrator: an emerging relationship, J. Nurs. Adm. **9**:11-13, February 1979.

Ganong, W.L., and Ganong, J.M.: Reducing organizational conflict through working committees, J. Nurs. Adm. **4**:50-57, November-December 1974.

Jacobs, B.C., and Rosenthal, T.T.: Managing effective meetings, Nurs. Econ. **2**:137-141, March-April 1984.

Jay, A.: The meeting chairperson: master or servant? J. Nurs. Adm. **11**:30-36, May 1981.

Jay, A.: How to run a meeting, J. Nurs. Adm. **12**:22-28, January 1982.

Lancaster, J.: Making the most of meetings, J. Nurs. Adm. **11**:15-19, October 1981.

Levenstein, A.: The art and science of supervision: talk—talk—talk, Supervisor Nurse **11**:13-14, January 1980.

Monson, T.: Mastering the art of planning by committee, J. Nurs. Adm. **11**:71-72, November-December 1981.

Price, G.M.: How to be a better meeting chairman, Harvard Business Rev. **47**:98-108, January-February 1969.

Stevens, B.J.: Use of groups for management, J. Nurs. Adm. **5**:14-22, January 1975.

Thier, L.: The committee. II. J. Nurs. Adm. **8**:10-15, April 1978.

Veninga, R.L.: Benefits and costs of group meetings, J. Nurs. Adm. **14**:42-46, June 1984.

Webber, J.B., and Dula, M.A.: Effective planning committees for hospitals, Harvard Business Rev. **52**:133-142, May-June 1974.

Zella, V.: Patient care policies: the professional approach, Nurs. Homes **18**:18+, April 1969.

Consultation

Anders, R.L.: Program consultation by a clinical specialist, J. Nurs. Adm. **8**:34-38, November 1978.

Archer, J.F.: Getting the most out of management consultants, Eur. Business **42**:34-41, Fall 1974.

Argyris, C.: Explorations in consulting-client relationships, Hum. Organization **20**:121-133, 1961.

Benne, K.D.: Some ethical problems in group and organizational consultation, J. Social Issues **15**:60-67, 1959.

Blake, P.: The clinical specialist as nurse consultant, J. Nurs. Adm. **7**:33-36, December 1977.

Blumberg, A.: A selected annotated bibliography on the consultant relationship with groups, J. Social Issues **15**:68-73, 1959.

Frankenhuis, J.P.: How to get a good consultant, J. Nurs. Adm. **11**:56-60, November-December 1981.

Gibb, J.R.: The role of the consultant, J. Social Issues **15**:1-4, 1959.

Glidewell, J.C.: The entry problem in consultation, J. Social Issues **15**:51-59, 1959.

Hayter, J.: So you need a consultant, Can. Nurse **58**:120-123, February 1962.

Knecht, A.A.: Evaluation of a nursing consultant, J. Nurs. Adm. **2**:46-51, March-April 1972.

Kolb, D.A., and Boyatzis, R.E.: On the dynamics of the helping relationship, J. Appl. Behav. Sci. **6**:267-289, 1970.

Lippitt, G.L.: A study of the consultation process, J. Social Issues **15**:43-50, 1959.

Lippitt, R.: Dimensions of the consultant's job, J. Social Issues **15**:5-12, 1959.

Norris, C.M.: A few notes on consultation in nursing, Nurs. Outlook **25**:756-761, December 1977.

Pankratz, D.: Effects of coaching nursing service personnel, Nurs. Res. **20**:517-521, November-December 1971.

Pati, B.: Nursing consultation: a collaborative process, J. Nurs. Adm. **10**:33-37, November 1980.

Stevens, B.J.: The use of consultants in nursing service, J. Nurs. Adm. **8**:7-15, August 1978.

Strombeck, R.D.: The client-consultant relationship: guidelines for the nursing administrator, J. Nurs. Adm. **12**:42-46, July-August 1982.

Purpose, philosophy, goals, and objectives

Cantor, M.M.: Philosophy, purpose, and objectives: why do we have them? J. Nurs. Adm. **3**:21-25, July-August 1973.

Lasagna, J.B.: Translating distant goals into immediate objectives, Supervisor Nurse **4**:32+, June 1973.

Moore, M.A.: Philosophy, purpose, objectives: why do we have them? J. Nurs. Adm. **1**:9-14, May-June 1971

Swansburg, R.C.: Planning: a function of nursing administration. I. Supervisor Nurse **9**:25-28, April 1978.

Swansburg, R.C.: Planning: a function of nursing administration. II. Supervisor Nurse **9**:76-80, May 1978.

Watkin, B.: Objectives, Nurs. Mirror **138**:49, March 29, 1974.

Policies

Ames, A.: Bylaws: one hospital's experience, J. Nurs. Adm. **15**:28-30, December 1985.

Bennett, A.C.: Department policies: guides for action focus on management methods, Hosp. Top. **45**:44+, November 1967.

Casanova, G.: Developing and writing policy, Supervisor Nurse **3**:62-64+, April 1972.

Cox, E.: A systematic approach to developing a dress code, Supervisor Nurse **12**:52-54, June 1981.

Feldman, J., and Hundert, M.: Determining nursing policies by use of the nursing home simulation model, J. Nurs. Adm. **7**:35-41, April 1977.

Hamelin, I., et al.: The nurses' role in policy-making, N.Z. Nurs. J. **65**:20-21, December 1972.

Hodgman, E.C.: Research policy for nursing services. II. J. Nurs. Adm. **11**:33-36, May 1981.

Milio, N.: The realities of policymaking: can nurses have an impact? J. Nurs. Adm. **14**:18-23, March 1984.

Moccia, P.: The nurse as policymaker: toward a free and equal health care system, Nurs. & Health Care **5**:481-485, November 1984.

Moccia, P., and Mason, D.J.: Poverty trends: implications for nursing, Nurs. Outlook **34**:20-24, January-February 1986.

Moore, M.: Standard III policies . . . guidelines for action, J. Nurs. Adm. **2**:29-33, May-June 1972.

Nardecchia, M.A., and Myers, M.T.: The policy manual: a basis for legal protection, Nurs. Adm. Q. **5**:(1)57-62, 1980.

Parker, A.: Consumer as policy maker: issue of training, Am. J. Public Health **60**:2139-2153, November 1970.

Phillips, A.: Regional health care planning: the policies of economic development, Nurs. Management **16**:37-41, December 1985.

Porter-O'Grady, T.: Credentialing, privileging, and nursing bylaws: assuring accountability, J. Nurs. Adm. **15**:23-27, December 1985.

Sauer, J.E.: Cost containment—and quality assurance, too. II. Hospitals **46**:63-69, November 16, 1972.

Schmied, E.: Allocation of resources: preparation of the nursing department budget, J. Nurs. Adm. **7**:31-36, September 1977.

Steel, J.L.: What manual?! getting policies and procedures on the line, Nurs. Management **13**:43-46, March 1982.

Stevens, B.J.: Nursing division budget: generation and control, J. Nurs. Adm. **4**:16-20, November-December 1974.

Stevens, B.J.: What is the executive's role in budgeting for her department? Hospitals **50**:83-86, November 16, 1976.

Swansburg, R.C.: The nursing budget, Supervisor Nurse **9**:40-47, June 1978.

Weber, H.I.: Written policies: insurance for quality control, Nurs. Homes **21**:20-22, February 1972.

Wessel, L.: Preparing the operating room budget, AORN J. **18**:525-527, September 1973.

Wilson, B.S.: Medication error policy, Supervisor Nurse **9**:53-56, May 1978.

Zegeer, L.J.: Calculating a nurse staffing budget for a 20 bed unit at 100% occupancy, J. Nurs. Adm. **7**:11-14, February 1977.

Procedures

Griffith, J., and Ignatavicius, D.: Procedure development: a simplified approach, J. Nurs. Adm. **14**:27-31, September 1984.

Guida, F.K.: The procedure book: a monstrous problem, Nurs. Management **13**:32-33, December 1982.

Niederbaumer, L.: Rethinking the procedure manual, Supervisor Nurse **8**:59-63, April 1977.

Poole, P.E.: Who benefits from hospital routines? Can. Hosp. **47**:43+, July 1970.

Stevens, B.: The playscript method of developing administrative procedures . . . Loma Linda University Medical Center, Supervisor Nurse **6**:40-45, June 1975.

Wright, M.L.: A lesson in procedure writing, Supervisor Nurse **8**:26-27, April 1977.

Budgets

Althaus, J.N., et al.: Decentralized budgeting: holding the purse strings. I. J. Nurs. Adm. **12**:15-20, May 1982.

Anderson, R.: Alternative revenue sources for nursing departments, J. Nurs. Adm. **15**:9-13, November 1985.

Barnyk, M.A.: Defending a capital budget item: an approach that works, Nurs. Management **17**:38J-38P, July 1986.

Bruhn, P.S., and Howes, D.H.: Service line management: new opportunities for nursing executives, J. Nurs. Adm. **16**:13-18, June 1986.

Bruttomesso, K.A.: Variable hospital accounting practices: are they fair for the nursing department? J. Nurs. Adm. **11**:8-13, October 1985.

Caterinicchio, R.P., and Smith, G.P.: The relationship between nursing activity and age: a reassessment of the nursing cost for routine inpatient care differential, Hosp. Top. **58**:46-50, July-August 1980.

Crookston, B., and Kirchhoff, K.T.: Financial management series: a comprehensive charge system for unit supplies, J. Nurs. Adm. **16**:31-34, April 1986.

Curtin, L.: Wound management: care and cost—an overview, Nurs. Management **15**:22-25, February 1984.

Davis, C.K.: The federal role in changing health care financing, Nurs. Econ. **1**:10-17 July-August 1983.

DeJoseph, J.F., Petree, B.J., and Ross, W.: Costing and charging: pricing care in OB, Nurs. Management 15:36-37, December 1985.

Elliott, K.: The cost of supervisory services, Nurs. Management 17:33-36, October 1986.

Ethridge, P.: The case for billing my patient acuity, Nurs. Management 16:38-41, August 1985.

Fagin, C.M.: The economic value of nursing research, Am. J. Nurs. 82:1844-1849, December 1982.

Fanning, J.A., and Lovett, R.B.: Decentralization reduces nursing administration budget, J. Nurs. Adm. 15:19-24, May 1985.

Fuller, M.E.: The budget, J. Nurs. Adm. 6:36-38, May 1976.

Gabrielson, R.C., and Lund, C.A.: Enhancing the financial and operational performance of the nursing department, J. Nurs. Adm. 15:28-32, November 1985.

Grandbouche, A.: Nursing's cash value: how it's hidden; why it must be revealed, RN 45:83-84, May 1982.

Hillestad, E.A.: Budgeting: functional or dysfunctional? Nurs. Econ. 1:199-201, November-December 1983.

Hoffman, F.M.: Developing capital expenditure proposals, J. Nurs. Adm. 15:32-34, September 1985.

Maher, A.B., and Dolan, B.: Determining costs of nursing services, Nurs. Management 13:17-21, September 1982.

Marriner, A.: Budgets, Supervisor Nurse 8:53-56, April 1977.

Marriner, A.: Budgetary management, J. Continuing Education Nurs. 11:11-14, June 1980.

Miller, R.T., Campbell, J.L., and Sherman, T.L.: Allocating your merit increases the SMART way, J. Nurs. Adm. 13:32-35, March 1983.

Morgan, D.M.: Budgeting for the nursing service, Can. Hosp. 49:35-44, July 1972.

Munch, J.: Let's involve nurses in budget planning, Hospitals 48:75-120, February 16, 1974.

Pan, L.: Planned program budgeting: a workshop report, Nurs. Outlook 19:656-658, October 1971.

Player, J.M.: The economic importance of nurses, Nurs. Management 13:52-54, November 1982.

Porter-O'Grady, T.: Financial planning: budgeting for nursing. I. Supervisor Nurse 10:35-38, August 1979.

Porter-O'Grady, T.: Financial planning: budget-

ing for nursing. II. Supervisor Nurse 10:25-30, September 1979.

Riley, W.J., and Schaefers, V.: Nursing operations as a profit center, Nurs. Management 15:43-46, April 1984.

Rotkovitch, R.: The nursing director's role in money management, J. Nurs. Adm. 11:13-16, November-December 1981.

Salvekar, A.: Variable budget for nursing service, Hospitals 47:70-76, 1973.

Schmied E.: Allocation of resources: preparation of the nursing department budget J. Nurs. Adm. 7:31-36, September 1977.

Stanton, L.J.: Nursing care and nursing products: revenue or expenses? J. Nurs. Adm. 16:29-32, September 1986.

Stevens, B.J.: Nursing division budget: generation and control, J. Nurs. Adm. 4:16-20, November-December 1974.

Stevens, B.J.: What is the executive's role in budgeting for the department? J. Nurs. Adm. 11:22-24, July 1981.

Swansburg, R.C.: The nursing budget, Supervisor Nurse 9:40-47, June 1978.

Tower, R.B.: Analyzing accounting reports, Nurs. Management 13:12-16, September 1982.

Trofino, J.: A reality-based system for pricing nursing service, Nurs. Management 17:19-24, January 1986.

Villemaire, M., and Lane-McGraw, C.: Nursing personnel budgets: a step-by-step guide, Nurs. Management 17:28-32, November 1986.

Walker, D.D.: The cost of nursing care in hospitals, J. Nurs. Adm. 13:13-18, March 1983.

Wessel, L.: Preparing the operating room budget, AORN J. 18:525-527, September 1973.

Zegeer, L.J.: Calculating a nurse staffing budget for a 20 bed unit at 100% occupancy, J. Nurs. Adm. 7:11-14, February 1977.

Cost containment

Andreano, R.L.: Health care cost containment: Wisconsin's experience, Nurs. Adm. Q. 3:1-15, Fall 1978.

Bahr, J., Badour, G., and Hill, H.L.: Innovative methodology enhances nurse deployment, cuts costs, Hospitals 51:104-109, April 16, 1977.

Belinotti, A.M.: Systems control: reducing lost central supply charges, Supervisor Nurse 11:40-42, August 1980.

Boland, L.S.: An interim stay unit reduces costs, Nurs. Management 16:42-45, August 1985.

Brubaker, K.M., and McGowan, M.B.: Open hospital beds open new opportunities, Nurs. Management 17:39-41, November 1986.

Clark, B.B., and Lamont, G.X.: Accurate census forecasting leads to cost containment, Hospitals 50:43-48, June 1, 1976.

Crabtree, M.: Application of cost-benefit analysis to clinical nursing practice, J. Nurs. Adm. 8:11-16, December 1978.

Davis, K.: Non-nursing functions: our readers respond, Am. J. Nurs. 82:1857-1860, December 1982.

Donabedian, A.: Quality, cost, and cost containment, Nurs. Outlook 32:142-145, May-June 1984.

Foster, K.D.: Nursing: cost containment, nursing's role dominate, Hospitals 47:143-149, April 1, 1973.

Fry, S.T.: Rationing health care: the ethics of cost containment, Nurs. Econ. 1:165-169, November-December 1983.

Goertzen, I.: Regulation of hospital rates and its implications for nursing, Nurs. Adm. Q. 3:59-65, Fall 1978.

Grimaldi, P.L.: DRGs and nursing administration, Nurs. Management 13:30-34, January 1982.

Haw, M.A., Claus, E.G., Durbin-Lafferty, E., and Iversen, S.M.: Improving nursing morale in a climate of cost containment. I. Organizational assessment, J. Nurs. Adm. 14:8-15, October 1984.

Higgerson, N.J., and Slyck, A.V.: Variable billing for services: new fiscal direction for nursing, J. Nurs. Adm. 12:20-27, June 1982.

Hoffman, F.M.: Financial management series: functional value analysis, J. Nurs. Adm. 14:25-28, December 1984.

Jennings, C.P., and Jennings, T.F.: Containing costs through prospective reimbursement, Am. J. Nurs. 77:1155-1159, July 1977.

Knowlton, H.C., and Dunn, M.D.: Stratification of nursing services and costs, Hosp. Prog. 52:34-46, January 1971.

Koerner, B.L., Cohen, J.R., and Armstrong, D.M.: Professional behavior in collaborative practice, J. Nurs. Adm. 16:39-43, October 1986.

Lehman, M.W., and Friesen, Q.J.: Centralized control system cuts costs, boosts morale, Hospitals 51:75-80, May 16, 1977.

Madsen, N.L., and Harper, R.W.: Improving the nursing climate for cost containment, J. Nurs. Adm. 15:11-16, March 1985.

Micheletti, J., and Toth, R.: Diagnosis-related groups: impact and implications, Nurs. Management 12:33-39, September 1981.

Morgan, D.: Cost-effective nursing, Dimens. Health Serv. 52:12-14, August 1975.

Norby, R.B., et al: Exploring nursing issues: cost containment, Oncology Nurs. Forum 7:27-34, Summer 1980.

Porter-O'Grady, T.: The nurse administrator's role in cost-effective facilities planning, Nurs. Adm. Q. 3:67-73, Fall 1978.

Porter-O'Grady, T.: Financial planning: budgeting for nursing. II. Supervisor Nurse 10:25-30, September 1979.

Prescott, P.A.: Cost-effectiveness: tool or trap? Nurs. Outlook 27:722-728, November 1979.

Prescott, P.A., and Sorensen, J.E.: Cost-effectiveness analysis: an approach to evaluating nursing programs, Nurs. Adm. Q. 3:17-39, Fall 1978.

Sauer, J.E.: Cost containment—and quality assurance too. I. Hospitals 46:78, 82-90, November 1, 1972.

Sauer, J.E.: Cost containment—and quality assurance too. II. Hospitals 46:62-69, November 16, 1972.

Schmied, E.: Living with cost containment, J. Nurs. Adm. 10:11-17, May 1980.

Shelton, J.: Can nursing options cut health care's bottom line? Nurs. Health Care 6:251-253, May 1985.

Slen M.: Less staff plus more work equals low cost, good care, Mod. Hosp. 113:115-117, September 1969.

Sloane, L.: Watching your finances: what can you do to contain hospital costs? Am. J. Nurs. 77:1352, August 1977.

Smeltzer, C.H., and Flores, S.M.: Preadmission discharge planning: organization of a concept, J. Nurs. Adm. 16:18-24, May 1986.

Sorensen, J.F., and Grove, H.: Cost-outcome and cost-effectiveness analysis: emerging nonprofit performance evaluation techniques, Accounting Rev. 52:658-675, July 1977.

Swansburg, R.C.: Cost control in nursing, Supervisor Nurse 9:51-57, July 1978.

Turley, R.M., and Edwardson, S.R.: Can ICUs be used more efficientiy? J. Nurs. Adm. 15:25-28, July-August 1985.

Watkin, B.: Management topics: cost-benefit analysis, Nurs. Mirror **139**:58, July 19, 1974.

Wellever, A.: Variance analysis: a tool for cost control, J. Nurs. Adm. **12**:23-26, July-August 1982.

Time management

Braun, A.: Twelve ways to save time in critical care, Dimensions Crit. Care Nurs. **1**:294-297, September-October 1982.

Craik, P.: Using an OR activity log, Dimensions Crit. Care Nurs. **1**:301-303, September-October 1982.

Dow, C.: Taming the time-eating tiger, RN **47**:19-22, November 1984.

Eliopoulos, C.: Time management: a reminder, J. Nurs. Adm.**14**:30-32, March 1984.

Feldman, E.S., Monicken, D., and Crowley, M.B.: A systems approach to prioritizing, Nurs. Adm. Q. **7**:57-62, Winter 1983.

Howes, B.R.: Breeding and feeding alligators, Clin. Manage. **3**:(2)13-14, 1983.

Hutelmyer, C.: Managing your time, Nursing 81 **11**:97-107, May 1981.

Huttman, B.: All about hectic situations, Nursing 84 **14**:34-35, July 1984.

Lakein, A.: How to better manage time so that you and the company benefit from your increased productivity . . . , Review No. 205, San Francisco, Calif., Pacific Telephone Co., October 2, 1975.

Lancaster, J.: Making the most of every minute: reminders for nursing leaders, Nurs. Leadership **5**:6-10, June 1982.

Levinson, R.: Management savvy: how to squeeze 70 minutes out of every hour, Flightime, pp. 10-16, February 1977.

Marriner, A.: Time management, J. Nurs. Adm. **9**:16-18, October 1979.

Marriner, A.: Time management for career development, Nurs. Success Today **1**:4-7, March-April 1984.

Marriner, A.: Time management through planning, J. Cont. Edu. Nurs. **14**:21-26, January-February 1983.

Marriner, A.: Work smarter—not harder—with time management, J. Cont. Edu. Nurs. **12**:10-13, November-December 1981.

Marriner, A., and Blake, P.J.: Seven easy ways to get more done in less time, RN **46**:32C-32G, January 1983.

McCarthy, M.J.: Managing your own time: the most important management task, J. Nurs. Adm. **11**:61-65, November-December 1981.

McConnell, E.: Ten tactics to help beat the clock, RN **46**:47-50, September 1983.

McNiff, M.A.: Getting organized—at last! RN **47**:23-24, June 1984.

Morano, R.A.: Executive time management. I. Organizational support for better time management, S.A.M. Adv. Management J. **43**:36-40, Winter 1978.

Morano, V.J.: Time management: from victim to victor, Health Care Supervisor **3**:1-12, October 1984.

Moskowitz, R.: Make the most of your time with simple techniques that work, Nurs. Life **2**:22-25, January-February 1982.

Nerone, B.J.: Managing your time, Imprint **28**(2):19, 82-83, 1981.

Norville, J.L.: Improving personal effectiveness through better management of time, Nurs. Homes **33**:8-17, March-April 1984.

Oncken, W., and Wass, D.L.: Management time: who's got the monkey? J. Nurs. Adm. **5**:26-30, July-August 1975.

Predd, C.S.: How to stay efficient in hectic nursing situations, Nurs. Life **2**(3):50-51, May-June 1982.

Schmidt, D.L.: Where did the day go? Tips on time management, Hosp. Prog. **58**:73-75, March 1977.

Schwartz, E.B., and Mackenzie, R.A.: Time management strategy for women, Am. Management Assoc. Management Rev. **66**:19-25, September 1977.

Schwartz, E.B., and Mackenzie, R.A.: Time management strategy for women, J. Nurs. Adm. **9**:22-26, March 1979.

Singleton, E.K.: Too much to do? Use 'mental triage,' RN **45**:101-106, March 1982.

Storlie, F., and Leon, J.: Make the most of your time by trusting yourself, Nurs. Life **2**:27-28, January-February 1982.

Volk-Tebbitt, B.: Time: who controls yours? Supervisor Nurse **9**:17-22, April 1978.

Marketing

Alder, L.: Systems approach to marketing, Harvard Business Rev. **46**:105-118, May-June 1967.

Alward, R.R.: A marketing approach to nursing administration. I. J. Nurs. Adm. **13**:9-12, March 1983.

Alward, R.R.: A marketing approach to nursing

administration. II. J. Nurs. Adm. **13**:18-22, April 1983.

Archer, S.E.: Marketing: public health nursing services, Nurs. Outlook **31**:304-309, November-December 1983.

Assael, H., and Roscoe, A.M., Jr.: Approaches to market segmentation analysis, J. Marketing **40**:67-76, October 1976.

Boulding, K.: The concept of need for health service, Milbank Memorial Fund Q. **44**:202-223, October 1966.

Campbell, J.P., and Williams, T.: Marketing to nurses through an incentive program, J. Nurs. Adm. **13**:9-12, October 1983.

Camunas, C.: Using public relations to market nursing service, J. Nurs. Adm. **16**:21-25, October 1986.

Chaney, H.S.: Practical approaches to marketing, J. Nurs. Adm. **16**:33-38, September 1986.

Connelly, J.A., and Strauser, K.S.: Managing recruitment and retention problems: an application of the marketing process, J. Nurs. Adm. **13**:17-22, October 1983.

Couser, S., Daly, G., Grisham, J., and Rieder, B.: Health in the balance, Nurs. Outlook **34**:25-27, January-February 1986.

Crawford, M., and Fisher, M.L.: Marketing: the creative advantage, J. Nurs. Adm. **16**:17-20, December 1986.

Ellwood, P.M., Jr., and Herbert, M.E.: Health care: should industry buy it or sell it? Harvard Business Rev. **51**:99-107, July-August 1973.

Ferrell, O.C., and Weaver, K.M.: Ethical beliefs of marketing managers, J. Marketing **42**:69-73, July 1978.

Hughes, G.D.: Can marketing help recruit and retain nurses? HCM Rev. 61-66, Summer 1979.

Kalisch, B.J., and Kalisch, P.A.: Nursing images: the TV news picture, Nurs. Management **16**: 39-48, April 1985.

Kotler, P., and Conner, R.A., Jr.: Marketing professional services, J. Marketing **41**:71-76, January 1977.

Kotler, P., and Zaltman, G.: Social marketing: an approach to planned social change, J. Marketing **35**:3-12, July 1971.

Luciano, K., and Darling, L.A.W.: The physician as a nursing service customer, J. Nurs. Adm. **15**:17-20, June 1985.

Meyers, J.H.: Benefit structure analysis: a new tool for product planning, J. Marketing **40**:23-32, October 1976.

Reve, T., and Stern, L.W.: Interorganizational relations in marketing channels, Acad. Management Rev. **4**:405-416, July 1979.

Sabin, S.: Rehab program's marketing plan was tailored to fit, Nurs. Health Care **6**:269-271, May 1985.

Shapiro, B.P.: Marketing for nonprofit organizations, Harvard Business Rev. **51**:123-132, September-October 1973.

Shearer, K.M.: Contingency nursing, Nurs. Management **13**:56-58, March 1982.

Sheridan, D.R.: The health care industry in the marketplace: implications for nursing, J. Nurs. Adm. **13**:36-40, September 1983.

Stahl, D.A.: Developing and marketing ambulatory care problems, Nurs. Management **15**:20-24, May 1984.

Stanton, M.P.: Patient and health education: lessons from the marketplace, Nurs. Management **16**:28-30, April 1985.

Turner, E.B.: Marketing professional services, J. Marketing **33**:56-61, October 1969.

Walter, C.M.: Auditing the hospital nursing market, Nurs. Management **16**:31-34, April 1985.

Zaltman, G., and Vertinsky, G.: Health service marketing: a suggested model, J. Marketing **35**:19-27, July 1971.

PART
2

ORGANIZE

—————— OBJECTIVES ——————

After completing this part, the reader will be able to:

List at least five principles of organization.

Differentiate among models of organization.

Explain organizational concepts.

Appraise resistance to change.

Plan for change.

Write a job description.

—————— STUDY QUESTIONS ——————

1
What are the principles of organization?
2
What are pros and cons of various models of organization?
3
What are the implications of organizational concepts?
4
What are common sources of resistance to change?
5
How can one plan to minimize resistance to change?
6
What are the relationships among job analysis, job evaluation, and job descriptions?

NATURE AND PURPOSE OF ORGANIZING

Organizing is the second managerial function. Having planned, the manager must now organize so that personnel can accomplish the plans with efficiency and effectiveness. Organizing involves establishing a formal structure that provides the coordination of resources to accomplish objectives and determines position qualifications and descriptions.

ORGANIZATIONAL PROCESS

Organization grows out of a need for cooperation. It is a process by which a manager develops order, promotes cooperation among workers, and fosters productivity. Activities analysis, decision analysis, and relations analysis are tools that can be used to determine the needed structure. Activities analysis is the study of the tasks to be done, their order of priority, and the relationship of tasks to one another. Decision analysis is the investigation of what decisions are to be made, where they should be made in the structure, and who should make them. Relations analysis looks at the contribution each person makes to the organization, with special attention to whom she works with, to whom she reports, and who reports to her.

Organization is a logical process that involves defining the agency's mission and objectives, establishing policies and plans, clarifying the activities necessary to meet the objectives, organizing the activities for best utilization of available human and material resources, delegating the responsibility and authority necessary to do the activities to appropriate personnel, and grouping personnel vertically and horizontally through information systems and authority relationships.

ORGANIZATIONAL DEVELOPMENT

Organizations progress through developmental stages—birth, youth, and maturity. The creation of a new organization and its survival as a viable system are primary concerns during the birth stage. Gaining stability and developing a reputation and pride are the focuses of the youth stage. The maturity stage involves achieving both uniqueness and adaptability and contributing to society.

As organizations are born and grow, they pass through increasingly complex stages of life. They must develop internally and generate new control processes to fit the amount of turbulence and complexity in the environment. At each stage, the environment can become more unknown, unsettled, and difficult. A crisis develops in each stage. The organization needs to change its organizational and decision-making structure to fit this new complexity. The new organization copes by developing job descriptions, programs, policies, and procedures.

However, as the organization grows and becomes more complex, these policies do not cover the exceptions. As a result, the organization develops a set of hierarchical positions to make judgments about the exceptions to the existing job descriptions and policies. As the organization becomes larger and more complex, the superiors in the hierarchy become overloaded. They do not have time to deal with all the exceptions and cannot make sense out of the situation.

Consequently, in the third stage, the organization needs to accomplish orderliness by developing broader goals. However, as the organization becomes increasingly complex, conflicts arise among factions, and the organization regresses to hierarchical referral again.

A decentralized system of departments reduces the interconnections between divisions and reduces the number of communications necessary to make decisions. But as the revolutionary cycle continues, conflict between decentralized departments develops.

In the last stage, a vertical information system is developed so that standardized accounting and statistical reporting systems from each department are consolidated at the top, and then resources are allocated among departments. Because all the complex information in turbulent systems cannot be reduced to numbers, human contacts made among department members become a major coping mechanism. Liaisons, teams, committees, task forces, and integrator roles are used.

ORGANIZATIONAL STRUCTURE

Although planning is the key to effective management, the organizational structure furnishes the formal framework in which the management process takes place. The organizational structure should provide an effective work system, a system of communications, identity to individuals and the organization, and should consequently foster job satisfaction. Agencies contain both informal and formal structures.

The informal organization comprises personal and social relationships that do not appear on the organizational chart. This might include a group that usually goes to coffee together, works together on a particular unit, or takes a class together. Informal organization is based on personal relationships rather than on respect for positional authority. It helps members meet personal objectives and provides social satisfaction. People who have little formal status may gain recognition through the informal structure. Informal authority is not commanded through organizational assignment. It comes from the follower's natural respect for a colleague's knowledge and abilities.

Informal structure provides social control of behavior. The control can be either internal or external. If pressure is intended to make a member conform to group expectancies, it is internal. Kidding a member about her dirty shoelaces would be an example. On the other hand, an attempt to control the behavior of someone outside the social group, such as the supervisor, is external control.

The informal structure also has its own channels of communication, which may disseminate information more broadly and rapidly than the formal communication system. Unfortunately, the "grapevine" may contain rumors that are not authentic. The best way to correct an invalid rumor is for the supervisor to give accurate information. It is better not to state that she is correcting the rumor, for in doing so she may strengthen the rumor, and the facts that she gives may be seen primarily as a subterfuge to refute the rumor.

The informal organizational structure is important to management. The supervisor should be aware of its existence, study its operating techniques, avoid antagonism, and use it to meet the agency's objectives.

The formal organizational structure is defined by executive decision as a result of planning. It can be diagramed to show the relationships among people and their positions. It describes positions, task responsibilities, and relationships. The two basic forms of formal organizational structure are the hierarchic or bureaucratic model and the adaptive or organic model.

Bureaucratic structure

A hierarchy or bureaucracy is an organizational design to facilitate large-scale administration by coordinating the work of many personnel. It is associated with subdivision, specialization, technical qualifications, rules and standards, impersonality, and technical efficiency. In Fig. 2-1, which illustrates a typical bureaucratic hierarchy, the supervisors are responsible to the director of nursing. She in turn must answer to the hospital administrator, who is accountable to the board of directors. The supervisor also has authority over those below her, and they are accountable to her.

Dual management. Dual management separates technical and administrative responsibilities. It has one hierarchy in which technical professionals make technical decisions and control technical matters and another hierarchy in which supervisory management makes decisions about issues such as personnel and budget. This dual hierarchy gives equal status to managers and technical professionals. It provides a set of titles and job descriptions for each hierarchy.

Principles of organization. Certain principles of organization help to maximize the efficiency of the bureaucratic structure. The organization should have clear lines of authority running from the highest executive to the employee who has the least responsibility and no authority over others. There should be unity of command with each person having only one boss. Each person should know

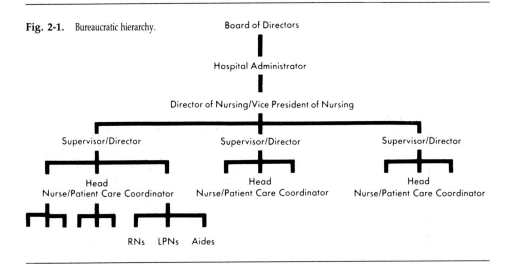

Fig. 2-1. Bureaucratic hierarchy.

to whom she reports and who reports to her. The authority and responsibility of every individual should be clearly defined in writing. This reduces role ambiguity. One knows what is expected of her and what her limitations are. This prevents gaps between responsibilities, avoids overlapping of authority, and helps to determine the proper point for decisions. Although many people do not feel it is necessary to have their responsibilities in writing, it can be revealing to have them write what they believe their functions are and to note the duplicated efforts and jurisdictional disputes. When someone leaves an agency, it is not uncommon for no one to know exactly what that person did. Under such circumstances, it can be difficult to justify replacement and to offer a meaningful orientation.

A clear definition of roles is necessary for effective delegation but does not guarantee it. Role clarity allows the employee to know what is expected of her, to whom she reports, and to whom she goes for help. In contrast, role ambiguity leads to anxiety, frustration, dissatisfaction, negative attitudes, and decreased productivity. Job descriptions increase productivity and satisfaction; however, they should not be so exact that innovation is discouraged.

Supervisors should delegate responsibility to the lowest level within the organization where there is enough competence and information for effective performance and appropriate decision making. Ordinarily, increased delegation and general rather than close supervision increase effective performance, production, and employee satisfaction.

The employee should be given formal authority commensurate with the responsibility delegated. It is not uncommon for supervisors to delegate authority and then undermine it by making decisions that were supposedly delegated. For example, if the head nurse is responsible for the quality of care given on her ward, she should not have to accept a member on her team who has been hired by the supervisor without consulting her. In turn, the head nurse should not tell a patient that he can have a bath at a certain time without consulting the person assigned to give that bath. Preferably, the nurse's aide and her patient will determine when various routines can be performed in accordance with the physician's orders and the team leader's rationale.

The delegation of responsibility should be accompanied by accountability. Most effective control systems are probably ones that provide feedback directly to the accountable person; this seems to increase motivation and provide direction. When feedback from a supervisor is given as performance evaluation rather than guidance, it tends to be nonfunctional and only infrequently contributes to improved performance. The delegation of functions with accompanying responsibility and accountability is particularly difficult for the supervisor, because she remains responsible for the actions of her subordinates. She is as responsible as her subordinates for their performance. Consequently, the span-of-control principle becomes important.

There is a limit to the amount of coordination that can be done by one person, and it depends on several factors. One can coordinate more similar than dissimilar positions. The more the positions are interdependent, the more coordination is involved. The span of control needs to decrease as the complexity of the subordinate's tasks increases. The stability of the agency should also be considered. If the agency has been functioning in a similar manner for a long time, the problems that arise have probably been solved before, and coordination is less difficult than in a changing situation where many new problems arise. The span of control is not likely to be uniform throughout an organization. Top-level managers of positions that are interdependent and dissimilar will probably have a smaller range of control than lower-level supervisors who are coordinating people doing similar tasks in a confined area. The span of control should not be so wide that the supervisor does not have time to deal with the human relations aspects, such as giving workers individual attention, communicating information about the agency's policies, and listening to suggestions, grievances, and problems. On the other hand, she needs a span of control large enough to keep her busy so she will not interfere with the delegated responsibilities of others.

Three types of divisions are commonly used to define span of control: (1) function or process, (2) product or service, and (3) region. Function is associated with specialization. Specialization may apply both to individuals and to departments or divisions. For example, one nurse may pass medications and do treatments, another may just start IVs, and the nurse's aides may give the baths and change linens. There may be a surgical nursing division with departments for specific types of surgery. It is preferable that if a person is responsible for more than one type of responsibility, they be similar. Efficiency is maximized if a person predominantly performs the tasks she does best and for which her proficiency will consequently continue to increase; she may, however, become bored. It is not uncommon to find individuals within an organization who are assigned several unrelated tasks. Although that may work for some people in given situations, it is not considered good organization, and their replacements are not as likely to be successful. It is more viable to hire personnel to fill the organizational structure than to change the structure to fit personnel.

Having individuals doing the same or similar tasks and having divisions with specific functions can help expand the range of control. Similarly, having departments that provide specific services, such as cardiac intensive care, or produce certain products can influence the structure. Organization by geographical location becomes increasingly viable when operations are scattered. Many agencies use a combination of these methods. For instance, a school of nursing may be organized according to campuses (regional division); according to undergraduate, graduate, and continuing education (product division); according to inpatient, outpatient, medical-surgical, maternal-child, or some other service division, and may have individual faculty members assigned to teach according to specialization (functional division).

The organizational structure should be flexible enough to permit expansion and contraction in response to changing conditions without disrupting the basic design. It should also be kept as simple as possible, because additional levels of authority complicate communications, and too many committees may impede progress.

Disadvantages of the bureaucratic structure. There are disadvantages to the bureaucratic model. It may be detrimental to healthy personality patterns by predisposing the authoritarian leadership style, increasing insistence on the right of authority and status, and fostering a pathological need for control. If the superior does not have the technical competence of her subordinates, she may feel insecure and fear them. Autocratic behavior may become a defense mechanism through the use of power and fear strategies over subservients and the enforcement of norms through arbitrary or rigid rules. The use of rewards and punishment to get desired behavior may alienate personnel. Self-serving behavior patterns may develop because of competition for the advancement of individual interests. A certain aloofness can result from the specialization that leads to impersonality. Personnel also may develop a ritualistic attachment to routine, become attached to subgoals, and show resistance to change.

Adhocracy organizational models

Adhocracy or organic models are newer organizational frameworks that are more free form, open, flexible or fluid models than are older bureaucratic models. Boundaries separating internal and external relationships are more easily penetrated. Temporary affiliations such as consultantships are used.

The underlying assumptions, aims, and structures of adaptive frameworks are different from those of the bureaucratic model. They have resulted from behavioral research to facilitate job satisfaction and creativity as well as efficiency. They give greater recognition to the informal structure and encourage the group to improve its own norms. Adaptive models recognize realities and are designed to meet them. They are less likely to use organizational charts, because the relationships are flexible. Job descriptions are also less meaningful. The models are ambiguous and consequently need to be staffed by independent, self-reliant people who have a high tolerance for ambiguity. They lend themselves to participative management. Motivation is derived from system needs, task-related factors, and peer pressure rather than from supervision. Rewards are based on individual and group results rather than subjective evaluations from supervisors.

Free form. Free-form organizational design is structured so that the parts can be operated flexibly. It stresses centralized control, decentralized operations, computerized evaluations, profit centers, and dynamic managers who are willing to take risks. The stable part of the organization is composed of planners and a center for control and evaluation. The decentralized operations consist of changing combinations of the various functions, talents, and material resources across lines within the agency. Profit centers rather than budgetary units are used. These centers foster teamwork by organizing all contributors to an objective into a unit so that all will gain or lose by the results. It is an organization that seeks change, development, and expansion by being opportunistic. Managers are expected to manage change. Open communication, consensus, independent judgment, and self-regulation are stressed. Organizational charts, manuals, job descriptions, and position titles are minimized to increase flexibility.

Collegial management. Collegial management restricts monocratic authority by maintaining a division and balance of power among the top management group through collective responsibility. It is most commonly used in Germany and Holland but is also used in Austria, Switzerland, and France. Consequently, it is also referred to as European-style management. The directors usually represent functional areas of the organization. They may or may not have a chairperson. If so, she may be the first among equals and merely speak for the directors, may coordinate the others, or may be recognized as the general manager or chief executive. The directors may have vice-directors.

The decision-making process varies from one country to another, but in every case, it is the board that makes policy decisions. Essentially, the directors need to persuade each other. Although the chairperson may not have strong decision-making powers, she does have strong veto powers.

Collegial management has several strengths. It limits autocratic leadership, breeds democratic management, and assures representation of each functional area. Because of their collective responsibility, directors are better informed about the other functional areas; this broadens the approach to problem solving. Collegial management prevents precipitous decisions, encourages long-range planning, and fosters objective appraisal of the functions. Camaraderie can exist.

Collegial management also has limitations. The need for consensus can slow down decision making. Consensus based on compromise may be an inferior solution. Logrolling results when directors give reciprocal support to programs that are not viable. Collegial management requires considerable, expensive executive time for what may be relatively minor matters or what may be others' functional affairs; this results in a diffusion of responsibility. The management process may even cease at times, especially when policies and programs are to be determined. Differences of opinions may smolder and lead to rudeness and cold wars. Communications are more likely to be vertical than horizontal. Consequently, coordination is a problem. The encouragement of group action may stifle a strong creative director. Because of the inherent problems in collegial management, some organizations are moving toward committee management with an executive to coordinate policy.

Project management. Project organizational design is used for large, long-range projects where a number of project groups are developed and administered through the various phases of their existence. This method is useful for one-time projects when the task is unfamiliar and complex; when considerable planning, coordination, high-risk research, and development are involved; and when there is a long lead time between planning and production.

There are several types of project units. The general or functional management type is the most common. Project activities are done within functional groups that are managed by department heads. The general manager coordinates the activities. With this type of arrangement there is no strong central project authority, and consequently decisions are likely to be made to the advantage of the strongest functional group rather than in the best interests of the project. Lead time and decision-making time are increased because the coordination and approval of all functional groups are required.

Aggregate management has an appointed manager who is given her own staff and full authority over her project. All people involved with the project report directly to that manager, giving her a high degree of control over each project. This allows a rapid reaction time and reduces the lead time. Project

83

management is highly regarded by outside sources, and the people involved tend to be loyal to the project because it is their only job at the time.

There are also disadvantages to aggregate management. The people involved are interested in the technology to do the project but do not develop technology as well as functional organizations that have to in order to survive. There tends to be little technical interchange between projects and inefficient use of production elements. Because she is managing just one project, the manager cannot keep all production elements in use at all times. With this management method, production elements are not shared with other projects, and there is consequently duplication of functional activities among projects. There is also a lack of career continuity. Anxiety may increase toward the completion of a project, because project personnel do not know where they will be assigned next. It is difficult to balance work loads as projects begin and reach completion. Aggregate management is not often used.

The matrix organization combines concepts from both functional and aggregate organizations. It departmentalizes functions and shares authority among functional heads and project managers. The project manager uses people assigned to functional areas to complete the project while they are still assigned to the functional area. Thus, the worker has two bosses. Reaction time is quite rapid. Matrix organization seems well received by outside contacts. It does not slow down the development of technology; it facilitates the interchange of technology between projects and provides career continuity, because personnel remain in their functional areas. However, conflicts can arise between project and functional managers. Workers have two bosses and accountability becomes diffuse.

In still another design the project manager may monitor the project but serves only in an advisory capacity to the general manager. The project director controls through influence. She has responsibility without authority, but the workers once again report to one boss, the general manager.

Project management offers several advantages. It visualizes projects and focuses on results. There is good control over the project, shorter development time, improved quality, and lower program costs. This yields higher profit margins and good customer relations. Project management facilitates coordination among functional areas and good mission orientation for people working on the project. It can help elevate morale and develop managers.

There are also numerous disadvantages to project management. It requires changes in patterns of interaction and disrupts the established patterns of hierarchy, span of management, unity of control, resource allocation, departmentalization, priorities, and incentives. Work groups are disrupted, and interfunctional groups develop. Duplication is common. Interdepartmental consensus is used and tends to increase fears of invasion from other departments.

Confusion may arise from authority's ambiguity as new patterns for control develop. Power is one's ability to affect the behavior of others. Authority is power derived from one's position. Influence may be power without authority. Sometimes a project manager uses authority; at other times she has to use influence. Personnel may report to more than one person with varying patterns of authority. Multiple levels of management are more likely to be problems for project than functional management. Authority's ambiguity frequently frustrates personnel.

Project managers tend to be dependent on functional managers for resources. This dependence can create a conflict over those resources. Hence, the project may deplete the functional department of premium professional talent, and the competition for talent may disrupt the stability of the organization and interfere with long-range interests by disrupting traditional business. Some professionals complain that incentives for higher-level ego needs are not met. Project personnel are more likely to be anxious about the loss of their jobs, frustrated by make-work assignments between projects, and confused by a lack of role definitions. They are concerned about setbacks in their careers and upset by the apparent lack of concern about their personal development. Conflicts of allegiance result and undermine loyalty to the organization. Shifting personnel can disrupt their training. What is learned may not be transferred from one project to another. Long-range planning suffers when people are more concerned with their temporary projects.

Several factors contribute to the failure of project management. The most common include an initially unsound basis for the project, poor selection of the project manager, lack of agency support, use of inappropriate management techniques, poor role and task definitions, and no projected termination date.

Precautions can be taken to prevent failure. Planning is always essential. The project needs to be well conceived with its scope outlined and the end results described. A well-qualified manager should be selected, and her role defined. It is helpful if her executive rank ensures responsiveness from others. She needs the authority to control funds, budgeting, and scheduling for the project; to select subcontractors; and to be able to select, add, or eliminate staff as necessary. She should participate in major managerial activities, especially in policy making and other decisions related to her project.

Because functional managers may not wish to take directions from a lesser executive who is suddenly a project manager, top management might select a person from a high position of responsibility, assign her an impressive title, support her dealings with functional managers, and have her report to a manager on the same or higher level than the functional managers.

One of the first responsibilities of the project manager is to staff the project. Sometimes several projects compete for the same talent. Functional managers may not be willing to release the requested personnel, or the person may not want to transfer. People may be hesitant to transfer because (1) there is a division of responsibilities between functional and project organizations, (2) the job is less desirable, or (3) they fear unemployment at the end of the project. Management can offer salary increases as incentives. Promotional opportunities may arise from the additional management structure required for the project. Special efforts should be made to relocate people as they are phased out of the project, thus maintaining security. All of these measures, however, are expensive.

Next, the project manager sets time controls. The manager determines what tasks are required from each department to complete the project and what their proper sequence is. Each department itemizes what it needs to know from other departments and then commits itself to an estimate of the time required to do its part. An overall schedule can be developed by use of critical-path scheduling. It should be checked frequently to compare actual progress against the projected deadlines. This network can be the focal point of project implementation. The manager develops information links that serve the project and help her prepare to replan jobs as project dynamics change.

The project manager also needs to determine cost controls. The most sound decisions can be made by dividing the comprehensive cost summary into work packages. Then technical decision makers can offer commitment reports, and the project manager can act on the approximate cost data. After reviewing the detailed estimated costs and current expenses, the manager can switch staff from less productive duties to duties that will reduce costs.

To maintain quality control, the manager defines the project objectives in quality standards, describes performance criteria, and monitors individual and project progress against the standards. It is helpful to reward responsibility and performance and to try to accommodate staff's personal goals while working toward the objectives of the project.

Task forces. Task forces are sometimes used for special projects. The task force has a mission, a leader, and a projected completion date. To be most successful, the project should be short range. There must be a pool from which to select talent, and task force members should be readily reabsorbed by the organization. Personnel are relieved of their usual tasks and given a temporary assignment, usually to investigate, analyze, research, and plan. They are less often used for decisions and actions. The task force allows personnel with special qualifications to combine their expertise and concentrate on a project in a manner that would not be possible while performing their usual duties. Structural flexibility is accomplished by adding members when their potential contribution is high and removing them when their specific talents are no longer required. It may be an efficient problem-solving method and can offer training opportunities for managers. It can unleash creative energies and introduce innovations.

On the other hand, it can be disruptive to the organization. Key personnel may be away from their jobs for unknown lengths of time. As members experience different qualities of supervision by moving from one team to another, they may become more critical of the less capable manager. Assignment to a task force may make an employee think she is special compared with peers. She may feel independent and detached from her usual work group. It is not uncommon for personnel to be promoted and removed from their original departments after the task force responsibilities are completed. Reabsorbing the task force member back into the organization is sometimes difficult, and that realization is almost certain to increase the employee's anxiety. Or what began as a short-range, problem-solving task force may become an unwanted permanent arrangement.

Matrix. Matrix organizational designs try to combine the advantages of project and functional structures. The functional line organization provides support for the project line organization. In a functional organization, the functional manager has the authority to determine and rate goals, select personnel, determine pay and promotions, make personnel assignments, and evaluate personnel and the project. The manager is responsible to her superior but works quite independently. In a matrix organization, the functional manager shares those responsibilities with the project manager, because management by project objectives is important to the matrix organization. Initially, the functional manager may experience a sense of loss in status, authority, and control. Therefore, it is important for the manager to be able to persuade others by using her personal qualities and knowledge of the program (Fig. 2-2). The functional and project managers need each other's cooperation for approvals and signoffs. The intent in the matrix organization is to have the decision making as far down in the organizational structure as possible. This encourages group consensus. Most decisions are made at the middle-management level, thus freeing top administration for long-range planning.

The matrix organization increases the amount of contact between individuals, and its complexity makes conflict inevitable. Increased communications are essential. Differences need to be recognized and dealt with, because collaborative behavior is needed. Team building between departments is encouraged, and consultants are used as connections between parts. Managers need human relations training. Organizational charts showing task responsibilities and levels of responsibility may reduce conflict.

Matrix organizations foster flexibility in dealing with change and uncertainty. They enable managers to balance conflicting objectives by maximizing technical

Fig. 2-2. Adaptive model: matrix for a school of nursing.

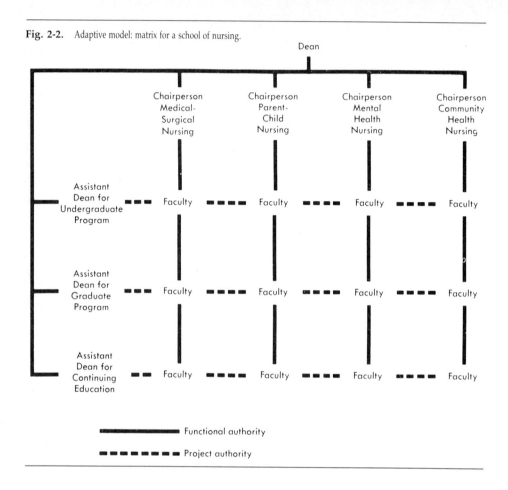

excellence through efficient use of resources. By moving decision making down in the organization, opportunities are provided for personal development and motivation. Commitment is improved, and top management is freed for long-range planning.

Because people are more familiar with bureaucratic structures, there is considerable need to orient personnel to the matrix structure and philosophy. Rigid lines of authority, inflexible boundaries separating jobs and divisions, unambiguous resource allocation to divisions, and specific loyalties that exist in bureaucracies are not appropriate in dynamic organizations with overlapping and sometimes contradictory interests and goals. But because of multiple and often ambiguous roles, some personnel may get frustrated and feel insecure.

Systems. Systems design is an adaptive organizational model. It has been facilitated by the use of computers. The systems approach can be applied to bureaucracies that are considered closed systems or to adaptive models viewed as open systems. The design develops from the flow of work and information. It considers relationships, time, and decision points.

Mixed model. A mixed model may be the most viable. Bureaucratic design can work very well for routine functions. Adaptive designs may be more useful for research and development. However, the success of any organizational design is largely dependent on the manager's skills.

ORGANIZATIONAL CONCEPTS
Charts

An organizational chart is a drawing that shows how the parts of an organization are linked. It depicts the formal organizational relationships, areas of responsibility, persons to whom one is accountable, and channels of communication.

Managers should consider actual working relationships when drawing an organizational chart. The formal organization may not be functioning as was outlined on an older chart. Rather, an alternate structure may have emerged that operates very effectively. It is essential, then, that the manager know what is happening in actual practice. The process of drawing the chart demands a review of current practices, discovery of relationships not previously examined, and clarification of vague associations.

The organizational chart may be used for outlining administrative control, for policymaking and planning (including organizational change) to evaluate strengths and weaknesses of the current structure, and for showing relationships with other departments and agencies. It also can be used to orient new personnel or to present the agency's structural design to others. The visual diagram of a chart is a more effective means of communicating the agency's organizational structure than a written description.

Organizational charts are not used by all managers. An autocratic manager who wishes to control and manipulate others may feel that her power would be diminished if subordinates understood the working environment. Adaptive structures are more difficult to chart because they are more fluid and subject to change.

Charts become outdated as changes are made. On charts, the informal structure has not been diagramed, the formal structure may be difficult to define, and duties and responsibilities are not described. Charts may foster rigidity in relationships and communications. People may be sensitive about their relative status in the organization and may not want their positions revealed. It can be expensive to develop, disseminate, and store the charts.

Vertical charts, depicting the chief executive at the top with formal lines of

Fig. 2-3. Vertical chart.

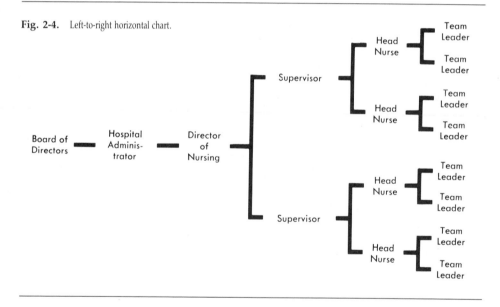

Fig. 2-4. Left-to-right horizontal chart.

authority down the hierarchy, are most common, but other modifications are available (Fig. 2-3). A left-to-right, or horizontal, chart depicts the chief executive at the left with lower echelons to the right (Fig. 2-4). It follows the normal reading habit, shows relative length of formal lines of authority, helps simplify the lines of authority and responsibility, and can reveal problems within the structure. A concentric or circular chart shows the chief executive in the center with suc-

Fig. 2-5. Circular chart.

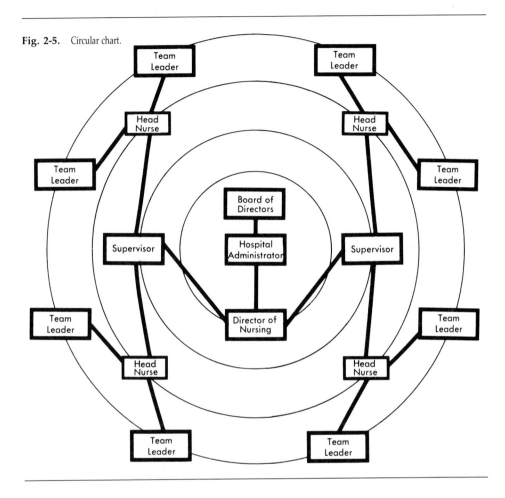

cessive echelons in concentric circles (Fig. 2-5). It helps depict the outward flow of formal authority from the top executive and supposedly reduces status implications.

The informal structure can be superimposed on the formal structure or charted through the use of sociograms. Sociograms analyze data on the choice of, communication between, and interaction among members of a small group. Each person may be asked with whom she prefers to work, or her interactions may be observed and charted. The person with the most relationships is often the leader. Members of the primary group are those most accepted by other group members. Managers should use this information to increase production, because work groups based on sociograms are generally more productive than those arbitrarily designed.

Span of management

Span of management has been of concern since biblical times. Exodus 18:13-26 is an account of how Moses had to deal with the problem of leading the Israelites out of Egypt. His father-in-law, Jethro, observed Moses counseling people all day long, while others had to wait long periods of time to tell Moses their problems. Jethro suggested that he delegate authority by selecting rulers of thousands, hundreds, fifties, and tens, who would teach the people laws and leave Moses free to deal only with the exceptions.

Initial work with span of management was quantitative and attempted to devise formulas for determining the most desirable number of subordinates. General Hamilton, a British officer in World War I, concluded that supervisors at the lower levels could direct more people than those at higher levels. He thought an effective span of control was three to six others, especially at upper levels. Henri Fayol, a French industrialist and early writer about scientific management, used a similar philosophy to develop a hierarchy.

Hamilton's principle has been elaborated on by A.V. Graicunas, a Lithuanian management consultant, whose mathematical analysis of potential relationships illustrates the complex social processes between a supervisor and her subordinates, and among the subordinates; the complexity especially increases with each additional subordinate. Graicunas demonstrated that as the number of subordinates responsible to a supervisor increases arithmetically, the number of potential interactions increases geometrically. The geometrical interactions can be classified as direct single relationships, direct group relationships, and cross relationships. If a supervisor has two subordinates, x and y, the supervisor may have two direct relationships, one with x and one with y. She may speak to either in the presence of the other, forming two group relationships. Two cross relationships exist between x and y and between y and x. Consequently, there are six possible interactions between one supervisor and two subordinates—two direct, two group, and two cross. If a third subordinate is added, one direct relationship, seven group relationships, and four cross relationships are added, making eighteen potential interactions.

Graicunas's formula is $R = n(2n/2 + n - 1)$. R equals all types of relationships and n equals the number of subordinates. The results are presented in Table 1.

Graicunas's formula calculates the number of potential relationships. It does not deal with the actual frequency or the importance of the various relationships. In reality, the number of relationships with which a supervisor must deal is probably not so great. One might question if the relationship in which the supervisor speaks to x in y's presence is different from speaking to y in x's presence. Graicunas considers them different psychological situations. It is unlikely that

Table 1. Variable number of subordinates and resulting number of potential relationships

Number of subordinates	Number of relationships
1	1
2	6
3	18
4	44
5	100
6	222
7	490
8	1,080
9	2,376
10	5,210
11	11,374
12	24,708
13	53,404
14	114,872
18	2,359,602

people will engage in all of the relationships that are theoretically possible. Nevertheless, Graicunas's formula illustrates how complex a situation can become as additional subordinates report to a manager.

The optimal span of management is dependent on many considerations that affect the time requirements for management. The manager's competence and qualifications and those of her subordinates affect her time requirement. Some managers, because of their education and personal qualities, can work with more people than others. The better prepared a subordinate is for her job, the less time a manager must devote to teaching, clarifying responsibilities, and correcting mistakes.

Rapidly changing technology, procedures, and policies increase training problems and the need for problem solving. Availability of expert advice and services to the manager can free her time and widen her span of management. However, a larger personal staff does not necessarily allow a broadening of the span of control because of the supervision required for those assistants. It may be more economical to increase the responsibilities of lower level management. The greater the clarity of delegated authority, the less time it will take for the manager to explain the responsibilities and tasks. There will be less need for her to make decisions subordinates can make. If the subordinate's task is not clearly defined, is unaccompanied by the necessary authority, or is beyond her competence, there will be an increase in time required for supervision.

Much of a manager's time is spent explaining plans, giving instructions, and receiving information about problems and progress. Clear and concise communications transmit information quickly and accurately. Much communication can be written. However, some situations cannot be handled with planning documents, policy statements, written reports, memoranda, or other written communications. These require personal contact. Some situations, which could be handled by written communications, may be better handled by personal contact. These might include delicate situations and instances where attitudes are involved. Personal contacts require considerable time.

If plans are clear, the subordinate will know what is expected of her without frequently checking with her supervisor. If the subordinate does her own planning, she will need more supervision. However, clear policies to guide her planning will reduce demands on the supervisor. Clear and complete policy statements can also simplify the supervisor's decision making and allow expansion of her span of management. Deciding every problem individually requires more time than making policy decisions that anticipate problems.

The demands on the supervisor vary according to the complexity of functions. Standardization reduces time requirements, because people know what is expected. Routine work requires less time than innovative work. But we can expect that as the degree of difficulty for performing a task satisfactorily increases, so does the demand on the supervisor. As the variability of functions increases, the supervisor must consider more factors and interrelationships; this takes more time. Interdependent functions require more management time than independent functions because of the increased need for coordination. The greater the geographical separation of personnel reporting to the supervisor, the more limiting the span of control. The greater the nonmanagerial responsibilities, the less time the supervisor has for management. Supervisors in flat organizational structures have a broader range of management than those in tall structures, and lower level managers have a broader range than top management.

Flat versus tall structures

The flat structure is developed along horizontal dimensions according to the number of organizational functions that are identified separately. There are few levels of supervision. The tall structure is developed along vertical dimensions by use of the scalar process to define relationships among levels in an organization. Because there are advantages and disadvantages to both the flat and tall structures, it is best to maintain a reasonable balance of dimensions. Changes within the organization bring imbalance over time, so the organizational structure should be reviewed periodically.

The flat structure shortens the administrative distance between top and bottom levels in the organization, thereby minimizing distortions through shorter lines of communication. Communications are direct, simple, fast, and clearly apparent to employees. Another advantage of the flat structure is that large groups have a greater variety of skills available and are capable of solving a greater variety of problems. This structure is believed to contribute to high employee morale and helps develop capable, self-confident subordinates. It lends itself to a democratic approach and general supervision, which are preferred by many people. This minimal social stratification is consistent with an egalitarian political and social philosophy, which is currently popular.

However, a flat structure may be impractical in large organizations. Large groups have more difficulty reaching a consensus and require more coordination. The flat structure places tremendous pressure on each manager because of the amount of authority and responsibility she has and the high penalties for failures. An overburdened manager may not have the time to select, evaluate, and teach subordinates, or the energy to think and plan. She may have difficulty making and communicating decisions. Socializing with subordinates may reduce her authority.

Tall structures lend themselves to authoritarianism, which is most effective in situations requiring rapid changes and precise coordination. In a tall structure, messages from superiors are given more attention than those from peers and consequently pass through levels quickly. The narrow range of management allows staff to evaluate decisions frequently. With small groups, decision making takes less time, and there is more opportunity for members to participate and to understand the goals. Such interaction facilitates group cohesiveness.

Levels are expensive because of the large number of executives needed with high salaries. Each additional level makes communication more cumbersome. The more levels that communications pass through, the greater the distortion. Therefore, a tall structure reduces the understanding between higher and lower levels and increases impersonality.

Decentralization versus centralization

Decentralization is the degree to which decision making is diffused throughout the organization. It is relative, for the degree of decentralization is larger when more important decisions affecting more functions are made at lower levels with less supervision. There are several factors to consider when determining the optimal degree of decentralization for an organization. Top management needs a positive attitude toward decentralization, and they need competent personnel to whom they can delegate authority. The latter need access to the information necessary for decision making.

The number of people who need to interact to solve a problem should be considered. In general, the larger the organization, the greater the number of complex decisions that must be made and that can overburden top management and delay decision making. Smaller, decentralized units reduce the number of decisions made by each manager and increase the time available to devote to each problem. Usually agencies tend to be more centralized during their early formative years. If the agency gradually expands from within, it is more likely to remain centralized. An organization that grows rapidly through acquisitions is more likely to be decentralized; thus, decentralization is more common in organizations with geographical dispersion of operations. Some functions lend themselves more readily to decentralization than do others; production, marketing, personnel, and some purchasing may be readily decentralized. In contrast, finances, accounting, data processing of statistics, and purchase of capital equipment are likely to remain centralized.

The profit center concept has developed from decentralization and has been quite popular since World War II. It is particularly characteristic of large organizations with multiple product lines. The organization is divided into manageable units called profit centers that are self-contained and have their own management and staff. Each unit competes with others for profits; this arrangement motivates managers to make decisions that will maximize profits. The manager has considerable freedom for making operational decisions. The profit center concept helps give meaning to decentralization by placing the responsibility for profit making on a number of managers instead of just top management.

The advantages of decentralization seem to outweigh the disadvantages. Decentralization increases morale and promotes interpersonal relationships. When people have a voice in governance, they feel more important and are more willing to contribute. This increased motivation provides a feeling of individuality and freedom that in turn encourages creativity and commits the individual to making the system successful. Decentralization fosters informality and democracy in management and brings decision making closer to the action. Thus, decisions may be more effective because people who know the situation and have to implement the decision are the ones who make it. Because managers do not have to wait for the approval of their superiors, flexibility is increased, and reaction time is decreased. Fewer people have to exchange information; consequently, communications are swift and effective. Coordination improves, especially for services, production with sales, and costs with income. Products or an operation that is minor to the total production receives more adequate attention. Plans can be tried out on an experimental basis in one unit, modified, and proven before used in other units. Risks of losses of personnel or facilities are dispersed.

Decentralization helps determine accountability. It makes weak management visible through semi-independent and often competitive divisions. Operating on the premise that people learn by doing, decentralization develops managers by allowing them to manage. A management pool can be developed that thereby eases the problem of succession. There is usually less conflict between top management and divisions. Decentralization releases top management from the burden of daily administration, freeing them for long-range planning, goal and policy development, and systems integration.

Nevertheless, several problems can also result from decentralization. An organization may not be large enough to merit decentralization, or it may be difficult to divide the organization into self-contained operating units. Top administrators may not desire decentralization. They may feel it would decrease their status, or they may question the abilities of the people to whom they would delegate. They may feel that most people prefer to be dependent on others and do not want decision-making responsibility. An increased awareness of division consciousness and a decrease in company consciousness may develop. Divisions may become individualized and competitive to the extent that they sacrifice the overall objectives for short-range profitability and work against the best interests of the whole organization. Because of conflicts between divisions, it may be difficult to obtain a majority vote, and compromises may result. If the majority vote is delayed, it may come too late to be effective.

Decentralization involves increased costs. It requires more managers and larger staffs. There may be underutilization of managers. Divisions may not adequately use the specialists housed at headquarters. Functions are likely to be duplicated between divisions and headquarters. Because decentralization develops managers, there are novice managers in the system who will make mistakes. Division managers may not inform top management of their problems. There are problems with control and nonuniform policies. Some restrictions on autonomy remain. Even with decentralization, top management remains responsible for long-range objectives and goals, broad policies, selection of key executives, and approval of major capital expenditures.

Delegation. Related to decentralization is the concept of delegation, for it is only through delegation that decentralization can be accomplished. Delegation is the process of assigning work from one organizational level to another, or from superior to subordinate. Delegation maximizes the utilization of the talents of subordinates. It uses latent abilities in personnel that contribute to their growth and development. Staff members learn by doing. Their involvement tends to increase their motivation and commitment to accomplish goals while freeing the manager to manage. This also reduces managerial costs.

Several conditions facilitate delegation. First, the manager needs to understand the concept of delegation and have a generally positive attitude toward people. She needs to overcome feelings of loss of prestige through delegation and to develop a positive atmosphere for her subordinates. She should help achieve results through effective communication instead of by doing the job herself. Thus, she concentrates on the accomplishment of overall goals and objectives rather than the day-to-day details.

Top management clarifies policies, goals, and objectives, and these are further developed by each succeeding lower level. For example, top management sets the overall budget, but each department then works with its own budget. Specifying goals and objectives directs personnel and determines priorities and the use of resources. Management by objectives promotes this.

Job descriptions provide a definition of the responsibility and authority involved with each position. Everything that must be done for the organization to meet its goals is part of someone's job. Consequently, job descriptions are based on the functional needs of the agency and clarify the responsibility of the individual's position and the objectives of the work.

Before writing job descriptions, management decides which assignments to delegate. In order to do so, the manager should be aware of the capabilities and characteristics of her subordinates. Testing of employees to learn what they can and cannot do and providing the necessary training helps overcome many personnel failures. Staff members are often asked to perform skills for which they are not qualified or in which they are not interested. People tend to put off tasks they find unpleasant and then do them poorly. It is not necessary to delegate equally. By knowing individual capabilities, the manager can delegate according to the subordinate's interests and abilities.

Job descriptions are not always advantageous in small or rapidly changing organizations, because those staffs often assume different roles at different times. Generalization is more common than the specialization required in larger, more stable organizations. Some employees outperform the requirements of their job descriptions, whereas others are not able to do some of the duties described. Job descriptions can be redefined according to the person's capability and organizational needs. If a person is unable to handle the required duties, she may be transferred to another area, given further training, supplied with an assistant to supplement her weak areas, or fired.

Controls based on goals, rather than means, are important. The manager checks on how well the delegated responsibilities are being performed, and the subordinates know if they are meeting their responsibilities. Performance standards clarify how the supervisor measures achievement. These standards cover the quantity and quality of work expected and the time allowed for its accomplishment. The standards should be broad enough to allow individuality. If the standards are perceived as reasonable and fair by both supervisor and subordinate, they will be both happier with their jobs. Subordinates like their work to be noticed and appreciated. The supervisor meets their need for recognition and appreciation by having a general knowledge of what is happening, using an open door policy, expressing willingness to give assistance and support, and taking a personal interest in their problems. A snoopervisor, however, is not appreciated.

It is the supervisor's responsibility to assess the results of delegation. One of the most satisfactory ways of being aware of what is happening is by being among the subordinates. Formal and informal meetings, systems of reporting, quality control, and statistical sampling are other means. Although inspection is perceived as unpleasant, most subordinates accept it as necessary. However, they do object to unnecessary inspections that disturb routines.

Even though a person may receive satisfaction by knowing that she is doing a good job, having those efforts recognized by others is appreciated. Supervisors err if they do not give praise for work well done. People should also be rewarded for their continued contributions to the agency through raises and promotions. If subordinates err, they should be corrected—the sooner the better. But when subordinates participate in goal setting, when the emphasis is on the goal rather than individual personalities, and when training is a continuous process, corrections that otherwise would have been made by the supervisor may be unnecessary. The system encourages self-correction.

Learning to live with differences may be difficult for a supervisor, especially if she once performed her subordinate's tasks and now finds that they are not done as she did them. It is even more threatening when the subordinate does a better job than the superior once did. It has to be recognized that there will be differences in quantity and quality of work accomplished and methods used between the supervisor and subordinates or among subordinates.

Assignment of responsibility, delegation of authority, and creation of accountability are the three concepts most often mentioned in relation to the delegation process. Responsibility denotes obligation. It refers to what must be done to complete a task and the obligation created by the assignment. The supervisor and the subordinate must understand what activities the subordinate is responsible for, what results are expected, and how performance is to be evaluated. The supervisor needs a clear idea of what she wants done before she can communicate that to others. To clarify them for herself, the supervisor may put her ideas in writing. By so doing, she is then less likely to give incomplete directions. The assignment of responsibility is not complete, however, until the subordinate decides to accept the obligation.

Authority is the power to make final decisions and give commands. The person to whom responsibility has been assigned needs the authority to direct the performance of delegated duties. She needs authority of sufficient scope to include all related activities without frequent consultation with her superior. The granting of too little authority is a common problem, because organizational policies and procedures are often limiting, and sometimes the person may have little control over the actions of others.

The person with delegated authority performs for the supervisor. Although authority is delegated so that the subordinate can fulfill her responsibilities, the supervisor maintains control over the delegated authority and may recall it.

Delegation of authority involves the subordinate's knowledge, abilities, skills, and potential contribution and the supervisor's guidance. During the initial phase of delegating authority, the subordinate presents her ideas and plans. The supervisor raises questions, explores alternatives, and helps identify potential problems and ways to prevent them. Then mutual agreement is reached. The supervisor offers continuing support by providing staff, resources, and information needed by the subordinate for the completion of the delegated responsibility.

Accountability refers to liability. The subordinate incurs an obligation to complete work satisfactorily and to utilize authority appropriately when she accepts delegated responsibility. She is accountable to her supervisor. The manager is accountable for the performance of the task, the selection of the person to complete it, and both the subordinate's and her own performances. Head nurses are responsible for delegation to team leaders, who are accountable for delegation to team members. Each remains accountable for the work delegated.

There are numerous reasons for underdelegating. The superior may think she can do the job quicker herself, resent interruptions to answer questions, or not want to take the time to check what has been done. She may get cooperation from other departments more easily than from subordinates or be unwilling to take risks for fear of being blamed for others' mistakes.

Some managers do not have confidence in their subordinates and they are afraid that their subordinates will not keep them adequately informed. Or they may not trust their subordinates and complain that they lack training and sufficient experience. They may argue that their subordinates lack an understanding of the organizational objectives and are specialists without the general knowledge needed for problem solving. In some cases, they may even be afraid that their subordinates will outperform them.

Therefore, a manager may like to do the work herself and feel that she can do it better. She receives personal recognition for and satisfaction from the work and prefers to do the real things instead of just plan with others. This sort of person often expects perfection, considers herself indispensable, and desires to dominate. She is afraid of losing power and prestige and is aware that her poor operating procedures and practices may be exposed.

Subordinates have their reasons for not accepting delegation. Some are dependent on their supervisor and find it easier to ask the boss. Others lack self-confidence and fear failure and criticism. This fear is often related to how mistakes have been handled. Emphasis on the mistake itself is more threatening than using the situation as a learning experience.

Lack of guidelines, standards, and control are additional problems. Duties are not always clearly defined, authority not specified, or necessary information and resources not readily available. Some subordinates are already overworked. The incentives are inadequate, and they do not want to perform work if their supervisor receives the credit.

Departmentalization. Departmentalization results from span of management, division of work, and a need for cooperation. Its primary purpose is to subdivide the organizational structure so that managers can specialize within limited ranges of activity. Organization of the agency influences group behavior and the effectiveness of the group. The objectives of the agency can be met most easily if the group is properly organized. Two common types of departmentalization are input and output. The input, or process orientation, includes function, time, and simple numbers as bases for departmentalization, whereas the output, or goal orientation, includes product, territory, and client divisions.

The input, or process-oriented structure, emphasizes specialization of skills. It reinforces professional skills by uniting people with similar expertise in the same department. For example, the focus may be on cardiac nursing, respiratory nursing, or transplant nursing, depending on the departmentalization. It is possible for a professional to advance within her field of expertise instead of advancing through the administrative hierarchy. Unfortunately, the process-oriented structure emphasizes professional skills over organizational goals. Conflicts increase as communication and cooperation decrease. Input organization provides less favorable training for general administrators than does a goal-oriented structure.

Departmentalization by function groups activities according to similarity of skills or a group of tasks necessary to accomplish a goal. Logical, simple, and commonly used, it facilitates specialization that contributes to economic operations. It groups functions that can be performed by the same specialists with the same type of equipment and facilities. Less demand for one product may be counteracted by a greater demand for another product. Consequently, staff, equipment, and facilities will have optimal utilization. The combination of administrative activities also is economical. One manager is responsible for all related activities; therefore, coordination is improved because it is more easily achieved. The agency benefits from a few people with outstanding abilities, for only top management is able to coordinate the major functions. For example, the hospital may be organized by medical, surgical, and pediatric units.

Functional departmentalization also has its disadvantages. As the size of the agency increases, centralization may become excessive, making effective control more difficult. The necessary additional organizational levels may slow down communications and delay decision making. It becomes more difficult to measure performance. Functional departmentalization does not provide good training for general managers. They become expert in their particular function, have little opportunity to learn about other functions, and may emphasize their previous function while deemphasizing others when they become general managers.

Time factors are another basis for organization. Acute care settings need coverage 24 hours a day, 7 days a week, whereas preventive services may only need coverage for 8 to 12 hours a day for 5 to 6 days a week at the most.

Grouping by numbers divides undifferentiated labor into manageable units. A certain number of workers is assigned to each supervisor. This method is common in underdeveloped countries but is disappearing in industrialized areas.

The output or goal structure emphasizes service to the client. It collects all the work for a project under one supervisor and reduces dependence on other units for needed resources. This allows considerable autonomy, and the client, workers, and goals are readily identified. Systems and procedures are highly standardized. Family planning, pregnancy counseling, and school health are examples of services available from some health departments.

Unfortunately, these units may stress their own goals while de-emphasizing agency goals. Duplication of equipment and services may develop. Equipment may not be fully utilized, or smaller-scale equipment may be less effective. The grouping of various skills into one unit can reduce the expertise as professional reinforcement is weakened.

A product or group of closely related products may be the basis of organization for autonomous departments. Emphasis is on the product instead of the process. Improvement, expansion, and diversification of the product is possible because one manager is responsible for all activities affecting that specific product. In a large agency this could result in small, flexible units where functional groupings would be too complex. This method identifies profit responsibilities for specific products. Organization on the basis of products has become increasingly popular. It is common for schools of nursing to organize according to the products produced—medical nurses, surgical nurses, obstetrical nurses, pediatric nurses, psychiatric nurses, and community health nurses.

Departmentalization by territories is particularly useful for physically dispersed activities where branches provide similar services at each location. This method serves the local clients with greatest efficiency. Supervisors consider local circumstances that might be overlooked by a central manager. It uses local people who are familiar with local conditions. It reduces delivery time and may reduce transportation costs related to raw materials and finished products. It is particularly useful for production and sales and when perishability is a problem. However, financial management works best if centralized.

Departmentalization by client makes sense when service is important and the welfare of the client is of primary interest. For example, a clinic may have obstetric, pediatric, and adolescent clinics. Clinics may be open nights and weekends for working people. Schools of nursing may offer night classes for working students. This better utilizes facilities and is more satisfactory to the client. However, pressure for special consideration and treatment of specific groups may exist, and coordination problems may increase.

Line-staff relationships

Line authority. Line organization is the oldest type of structure. It is a chain of command, a superior-subordinate or leader-follower relationship. The superior delegates authority to a subordinate, who in turn delegates authority to her subordinate. This progression is the basis for the name "line authority." The command relationship is a direct line between superior and subordinate and is depicted by a solid line on organizational charts. The line positions are related to the direct achievement of organizational objectives. This arrangement fosters quick decision making because the manager is given complete charge of her area and at most would need to consult only with her direct supervisor. Buck-passing is reduced, and authority relationships are clearly understood. The superior has the right to give orders, demand accountability, and discipline violators.

Staff authority. Staff supports line-authority relationships and is advisory or service in nature. They handle details, locate required data, and offer counsel on managerial problems. Staff functions through influence, for they do not have authority to accept, use, modify, or reject plans. Staff makes the line more effective, but organizations can function without staff authority.

The two major categories of staff authority are personal and specialist. The personal category includes the assistant and general staff. The specialist staff is composed of advisory, service, control, and functional personnel.

Assistant staff. A personal staff member may be called an assistant to, a staff assistant, or an administrative assistant and is responsible to one line manager. Her chief purpose is to extend the line manager's capacity for completing a large amount of work by doing the more routine tasks that the manager would otherwise have to perform herself. The duties vary widely from one manager to another but might include such activities as answering mail, data collection for decision making, consolidation of information from various reports, preparation of documents, development of budgets, interpreting plans to others, and substituting for the manager at various meetings and functions.

The personal staff member has no specific function. Her duties vary with the assignments. She does not act on her own behalf but rather as a personal representative of her superior. The only specific authority she has comes from her supervisor on a limited basis, usually for a specific job over a brief time span. With delegated authority, the personal staff member can give instructions in her superior's name and make decisions that affect the organization. It is important for the assistant and the people with whom she works to know the extent of her influence. Misuses of and misunderstanding about the assistant are all too common. Some feel that the assistant is unnecessary and that the duties should be delegated to other line managers. When the assistant takes over tasks that belong to others, misunderstanding and poor cooperation result. Some assistants give the impression that they are the superior instead of just acting for one.

General staff. The general staff is composed of top administrators. The top administrator makes the decision after receiving input from these key people who together have the necessary expertise to make sound decisions for the agency. This is a coordinated group performing to maximize results. They serve in an advisory capacity by collecting and sharing information and are functional through their supervisory activities. The military has used this concept extensively, but it is relatively uncommon in business. Rotating general staff members to various areas and levels within the organization fosters an understanding of line problems.

Advisory staff. Advisory staff counsels line managers. They study problems, collect and analyze data, offer alternatives, and prepare plans. Their work may be accepted, rejected, or modified by the line manager. Although ideas are heard, they are not always implemented. This puts staff on the defensive, because they must sell their ideas. It is important that they counsel rather than suggest or confirm just what the line manager wants. Chances of an idea being approved are increased when staff has discussed proposed recommendations with line managers who will be affected by the decision and has received their approval before presenting the plan to the top administrator. Careful evaluation of the plan is important. The better prepared the advice, the more likely the staff will be heard and their suggestions implemented. If staff works in seclusion, secretly preparing reports without listening to, or discussing them with, line managers, they are likely to get a suspicious and negative reception from others.

Service staff. Service staff is not advisory. They perform a centralized service that has been separated from the line to prevent duplication and to allow more economical performance and good control. This includes dietary and laundry services in a hospital. Line relies on staff to get the job done. They do not do it themselves.

Control staff. Control staff also does not advise. They control by restraining line authority. They have direct or indirect control over certain line performance. They control directly by acting as an agent for a line manager or indirectly through procedural compliance and interpretation of policies and reports. Quality control personnel and the affirmative action officers are members of the control staff.

Functional staff. Functional authority exists when a specialist is given decisionmaking authority for specific activities outside the formal chain of command.

This authority may be delegated to line, staff, or service managers and may be exercised over line, staff, and service personnel. The functional staff has limited line authority with power to determine standards in their areas of specialization and to enforce them. This authority is usually of an impersonal nature in the form of schedules, inspection reports, and written orders. It breaks the scalar chain and violates the principle that personnel should only be accountable to one superior. Although done in the interest of convenience and efficiency, it should be restricted, because it can damage line authority, destroy departmentalization, and create confusion.

Line-staff conflict. Conflict is likely to arise in any situation where two or more people must interact to get results. Line-staff conflicts occur when there is a lack of understanding of the roles and functions of others and when their lines of responsibility, accountability, and authority are not clear. Line and staff have different responsibilities and goals. Line is generalized, whereas staff is specialized. The line manager is likely to be a pragmatist who has received her position through competent service. She may not have much formal education but prides herself on common sense. The staff manager probably considers herself an expert by virtue of her extensive formal education or experience in her area of competence, or both. In addition to their differences in responsibilities and backgrounds, they also have different loyalties. Line managers identify with their work group; staff managers are inclined to be loyal to their professional colleagues and the company as a whole.

Line may complain that staff is impractical and too academic. Specialists sometimes are not aware of the total picture. Offered from a specialized, narrow viewpoint, their advice is impractical because it ignores the ramifications of a given situation. Staff managers may be viewed as outside interference who do not understand line or technical problems. Consultation causes delay. Line may accuse staff of not keeping them informed in an effort to keep them off balance and to claim credit for good ideas that turn out well, while blaming line for failures. Line may believe that staff lacks responsibility or assumes too much authority and runs the show.

On the other hand, staff complains that line ignores them, resists staff assistance, or does not use them properly. Line may make decisions in specialized situations without consulting them or may seek their consultation too late. Line is often viewed as cautious, conservative, and resistant to new ideas. They want to do things as they have always done them. Staff may feel that line managers do not give them enough authority in their area of expertise and may be concerned about the way line implements staff's ideas and plans.

Improving line-staff relationships. Certain conditions can be created to foster the integration of line-staff efforts. It is helpful if both line and staff have participated in determining objectives and plans and their implementation. Participation increases everyone's awareness of the overall goals to be accomplished. Each should be briefed on the roles and functions of other team members. The lines of responsibility, accountability, and authority should be clearly established and publicized. A team-effort atmosphere is more likely to prevail in structures that allow line and staff to interact with open communications and that have a problem-solving focus.

BEHAVIORAL ASPECTS OF ORGANIZATIONAL CHANGE

Many people are unaware of the factors that initiate change or influence its direction. Even when known, some forces are beyond their control. Some factors that effect change in an agency stem from society, such as new knowledge and technology, new social requirements, changing client needs and demands, and increased competition. Even when known in advance and anticipated, they cannot be controlled by an agency.

The efficiency of an organizational structure is hard to measure, and the factors contributing to success or failure may be impossible to isolate. Organizational structure may not be the problem. A few ineffective people can disrupt an otherwise sound structure, and good people can make a bad structure work. High labor costs, inadequate equipment, ineffective advertising, changing client needs, and increased competition may contribute to inadequate profits.

Some symptoms reflect inefficiencies within the organization and indicate a need for change. If slow and erroneous decision making is a problem, one may question the qualiflcations of the person making decisions, the level at which responsibility is placed, and access to necessary information. Poor communications, a dearth of innovation, and failure in functional areas are other symptoms indicating a need for change. Diagnosis of the problem is extremely important for planned change. Some problems may be corrected by minor adjustments rather than major reorganizations. However, even a small change in one part of an organization can cause a chain reaction throughout the agency. This domino effect creates problems with coordination and control and brings about a need for comprehensive planning.

Change disrupts equilibrium. Equilibrium can be maintained only when opposing forces are equal. Production may be maintained when the forces fostering production, such as pressure of the supervisor to produce, desire for favorable attention from the supervisor to foster one's own gain, and desire to earn more through the incentive plan, equal the forces limiting production, such as the informal group's standard against rate busting, resistance to training from the supervisor, and the feeling that the job and product are not important. However, when the forces in one direction or the other change in relation to each other, a new grouping forms, and change is inevitable.

Resistance to change

Caution should be used when making organizational changes. Changes are disturbing to those affected, and resistance often develops. Giving the structure a chance to work may be better than changing it. Although changing the organizational structure may appear easy on paper, it is quite complicated in reality. It affects the attitudes and effectiveness of personnel whose prestige and status are threatened. Resistance to change is a common phenomenon whether it is initiated by positive stimuli— such as growth or promotion of an employee— or negative forces—such as poor management. Personnel develop vested interests, preferences, habits, and rigidities that attract them to the existing structure. People tend to consider the effects of the change on their personal lives, status, and future more than on the welfare of the agency. Change introduces the risk of error, fear of failure when trying something new, resistance to admission of weakness, fear of losing a current satisfaction, or a fatalistic expectation based on previous unsuccessful attempts to change. Change is most threatening in the presence of insecurity. Even logical, needed changes produce resistance.

Gradual changes made in progressive phases are usually less disturbing than radical, sweeping, unpredicted changes. Changes in the structure resulting from sharply defined events that have already been planned—such as changes in size, scope, or objectives—are easier to execute than shifts in personnel, which involve infinitely complex human relations. Careful planning, appropriate timing of communications, adequate feedback, and employee confidence in management can reduce resistance to change.

Resistance can be further reduced by informing personnel of the reasons for change, especially when the advantages of the change are stressed. Personnel can be involved by requests for their input, including feelings, suggestions, and talents; their negative as well as positive feelings should be respected. Communicating honestly about the changes, giving specific feedback, asking what assistance is needed to help them cope, and recognizing their contributions to the implementation of the change can further minimize resistance.

Types of change

Organizational structure usually grows vertically, then horizontally, and from functional to divisionalized type. Initially there is vertical growth, but as the amount of work and its complexity increases, horizontal growth develops. Usually organizations develop from a functional type, which is departmentalized by major functions, to one divisionalized by product or territory.

Planning for change

Plans for change begin with an evaluation of the existing organization. An organizational audit provides a detailed analysis of the organization, reveals the extent to which goals are accomplished, and examines the utilization of personnel and the growth of individuals. One begins an organizational audit by collecting and reviewing all available written material about the organization, including statement of the mission or purpose, scope of the agency, goals and objectives, organizational chart, job descriptions, annual reports, performance appraisals, and qualiflcations needed and not needed by personnel in their present positions. The planner notes if the reviewed materials are consistent, looks for gaps and overlapping of functioning, and determines if all activities contribute to the major goals of the agency.

Departmentalization, span of management, and balance and emphasis are analyzed. Authority relationships are studied. Leadership patterns, delegation, decentralization, utilization of committees, and provision of controls are considered. The agency may be compared with what is visualized as an ideal agency or with competitors to identify areas of need and to propose recommended changes. Personnel may be surveyed to identify areas needing improvement. The quantitative approach may be used where ratios are appropriate, such as figuring range of management. Then various organizational patterns are designed, and position breakdown using existing personnel is developed. Personnel needed who are not presently available and people available who are not qualified or needed are identified.

A job description and requirements are necessary for each position. Each person's qualifications can be compared with her job requirements. Notations are made of job requirements for which skills are not possessed. Those qualities that can be developed on the job within reasonable time limits should be separated from required skills that cannot be acquired. Unused abilities should be related to requirements of other jobs for which the individual may be better qualified.

Changes in personnel are normal, but they are accelerated during organizational changes. Unless managers are to become obsolete, they must change with the times. Some quickly increase their managerial knowledge and skills. Unfortunately, others are inflexible, overly conservative, and negative. Executive obsolescence is increasingly common with the rapid changes in our society. The manager who previously performed competently may be overwhelmed with increasingly complex duties, or she may have been promoted during an emergency to a position for which she was inadequately prepared.

What can one do about an unqualified incumbent? In developing a strategy, one should consider the ramifications of the action on the individual and on the group. The strategy should be dependent on the particular circumstances. An incompetent subordinate may be counseled toward satisfactory performance. Weaknesses should be identified and means to overcome them defined. On-the-job training, in-service education, college courses, and independent study may be explored. A contract may be written between the employer and the incompetent subordinate, specifying what skills are to be developed to what level of achievement and in what time frame.

An incompetent executive may be transferred to another position for which she is more qualified. She may be moved from line to staff authority. The change is most attractive when the advisory staff position is at a higher organizational level than the present line responsibilities, carries prestige, and maintains the current salary. The executive may be told there is a problem in the new area that she is to solve. This method fosters high morale and loyalty. It removes incompetence from line authority when damage could be done but uses the executive's knowledge and skills to solve specific problems. This is an expensive method.

Termination is the most extreme way to handle incompetence. It is either direct or indirect. In the direct method the person is informed that her work does not meet the minimal criteria and she is expected to leave the agency. The indirect method may involve giving the person nothing to do, withholding information from her, leaving her name off memoranda, excluding her from conferences, and generally making her so miserable she will voluntarily resign.

New managers may be hired, particularly when new positions become available during reorganization. They often bring new ideas, objectivity, and enthusiasm to the job. Recruitment is important for development of an executive pool. The best managers do not need to hunt for jobs. The jobs hunt for them. The agency needs to let its need be known and to seek good managers aggressively. Similar agencies may be a resource for managers with new ideas and different approaches. Graduates may be recruited from university programs. Recruiting advertisements in professional journals and through employment agencies are useful for locating potential managers and well-qualified staff.

Promotions within the agency provide incentives and supply the executive pool. However, some personnel may not be interested in managerial work, and competent, satisfied employees may lack managerial potential.

After the revised organization is decided, operational procedures to expedite changes need to be developed. They define activities that are necessary for specific work and identify changes needed. The revised operational procedures should be inclusive, show all details, and ensure coordinated change. Work flow should be maintained and standards upheld. Special activities are likely to be needed during a transitional period. The revised operational procedures should be perceived as carefully thought-out planned change and not just a stopgap action.

Strategies for change

Visions of what the organization can become, instead of what it is or has been, allow for organizational change. To this end, managers need to create an open atmosphere where questions can be asked. Welcoming criticism instead of forbidding it helps personnel be adequately self-critical. Denying problems has serious consequences. A good recruitment plan is needed for hiring competent, highly motivated personnel. Career development programs should be provided. Each person needs to feel that what she achieves is important to the agency and that needed change for the continuing vitality of the organization overrides her vested interests.

Job analysis

Job analysis affects employee recruitment, hiring, orientation and training programs, performance appraisal, placement, transfers, and promotions; it consequently influences nursing care. It can determine equitable rates of pay and grade nursing positions within the total agency personnel system. By reviewing national, state, regional, and local wage surveys and using wage scales and performance appraisal, nursing personnel can be compensated satisfactorily for performance. It is the nurse administrator's responsibility to inform the analyst of the scope of authority in nursing positions so that they might be upgraded. This is especially pressing in the nursing profession, because nursing positions have long been rated lower than those of other professionals with comparable education, experience, and responsibility.

Job analysis is the study of a position to determine what knowledge, skill, aptitude, and personal characteristics are needed to perform certain responsibilities successfully. Analysis does not include any attempt to change the task. Rather, one starts by locating or developing a job description and position requirements. Questionnaires, interviews, observation, and logs furnish information about the job title and summary, duties performed, type of supervision given and received, equipment used, working conditions, and relationship to other positions. Job analysis determines minimum requirements (type and level of knowledge, skill, aptitude, and personal characteristics) and consequently sets standards for such factors as education, experience, intelligence, personality, and physical strength.

Job evaluation

Job evaluation is a process of measuring the remunerative worth of a job in relation to other positions, both internal and external to the organization. Based on the assumption that workers will be more satisfied if they perceive pay rates as consistent, the objective of evaluation is to compare jobs and establish a consistent pay base, providing employees in responsible positions with more pay than those with less demanding jobs. A point system, ranking of jobs, job grading, and job-to-job comparison are used. Consideration is given to education, mental and manual skills, responsibility for resources (personnel, materials, and finances), mental and physical effort, and working conditions, such as exposure to dangerous or disagreeable elements.

With the point system the nurse manager assigns numerical values to specific qualifications. For instance:

Qualifications	Points
Education	
Less than a high school diploma	10
High school diploma	20
High school diploma plus a special training course	30
Associate degree or three years in work study program and passage of accrediting examinations	40
Baccalaureate degree and passage of accrediting examinations	50
Master's degree in area of specialty needed for the position	60
Doctorate in area of specialty appropriate for the position	70
Mental skills	
Work is simple and repetitive and is performed according to instructions	10
Work involves a variety of duties that are performed according to procedures but require alertness to identify needed changes	20
Work involves a variety of complicated duties and some independent actions in adapting procedures to specific situations	30
Work involves planning, organization, implementing, and evaluating actions related to patient care	40
Work involves development of policies and procedures, organization of functions, development of staffing patterns, and budget preparations	50
Manual skills	
Work involves the normal manual skills, such as lifting, pushing, folding, writing, filing	10
Work involves about-normal manual skills, such as accurate measurements, administration of medications and treatments, manipulation of instruments, typing, bookkeeping	40
Work involves considerable manual skill, such as administering complex treatments and manipulation of complex equipment	50
Responsibility for resources	
Personnel	
Supervises no one	10
Supervises fewer than 10 people	20
Directs up to 25 people	30
Directs up to 50 people	40

Qualifications	Points
Directs up to 100 people	50
Directs more than 100 people	60
Finances	
No responsibility for budget	10
Responsible for budget up to $10,000	20
Responsible for budget up to $25,000	30
Responsible for budget up to $100,000	40
Responsible for budget over $100,000	50
Effort	
Mental	
Requires little thinking or judgment	10
Requires some alertness while performing repetitious tasks according to directions	20
Requires mental effort for problem solving	30
Requires considerable mental effort for decision making and problem solving	40
Requires continuous mental effort for dealing with the most difficult situations	50
Physical	
Light work requiring little physical effort, usually seated	10
Light physical effort, use of light materials, frequently seated	20
Sustained physical effort, seldom seated, continuous activity	30
Considerable physical effort, continuous activity, lifting	40
Working conditions	
Good working conditions—light, ventilation, freedom from disagreeable elements such as dirt, heat, wetness, odors, noise	10
Average working conditions with occasional exposure to disagreeable elements and danger	20
Fair working conditions with frequent exposure to disagreeable elements and danger	30
Poor working conditions with continuous exposure to disagreeable elements and danger	40

Once point values have been assigned to various job factors, they can be added to determine a grade. The grades for various jobs can be ranked, and job-to-job comparisons can provide a basis for determining pay.

Job evaluation is a systematic rather than a scientific process, and its high reliability does not ensure validity. The management values used to choose and weigh factors may not be consistent with the values of other personnel, or the selected values may be different among work groups. Although relative pay rates can be determined by job evaluation, the absolute levels are often negotiated by the individual or unions.

The number of grievances related to pay rates commonly increases after the introduction of job evaluation because personnel now have an objective basis for a grievance. Before job evaluation, an employee had little concrete justification on which to file a grievance. She complained that she was not getting paid enough; management insisted that she was. With job evaluation, the employee has criteria on which to base her grievance.

The transition period is especially troublesome. Problems related to adjusting the worker's present pay to the new pay structure may interfere with traditional lines of promotion. Adjusting a worker's pay upward to the new rate is acceptable to employees, but some may then file grievances for back pay. Back pay, however, could undermine the agency's budget. Therefore, management may decide that back pay is retroactive only to a specified date. The case of an employee who has previously been overcompensated creates a more difficult situation. To avoid dissatisfaction, personnel can be assured that no one's pay will be reduced as a result of the new pay schedule. However, it is possible to deny any pay increase to the individual who was overcompensated until others' salaries have been raised and all have been realigned to the new pay schedule. That, of course, can be demoralizing to the overpaid individual, but her previous situation is quite demoralizing to other employees. More acceptable options may be to promote the individual to a job commensurate with her pay or give her additional responsibilities in her present position to make her current job commensurate with her salary. After the individual vacates the position, the salary for the job can be realigned at a lower salary level according to the pay schedule.

Job design

Job design specifies the job content (what the job requires), job methods (how to do it), and the relationship between the organizational, social, and personal needs of the worker. It involves observation, recording, and analysis of current jobs to make work more efficient and to provide incentives for the workers, thereby reducing costs and improving job satisfaction.

Time-and-motion studies were the first techniques used to study job designs. Time studies are observations that determine the amount of time it takes to do a job under certain circumstances. After the activity is timed with a stopwatch and the times recorded, the normal time and the standard time are determined. In this way the most expedient way to do a job and a fair day's work are calculated.

Motion studies help to determine the one best way to do a job. Process charts are useful in recording movements so the analyst can identify wasteful activity. Micromotion study utilizes a slowly projected movie to allow one to analyze and time each motion. Sociotechnical studies, which analyze the relationship between social needs and task performance, became popular after World War II. Suggestive and detailed questions asking who, what, when, where, why, and how became a method for analysis.

Methods improvement is an organized approach to determine better ways to accomplish a goal in less time, with less effort, and at a lower cost, while maintaining or improving the results. It is also called job improvement, work simplification, and methods engineering.

First one selects the job to improve and then collects related information such as policies, procedures, statistical reports, accounting data, work schedules, pertinent records, and architectural drawings. Next the manager analyzes how the task is currently being done.

A flow process chart helps analyze how a task is being performed (Fig. 2-6). Flow process chart symbols include ◯ for operation, → for transportation, □ for inspection, D for delay, and △ for storage. An operation is the actual performance of the work, such as giving an injection. Transportation represents physical movement—the relocation of a person or thing from one place to another, such as movement of the syringe from the medication room to the patient's bedside. Inspection is to determine if the necessary work has been properly performed. The nurse makes sure that she is giving the right medication and using the right mode at the right time, to the right patient. A delay is an unplanned interruption in the flow of the process. Storage is an anticipated interruption in the process or at the end of it.

When doing a flow process chart, one must decide whether to follow the flow of material or the activities of the worker, because they may not be the same. A flow diagram is an architectural drawing to scale. Lines are used to show material flow or paths of personnel movement (Fig. 2-7).

As a result of methods improvement, one should eliminate activities or combine steps when possible and change the sequence of activities as necessary to improve the performance of various steps. The proposed method is then analyzed using flow charting. The potential impact on people is considered. Trial runs are conducted, and debugging is done.

To reduce the boredom of workers, management turns to job enlargement— a horizontal approach to job design that makes a job structurally larger and challenges the employee. If a nurse has been taking care of an average of five patients, she is asked to attend seven. Similarly, the nursing educator might be challenged to teach an additional two hours a week or to add three more students to her clinical group. Not surprisingly, this method frequently fails. Nurses commonly respond, "Why should I?" Many employees are already doing large amounts of work or do not like their work in the first place.

Another technique, job simplification, removes the more difficult parts of the job so that the worker can do more of what remains. For example, a nurse can be hired to start all IVs. The treatment nurse, team leader, and primary nurse, then, do not have to start any IVs but can give other medications and treatments to more patients. Work simplification, however, tends to lead to further boredom.

Personnel may also be assigned more tasks. For instance, staff nurses can teach aides to do additional treatments. This may relieve some monotony, but many workers are already very busy, and the new tasks may prove to be no more meaningful than the others.

Job rotation is another horizontal job-enlargement technique. Nurses may rotate shifts and assignments among different units and different patients on the units, but this practice complicates continuity of care and often leads to additional frustration. Community health nurses may be rotated through clinic assignments. For instance, a nurse may work well-baby clinics one month; family planning the next; and immunization, tuberculosis, or venereal disease clinics at other times. Again, this can disrupt continuity of care.

Job enrichment is a vertical approach to job design that uses a fuller range of abilities and skills of the personnel. Each community health nurse may have "her own" assortment of clinics in addition to her family case load. Continuity is preserved as the nurse is always at that clinic. She needs to develop her expertise, knowledge, and skill in all of the clinical areas. A hospital unit may switch from functional or team nursing to primary nursing so each nurse can give total patient care and consequently assume additional responsibility and accountability.

Job enrichment is intended to increase motivation and productivity while reducing absenteeism and turnover. It can, however, increase anxiety, conflict, and feelings of exploitation. Skill levels of personnel limit the amount of job enrichment possible, since some workers lack managerial skills and may not be able or willing to plan and control their jobs. Supervisors may not be willing to trust workers, and personnel may feel they are being exploited.

Job descriptions

Job descriptions are derived from job analysis and are affected by job evaluation and design. They generally contain specifications that are the requirements for the job, major duties and responsibilities, and the organizational relationships of a given position. The title of the job indicates the major responsibilities and sets that job apart from others. The job description is a summary of primary duties in a complete but not detailed fashion. Job relationships and professional affiliations may be cited. Education, experience, and worker traits such as aptitude, interests, and temperament may be included. The physical demands and working conditions of the job may be mentioned. Job descriptions should be up to date, accurate, and realistic in terms of the resources available. Standard forms for all jobs within a category facilitate comparison.

Job descriptions should arrange duties in a logical order, state them separately and concisely, and use verbs to describe the action. They should be specific rather than vague and should avoid generalizations by using quantitative words whenever possible. To indicate frequency, one can note "daily," "periodically," or "occasionally" when the percentage of total time spent on a specific activity cannot be determined.

Job descriptions are useful for recruitment, placement, and transfer decisions.

Fig. 2-6. Flow process chart.

Procedure: Injection   Distance traveled   Present ☐ Proposed ☐

Person ☐

Material ☐

	Present		Proposed		Savings	
	No	Hr	No	Hr	No	Hr
Operation	8					
Transportation	2					
Inspection	2					
Delay	0					
Storage	1					

Steps in procedure	◯ → ☐ D △	Distance (ft)	Time (hr)	Remarks
Read medication order	◯ → ☐ D △			
Collect vial and syringe	◯ → ☐ D △			
Open vial	◯ → ☐ D △			
Open disposable syringe	◯ → ☐ D △			
Draw up solution	◯ → ☐ D △			
Recheck medication order	◯ → ☐ D △			
Put vial in medication drawer	◯ → ☐ D △			
Take shot to patient	◯ → ☐ D △			
Check patient identification	◯ → ☐ D △			
Administer shot	◯ → ☐ D △			
Return to medicine room	◯ → ☐ D △			
Dispose of syringe	◯ → ☐ D △			
Chart medication	◯ → ☐ D △			
Store chart	◯ → ☐ D △			

Fig. 2-7. Flow diagram.

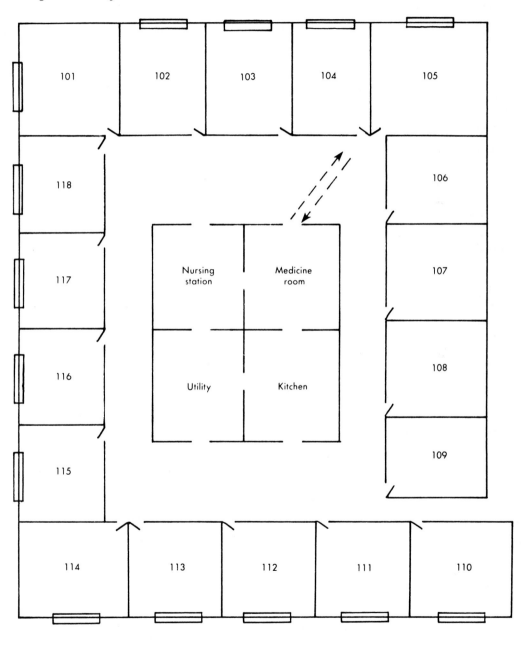

They can also be used to guide and evaluate personnel. Job descriptions help prevent conflict, frustration, and overlapping of duties.

SAMPLE JOB DESCRIPTIONS*

Nursing service director
DESCRIPTION OF WORK

General statement of duties: Performs administrative work in planning, coordinating, and directing the nursing service.

Supervision received: Works under general direction of the hospital administrator.

Supervision exercised: Supervises assigned personnel as a significant part of the duties.

EXAMPLES OF DUTIES

(Any one position may not include all of the duties listed, nor do the listed examples include all tasks that may be found in positions of this class.)

Directs and administers the nursing service, including inpatient and ambulatory care; develops and implements policies and patient care standards for all nursing service areas.

Participates in the planning and development of hospital policies and practices; works closely with administrative and medical personnel in coordinating nursing service functions with those of all other hospital departments and services.

Develops and implements staffing and ratio patterns to meet patient care and medical service needs; directs the broad planning of in-service training and orientation programs for nursing staff; directs research activities for continuing education and coordinates the clinical experience of nursing students.

Develops nursing service philosophies and goals in accordance with hospital policies; encourages and provides channels for staff participation in achieving these goals; interprets nursing service objectives to administrative and medical staff.

Serves on various hospital and community committees for the coordination of nursing services with other patient care and educational services; participates in professional organizational activities and represents the hospital in working with various service agencies and volunteer groups.

Directs the preparation of budget for nursing service staffing, equipment, and supplies; develops systems and standards for patient care records and reports.

Directs the recruitment, selection, transfer, and promotion of nursing personnel and the maintenance of personnel records.

Performs related work as required.

QUALIFICATIONS FOR APPOINTMENT

Knowledges, skills, and abilities. Extensive knowledge of professional nursing theory and practice. Extensive knowledge of modern principles and practices of hospital operation and nursing administration. Ability to plan, organize, and direct large-scale and comprehensive nursing activities. Ability to supervise, train, and motivate employees. Ability to communicate effectively orally and in writing. Ability to establish and maintain effective working relationships with administrative and medical personnel, employees, the public, and other agencies.

Education. Graduation from a four-year college with attainment of a Master's degree in

---

*Adapted from Job Descriptions, Denver General Hospital, Denver, Colo.

nursing and major course work in nursing administration or education.

Experience: Five years' professional nursing experience including three years in an administrative capacity.

Necessary special requirement: Possession of a license or permit to practice as a registered nurse as issued by the State Board of Nursing, permit to be used only until such time as a decision on licensure is made.

• • •

Clinical specialist I
DESCRIPTION OF WORK

General statement of duties: Performs advanced professional nursing work in a recognized medical specialty field.

Supervision received: Works under the general supervision of an administrative superior.

Supervision exercised: Supervises personnel as assigned, or full supervision incidental to the other duties.

EXAMPLES OF DUTIES

(Any one position may not include all of the duties listed, nor do the listed examples include all tasks that may be found in positions of this class.)

Performs advanced professional nursing work in specialized medical fields such as mental health, respiratory care, and other recognized medical specialities in accordance with standard nursing procedures and medical direction.

Interviews patient to obtain general background information and problem identification; evaluates patient's behavior and assesses immediate and long-range needs; schedules and conducts individual and group psychotherapy sessions.

Participates as a member of a professional medical, psychiatric, social public health team in evaluating, developing, and implementing health care plans.

Makes rounds with physician to review condition of patients; develops nursing care plans; participates in the care of the critically ill.

Participates in the orientation and in-service training of professional nursing personnel in teaching new, advanced, or complicated methods and procedures; interprets nursing services to patients and hospital personnel.

Performs related work as required.

QUALIFICATIONS FOR APPOINTMENT

Knowledges, skills, and abilities: Thorough knowledge of professional nursing theory and practice. Thorough knowledge of modern nursing care principles and practices in a recognized medical specialty. Ability to motivate and train employees. Ability to communicate effectively orally and in writing. Ability to establish and maintain effective working relationships with patients, employees, the public, and other agencies.

Education: Attainment of a Master's degree in nursing.

Experience: Two years' experience in an appropriate nursing clinical specialty.

Necessary special requirement: Possession of a license or permit as a registered nurse by the State Board of Nursing, permit to be used only until such time as a decision on licensure is made.

• • •

Graduate nurse I

DESCRIPTION OF WORK

General statement of duties: Performs professional general duty nursing work.

Supervision received: Works under direct supervision of a higher level nurse.

Supervision exercised: Supervises personnel as assigned, or full supervision incidental to the other duties.

EXAMPLES OF DUTIES

(Any one position may not include all of the duties listed, nor do the listed examples include all tasks that may be found in positions of this class.)

Performs professional nursing care in accordance with standard nursing procedures and medical direction.

Evaluates patient care needs; initiates nursing care plans; coordinates patient services.

Takes temperature, pulse, respiration, and blood pressure; administers prescribed medication and reports symptoms, reactions, and condition of patients; assists physicians with examinations, treatments, and diagnostic tests; prepares and applies dressings, compresses, and bandages; instructs patients in health measures and self-care; instructs nonprofessional nursing personnel and hospital attendants.

Performs related work as required.

QUALIFICATIONS FOR APPOINTMENT

Knowledges, skills, and abilities: Working knowledge of professional nursing theory and practice. Ability to communicate effectively orally and in writing. Ability to establish and maintain effective working relationships with patients, employees, the public, and other agencies.

Education: Graduation from a school of nursing.

Experience: None.

Necessary special requirement: Possession of a license or permit to practice as a registered nurse as issued by the State Board of Nursing, permit to be used only until such time as a decision on licensure is made.

Using the case study in the appendix:

Decide what new units will be added to Lake View Hospital and develop a new organizational chart. Note span of management, flat or tall structure, decentralization or centralization, and line authority. Discuss the advantages and disadvantages of the new organization with your classmates.

Write job descriptions for the personnel on one of the new units.

Write a procedure for a new unit.

Draw a floor plan for a nursing unit and discuss the advantages and disadvantages of the arrangement.

BIBLIOGRAPHY

Books

Albers, H.H.: Principles of management: a modern approach, New York, 1974, John Wiley & Sons, Inc.

Alexander, E.L.: Nursing administration in the hospital care system, ed. 2, St. Louis, 1978, The C. V. Mosby Co.

Althaus, J.N., et al.: Nursing decentralization: the El Camino experience, Wakefield, Mass., 1981, Aspen Publishing Co.

Barrett, J.: The head nurse: her changing role, New York, 1962, Meredith Publishing Co.

Beckhard, R., and Harris, R.T.: Organizational transitions: managing complex change, Reading, Mass., 1977, Addison-Wesley Publishing Co.

Belcher, D.W.: Compensation administration, Englewood Cliffs, N.J., 1974, Prentice-Hall, Inc.

Bennis, W.G., Benne, K.D., and Chin, R.: The planning of change, ed. 2, New York, 1985, Holt, Rinehart & Winston, Inc.

Blum, M.L., and Naylor, J.C.: Industrial psychology: its theoretical and social foundations, New York, 1968, Harper & Row, Publishers, Inc.

Brooten, D.A.: Managerial leadership in nursing, Philadelphia, 1984, J.B. Lippincott Co.

Charns, M.P., and Schaefer, M.J.: Health care organizations: a model for management, Englewood Cliffs, N.J., 1983, Prentice-Hall, Inc.

Christian, W.P., and Hannah, G.T.: Effective management in human services, Englewood Cliffs N.J., 1983, Prentice-Hall, Inc.

Connor, P.E.: Dimensions in modern management, ed. 3, Boston, 1982, Houghton Mifflin Co.

Dale, E.: Management: theory and practice, ed. 4, New York, 1978, McGraw-Hill Book Co.

Davis, K., and Newstrom, J.: Human behavior at work: organizational behavior, ed. 7, New York, 1985, McGraw-Hill Book Co.

Davis, S.M., and Lawrence, P.R.: Matrix, Reading, Mass., 1977, Addison-Wesley Publishing Co.

DiVincenti, M.: Administering nursing service, ed. 2, Boston, 1977, Little, Brown & Co.

Donnelly, J.H., Gibson, J.L., and Ivancevich, J.M.: Fundamentals of management: functions, behavior, models, Austin, Tex., 1971, Business Publications, Inc.

Donovan, H.M.: Nursing service administration: managing the enterprise, St. Louis, 1975, The C. V. Mosby Co.

Eckles, R.W., Carmichael, R.L., and Sarchet, B.R.: Essentials of management for first-line supervision, New York, 1974, John Wiley & Sons, Inc.

Filley, A.C., and House, R.J.: Managerial process and organizational behavior, Glenview, Ill., 1969, Scott, Foresman & Co.

Flippo, E.B.: Management: a behavioral approach, Boston, 1970, Allyn and Bacon, Inc.

French, W.L.: The personnel management process, ed. 5, Boston, 1982, Houghton Mifflin Co.

Gibson, J.L., Ivancevich, J.M., and Donnelly, J.H.: Organizations: behavior, structure, processes, Plano, Tex., 1985, Business Publications, Inc.

Gillies, D.A.: Nursing management: a systems approach, Philadelphia, 1982, W.B. Saunders, Co.

Haimann, T., and Scott, W.G.: Management in the modern organization, Boston, 1974, Houghton Mifflin Co.

Hall, R.H.: Organizations: structure and process, ed. 3, Englewood Cliffs, N.J., 1982, Prentice-Hall, Inc.

Hampton, D.R., Summer, C.E., and Webber, R.A.: Organizational behavior and the practice of management, ed. 2, Glenview, Ill., 1981, Scott, Foresman & Co.

Hand, L.: Nursing supervision, Reston, Va., 1980, Appleton & Lange.

Hicks, H.G.: The management of organizations: a systems and human resources approach, New York, 1972, McGraw-Hill Book Co.

Holle, M.L., and Blatchley, M.E.: Introduction to leadership and management in nursing, ed. 2, Monterey, Calif., 1987, Wadsworth Health Sciences Division.

Jernigan, D.K., and Young, A.P.: Standards, job descriptions, and performance evaluations for nursing practice, Norwalk, Conn., 1983, Appleton & Lange.

Joos, I.M., Nelson, R., and Lyness, A.: Man, health, and nursing: basic concepts and theories, Reston, Va., 1985, Appleton & Lange.

Kaluzny, A.D., et al.: Management of health services, Englewood Cliffs, N.J., 1982, Prentice-Hall, Inc.

Kast, F.E., and Rosenzweig, J.E.: Organization and management: a systems and contingency approach, ed. 4, New York, 1985, McGraw-Hill Book Co.

Katz, D., and Kahn, R.L.: The social psychology of organizations, ed. 2, New York, 1978, John Wiley & Sons, Inc.

Kazmier, L.J.: Principles of management: a programmed-instructional approach, New York, 1974, McGraw-Hill Book Co.

Koontz, H., and O'Donnell, C.: Principles of management: an analysis of managerial functions, New York, 1972, McGraw-Hill Book Co.

Laliberty, R., and Christopher, W.I.: Enhancing productivity in health care facilities, Owings Mills, Md., 1984, National Health Publishing.

Lancaster, J., and Lancaster, W.: Concepts for advanced nursing practice: the nurse as a change agent, St. Louis, 1981, The C. V. Mosby Co.

Langford, T.L.: Managing and being managed, Englewood Cliffs, N.J., 1981, Appleton & Lange.

Lawrence, P.R., and Lorsch, J.W.: Developing organizations: diagnosis and action, Reading, Mass., 1969, Addison-Wesley Publishing Co.

Lippitt, R., Watson, J., and Westley, B.: The dynamics of planned change, New York, 1958, Harcourt, Brace & World, Inc.

Litterer, J.A.: The analysis of organizations, New York, 1973, John Wiley & Sons, Inc.

Longest B.B.: Management practices for the health professional, ed. 3, Reston Va., Appleton & Lange.

Magula, M.: Understanding organizations, Wakefield, Mass., 1982, Nursing Resources, Inc.

Margulies, N., and Wallace, J.: Organizational change: techniques and applications, Glenview, Ill., 1973, Scott, Foresman & Co.

Marriner, A.: Contemporary nursing management: issues and practice, St. Louis, 1982, The C. V. Mosby Co.

Mauksch, I.G., and Miller, M.H.: Implementing change in nursing, St. Louis, 1981, The C. V. Mosby Co.

McConnell, C.R.: The effective health care supervisor, Germantown, Md., 1982, Aspen Systems Corp.

McConnell, E.A.: Burnout in the nursing profession, St. Louis, 1982, The C. V. Mosby Co.

McFarland, D.: Management principles and practices, New York, 1974, Macmillan, Inc.

McQuillan, F.: Realities of nursing management: how to cope, Bowie, Md., 1978, Robert J. Brady Co.

Mintzberg, H.: The structuring of organizations, Englewood Cliffs, N.J., 1979, Prentice-Hall, Inc.

Newman, W.H., Summer, C.E., and Warren, E.K.: The process of management, ed. 5, Englewood Cliffs, N.J., 1981, Prentice-Hall, Inc.

Osborn, R.N., Hunt, J.G., and Jauch, L.R.: Organization theory: an integrated approach, New York, 1980, John Wiley & Sons, Inc.

Porter-O'Grady, T., and Finnigan, S.: Shared governance for nursing: a creative approach for professional accountability, Rockville, Md., 1984, Aspen Systems Corp.

Price, M., Franck, P., and Veith, S.: Nursing management: a programmed text, ed. 2, New York, 1980, Springer Publishing Co.

Robbins, S.P.: Organizational behavior: concepts, controversies, and applications, Englewood Cliffs, N.J., 1983, Prentice-Hall, Inc.

Robbins, S.P.: Organizational theory: the structure and design of organizations, ed. 3, Englewood Cliffs, N.J., 1986, Prentice-Hall, Inc.

Rowland, H.S., and Rowland, B.L.: Nursing administration handbook, ed. 2, Germantown, Md., 1985, Aspen Systems Corp.

Rubin, I.M., Fry, R.E., and Plomick, M.S.: Managing human resources in health care organizations: an applied approach, Reston, Va., 1978, Reston Publishing Co., Inc.

Scanlan, B.K.: Principles of management and organizational behavior, New York, 1973, John Wiley & Sons, Inc.

Schmied, E., editor: Organizing for care: nursing units and groups, Wakefield, Mass., 1982, Aspen Publishing Co.

Schweiger, J.L.: The nurse as manager, New York, 1980, John Wiley & Sons, Inc.

Sheridan, R.S., Bronstein, J.E., and Walker, D.D.: The new nurse manager: a guide to management development, Rockville, Md., 1984, Aspen Systems Corp.

Simms L.M., Price, S.A., and Ervin, N.E.: The professional practice of nursing administration, New York, 1985, John Wiley & Sons, Inc.

Sisk, H.L.: Management and organization, Cincinnati, 1973, South-Western Publishing Co.

Stone, S., et al., editors: Management for nurses: a multidisciplinary approach, ed. 3, St. Louis, 1986, The C. V. Mosby Co.

Sullivan, E.J., and Decker, P.J.: Effective management in nursing, Reading, Mass., 1985, Addison-Wesley Publishing Co.

Terry, G.R.: Principles of management, ed. 8, Homewood, Ill., 1982, Richard D. Irwin, Inc.

Veninga, R.L.: The human side of health administration, Englewood Cliffs, N.J., 1982, Prentice-Hall, Inc.

Voich, D., and Wren, D.A.: Principles of management . . . resources and systems, New York, 1968, Ronald Press Co.

Weick, K.E.: The social psychology of organizing, ed. 2, Reading, Mass., 1986, Random House.

Journals
Organizational process

Cohen, M.D., March, J.G., and Olsen, J.P.: A garbage can model of organizational choice, Adm. Sci. Q. 17:1-25, March 1972.

Miller, D.I.: Organization is a process, J. Nurs. Adm. 2:19-24, March-April 1972.

Muther, R., and De Moor, R.J.: Planning an organization structure, S.A.M. Adv. Management J. 38:28-33, January 1973.

Scott, W.G.: Organization theory: an overview and an appraisal, J. Acad. Management 4:642-666, April 1961.

Smith, D.: Organizational theory and the hospital, J. Nurs. Adm. 2:19-24, May-June 1972.

Tersine, R.J., and Jones, M.B.: Models for examining organizations, J. Systems Management 24:32-37, September 1973.

Organizational structure

Ansoff, H.I., and Brandenburg, R.G.: A language for organization design. I. Management Sci. 17:B705-B731, August 1971.

Ansoff, H.I., and Brandenburg, R.G.: A language for organization design. II. Management Sci. 17:B705-B731, August 1971.

Cherns, A.B.: Can behavioral science help design organizations? Organizational Dynamics 5:44-64, Spring 1977.

Forrester, J.W.: A new corporate design, Industrial Management Rev. 7:5-17, Fall 1965.

Georgopoulous, B.: The hospital system—nursing—some basic problems and issues, Nurs. Forum 5:8-35, Winter 1966.

Gerwin, D., and Christoffel, W.: Organizational structure and technology: a computer model

approach, Management Sci. 20:1531-1541, August 1974.

Hilgar, E.: Unit management systems, J. Nurs. Adm. 2:43-49, January-February 1972.

Jaques, E.: Organizational structure and role relationships, Nurs. Times 67:154-157, February 4, 1971.

Lawrence, P.R., and Lorsch, J.W.: Differentiation and integration in complex organizations, Adm. Sci. Q. 12:1-47, June 1967.

Rehn. D.A.: Design for staff growth, Am. J. Nurs. 70:1930-1933, September 1970.

Salvatore, T.: Lessons from a failed consolidation: how two home health agencies never became one, Nurs. Health Care 7:31-34, January 1986.

Schaefer, M.: How should we organize? J. Nurs. Adm. 6:12-14, February 1976.

Schollhammer, H.: Organization structures of multinational corporations, Acad. Management J. 14:345-365, September 1971.

Sheedy, S.G.: Vice-president of medicine/vice-president of nursing: collaboration or conflict? J. Nurs. Adm. 14:38-41, June 1984.

Shetty, Y.K.: Is there a best way to organize a business enterprise? S.A.M. Adv. Management J. 38:47-52, April 1973.

Smith, D.: Organizational theory and the hospital, J. Nurs. Adm. 2:19-24, May-June 1972.

Stevens, B.J.: Nursing management and the sense of structure, J. Nurs. Adm. 4:57-59, July-August 1974.

Informal organization

Graham, G.: Interpersonal attraction as a basis of informal organization, Acad. Management J. 14:483-495, December 1971.

Hamm, S.R.: The influence of formal and informal organization within a modern hospital, Supervisor Nurse 11:38-42, December 1980.

Odiorne, G.S.: Put cliques to work for you, Nation's Business 46:50-53, August 1958.

Schuldt, S.: Supervision and the informal organization, J. Nurs. Adm. 8:21-25, July 1978.

Bureaucratic structure

Athanassiades, J.C.: The distortion of upward communication in hierarchical organizations, Acad. Management J. 16:207-225, June 1973.

Bennis, W.: Organizational developments and the fate of bureaucracy, Industrial Management 7:41-55, Spring 1966.

Bennis, W.: The coming death of bureaucracy, Think **32**:30-35, November-December 1966.

Brinkerhoff, M.B.: Hierarchical status, contingencies, and the administrative staff conference, Adm. Sci. Q. **17**:395-407, September 1972.

Graves, H.H.: Can nursing shed bureaucracy? Am. J. Nurs. **71**:491-494, March 1971.

Landsberger, H.A.: The horizontal dimension in bureaucracy, Adm. Sci. Q. **6**:299-332, December 1961.

Maniha, J.K.: Universalism and particularism in bureaucratizing organizations, Adm. Sci. Q. **20**:177-190, June 1975.

Maritz, D.G.: Management principles and nursing: the inefficiency of efficiency, Supervisor Nurse **11**:40-41, March 1980.

Marriner, A.: Organizational process and bureaucratic structure, Supervisor Nurse **8**:54-58, July 1977.

Read, W.H.: The decline of the hierarchy in industrial organizations, Business Horizons **8**:71-75, Fall 1965.

Dual management

Aleksandrowicz, L.I., and Dickau, S.G.: A clinical ladder, Nurs. Health Care **4**:510-514, November 1983.

Andrews, M., et al.: A nursing management model, Supervisor Nurse **10**:28-30, December 1979.

Colavecchio, R., Tescher, B., and Scalzi, C.: A clinical ladder for nursing practice, J. Nurs. Adm. **4**:54-58, September-October 1974.

Deckert, B., Oldenburg, C.J., Pattison, K.A., and Swartz, S.L.: Clinical ladders, Nurs. Management **15**:54-62, March 1984.

del Bueno, D.J.: A clinical ladder? Maybe! J. Nurs. Adm. **12**:19-22, September 1982.

Evans, P.B.: Multiple hierarchies and organizational control, Adm. Sci. Q. **20**:250-259, June 1975.

Gassert, C., Holt, C., and Pope, K.: Building a ladder, Am. J. Nurs. **82**:1527-1530, October 1982.

Huey, F.L.: Looking at ladders, Am. J. Nurs. **82**:1520-1526, October 1982.

Knox, S.L.: A clinical advancement program, J. Nurs. Adm. **10**:29-33, July 1980.

O'Connor, A., and Fralic, M.F.: A management progression system for nurse administrators. III. J. Nurs. Adm. **13**:7-12, June 1983.

Ritti, R.R.: Dual management: does it work? Res. Management **14**:19-26, November 1971.

Weeks, L.C., and Vestal, K.W.: PACE: a unique career development program, J. Nurs. Adm. **13**:29-32, December 1983.

Wieczorek, R.R., Weissman, G.K., and Devereux, P.M.: Clinical career pathway: the Mount Sinai experience, Nurs. Health Care **6**:143-145, March 1985.

Williams, L.B., and Cancian, D.W.: A clinical nurse specialist in a line management position, J. Nurs. Adm. **15**:20-26, January 1985.

Woldrum, K.M., et al.: The professional development program: an alternative to clinical ladders, Nurs. Adm. Q. **7**:87-93, Spring 1983.

Zimmer, M.J.: Rationale for a ladder for clinical advancement, J. Nurs. Adm. **2**:18-19, November-December 1972.

Adhocracy

Bishop, J.K.: Adhocracy as an organizational structure in a psychiatric institution, J. Nurs. Adm. **13**:20-24, January 1983.

Fuszard, B.: "Adhocracy" in health care institutions? J. Nurs. Adm. **13**:14-19, January 1983.

Free form

Carlisle, H.M.: Developing the adaptive organization, Management Advisor **9**:40-43, May-June 1972.

Marriner, A.: Adaptive organizational models, Supervisor Nurse **8**:44-49, August 1977.

McKelvey, B., and Kilmann, R.H.: Organization design: a participative multivariate approach, Adm. Sci. Q. **20**:1-36, March 1975.

Pascucci, J.J.: The emergence of free form management, Personnel Adm. **31**:33-39, September-October 1968.

Collegial management

Parks, F.N.: Group management, European style, Business Horizons **9**:83-90, Fall 1966.

Project management

Avots, I.: Why does project management fail? California Management Rev. **12**:77-82, Fall 1969.

Butler, A.G.: Project management: a study in organizational conflict, Acad. Management J. **16**:84-101, March 1973.

Cleland, D.I.: Why project management? Business Horizons 7:81-88, Winter 1964.

Cleland, D.I.: Understanding project authority, Business Horizons 10:63-70, Spring 1967.

Hodgetts, R.M.: Leadership techniques in the project organization, Acad. Management J. 11:211-219, June 1968.

Killian, W.P.: Project management as an organizational concept, Office 73:14-17+, April 1971.

Meinhart, W.A., and Delionback, L.M.: Project management: an incentive contracting decision model, Acad. Management J. 11:427-434, December 1968.

Middleton, C.J.: How to set up a project organization, Harvard Business Rev. 45:73-82, March-April 1967.

Reeser, C.: Some potential human problems of the project form of organization, Acad. Management J. 12:459-467, December 1969.

Stewart, J.M.: Making project management work, Business Horizons 8:54-68, Fall 1965.

Task force

Wickesberg, A.K., and Cronin, T.C.: Management by task force, Harvard Business Rev. 40:111-118, November-December 1962.

Matrix

Anders, R.L.: Matrix organization: an alternative for clinical specialists, J. Nurs. Adm. 5:11-14, June 1975.

Galbraith, J.R.: Matrix organization designs: how to combine functional and project forms, Business Horizons 14:29-40, February 1971.

Gray, J.L.: Matrix organizational design as a vehicle for effective delivery of public health care and social services, Management Int. Rev. 14:73-83, 1974.

Johnson, G.V., and Tingey, S.: Matrix organization: blueprint of nursing care organization for the 80s, Hosp. Health Services Adm. 21:27-39, Winter 1976.

Knight, K.: Matrix organization: a review, J. Management Stud. 13:111-130, May 1976.

Lawrence, P.R., Kolodny, H.F., and Davis, S.M.: The human side of the matrix, Organizational Dynamics 6:43-61, Summer 1977.

Mee, J.F.: Matrix organization, Business Horizons 7:70-72, Summer 1964.

Moore, T.F., and Simendinger, E.: The matrix organization: its significance to nursing, Nurs. Adm. Q. 3:25-31, Winter 1979.

Porter-O'Grady, T.: The organization of nursing services, Supervisor Nurse 9:30-38, July 1978.

Ryan, J.E.: Better style for change: matrix management, Hospitals 54:105-108, November 16, 1980.

Sayles, L.R.: Matrix management: the structure with a future, Organizational Dynamics 5:2-17, Fall 1976.

Shull, F.A., and Judd, R.J.: Matrix organizations and control systems, Management Int. Rev. 11:65-73, 1971.

Tytler K.: Making matrix management work—and when and why it's worth the effort, Training H.R.D. 15:78-82, October 1978.

Charts

Murdick, R., Ross, J.E., and Westmoreland, J.E.: Linear organization chart clears away confusion, J. Systems Management 22:23-25, August 1971.

Patton, J.A.: Make and use an organization chart, Business Management 24:55-57, May 1963.

Prouty, M.P.: Making an organization chart, J. Nurs. Adm. 4:32-35, 1974.

Tsaklanganos, A.A.: The organization chart: a managerial myth, S.A.M. Adv. Management J. 38:53-57, April 1973.

Span of management

Koontz, H.: Making theory operational: the span of management, J. Management Stud. 3:229-243, October 1966.

Nelson, E.A.: Economic size of organizations, California Management Rev. 10:61-70, Spring 1968.

Suojanen, W.: The span of control—fact or fable? Adv. Management 20:5-13, November 1955.

Tosi, H., and Patt, H.: Administrative ratios and organizational size, Acad. Management J. 10:161-168, June 1967.

Urwick, L.F.: The manager's span of control, Harvard Business Rev. 34:39-47, May-June 1956.

Flat versus tall structures

Ghiselli, E.E., and Siegel, J.P.: Leadership and managerial success in tall and flat organization structures, Personnel Psychol. 25:617-624, 1972.

Jones, H.R.: A study of organization for experimental structures of two, three, and four levels, Acad. Management J. **12**:351-365, September 1969.

Decentralization versus centralization

Burlingame, J.F.: Information technology and decentralization, Harvard Business Rev. **39**: 121-126, November-December 1961.

Burns, R.K.: Technics for strengthening intra- and interdepartmental cooperation and coordination, Hosp. Top. **53**:30-39, March-April 1975.

Cox, C.L.: Decentralization: uniting authority and responsibility, Supervisor Nurse **11**:28-35, March 1980.

Dale, E.: Centralization versus decentralization, Adv. Management **20**:11-16, June 1955.

Ehrle, R.A.: Management decentralization: antidote to bureaucratic ills, Personnel J. **49**:396-397, May 1970.

Elpern, E.H., White, P.M., and Donahue, M.F.: Staff governance: the experience of one nursing unit, J. Nurs. Adm. **14**:9-15, 27, June 1984.

Gill, W.C.: Key concepts in management for nursing, Supervisor Nurse **3**:13-16, 1972.

Howe, E.: Decentralization aids coordination of patient care services, Hospitals **43**:53-55, March 1, 1969.

Johnson, L.M., Happel, J.R., Edelman, J., and Brown, S.J.; NAQ forum: a model of participatory management with decentralized authority, Nurs. Adm. Q. 30-46, Fall 1983.

Mahowald, J.F., Freeman, J.F., and Dietsche, B.: Decentralization of nursing authority, Supervisor Nurse **5**:40-46, March 1974.

Marciniszym, C.: Decentralization of nursing service, J. Nurs. Adm. **1**:17-24, July-August 1971.

McKellop, M.: Decentralized nursing service, Can. Nurse **66**:36-37, June 1970.

Moving decision down to where the action is, Business Week **2001**:138-144, December 6, 1969.

Munschauer, B.J.: Decentralizing management, Nurs. Management **14**:21-22, April 1983.

Peterson, M., and Allen, D.G.: Shared governance: a strategy for transforming organizations. I. J. Nurs. Adm. **16**:9-12, January 1986.

Peterson, M., and Allen, D.G.: Shared governance: a strategy for transforming organizations. II. J. Nurs. Adm. **16**:11-16, February 1986.

Probst, M.R., and Noga, J.J.M.: A decentralized nursing care delivery system, Supervisor Nurse **11**:57-60, January 1980.

Simons, B.J.A.: Decentralizing nursing service: six months later, Supervisor Nurse **11**:59-64, October 1980.

Spitzer R.: Decentralization: cardiac care as a case in point, Nurs. Management **17**:42A-42F, June 1986.

Starkweather, D.B.: The rationale for decentralization in large hospitals, Hosp. Adm. **15**:27-45, Spring 1970.

Wellington, M.: Decentralization: how it affects nurses, Nurs. Outlook **34**:36-39, January-February 1986.

Zald, M.N.: Decentralization: myth vs. reality, Personnel **41**:19-26, July-August 1964.

Delegation

Brown, D.S.: Why delegation works—and why it doesn't, Personnel **44**:44-52, January-February 1967.

Diekelmann, N.L., and Broadwell, M.M.: How to get the job done . . . by someone else, Nursing 77 **7**:110-116, September 1977.

Ewing, J.E.: Patterns of delegation, Harvard Business Rev. **39**:32-40, July-August 1961.

Murphy, E.C.: Practical management course: module 8: delegation—from denial to acceptance, Nurs. Management **15**:54-56, January 1984.

Newman, W.H.: Overcoming obstacles to effective delegation, Management Rev. **45**:36-41, January 1956.

Pellet, J.: Are you making delegation work for you? AORN J. **25**:865-868, April 1977.

Poteet, G.W.: Delegation strategies: a must for the nurse executive, J. Nurs. Adm. **14**:18-21, September 1984.

Russell, C.J.: Maintaining control: delegating responsibility presents real opportunities for a better kind of managerial control, Nurs. Management **14**:51-52, March 1983.

Vekteris, T.: Five easy steps from do-it-yourselfer to delegator, Nurs. Success Today **1**:16-17, December 1984.

Volante, E.M.: Mastering the managerial skill of delegation, J. Nurs. Adm. **4**:20-22, January-February 1974; also published in Nurs. Digest **5**:33-35, Fall 1977; and in The techniques of nursing management, Wakefield, Mass., 1975, Contemporary Publishing Co., Inc., pp. 21-23.

Watkin, B.: Management topics: delegation, Nurs. Mirror **138**:75, June 7, 1974.

Wickesberg, A.K.: Determining relative degrees in the delegation of executive authority, J. Acad. Management **1**:18-22, April 1958.

Wilkes, J.B.: Delegation and control, Nurs. Times **68**:1619, December 21, 1972.

Line-staff relationships

Browne, P.J.: The line-staff concept revisited: an empirical study of organizational images, Acad. Management J. **17**:406-417, September 1974.

Browne, P.J., and Cotton, C.C.: The topdog/ underdog syndrome in line-staff relations, Personnel J. **54**:443-444, August 1975.

Gemmil, G.R.: How managers use staff advice, Personnel **45**:48-52, September-October 1968.

Get line and staff to pull together, Industry Week **172**:30-33, February 7, 1972.

Marriner, A.: Line-staff relationships, Supervisor Nurse **8**:27-29, November 1977.

Toussaint, M.N.: Line-staff conflict: its causes and cure, Personnel **39**:8-20, March-April 1962.

Behavioral aspects of organizational change

Daniel, D.R.: Reorganizing for results, Harvard Business Rev. **44**:96-104, November-December 1966.

deLodzia, G.: Recognizing change and conflict in a nursing environment, Supervisor Nurse **4**:14-25, June 1973.

deLodzia, G., and Greenhalgh, L.: Creative conflict management in a nursing environment, Supervisor Nurse **4**:33-41, July 1973.

Glueck, W.F.: Organization change in business and government, Acad. Management J. **12**:439-448, December 1969.

Labovitz, G.H.: How to improve your management effectiveness in coping with change, Hosp. Top. **52**:24-41, July-August 1974.

Nehls, D., et al.: Planned change: a quest for nursing autonomy, J. Nurs. Adm. **4**:23-27, January-February 1974.

Poulin, M.A.: Nursing service: change or managerial obsolescence, J. Nurs. Adm. **4**:40-43, July-August 1974.

Schwier, M.E., and Gardella, F.A.: Identifying the need for change in nursing service, Nurs. Outlook **18**:56-62, April 1970.

Job analysis

Carey, J.F.: Participative job evaluation, Compensation Rev. **9**:29-38, Fourth Quarter 1977.

Creighton, H.: Comparable worth cases. I. Nurs. Management **15**:21-22, October 1984.

Creighton, H.: Comparable worth cases. II. Nurs. Management **15**:20-22, November 1984.

Davis, K.: Non-nursing functions: our readers respond, Am. J. Nurs. **82**:1857-1860, December 1982.

Disch, J.M., and Feldstein, P.J.: Financial management series: an economic analysis of comparable worth, J. Nurs. Adm. **16**:24-31, June 1986.

Hackman, J.R., and Oldham, G.R.: Development of the job diagnostic survey, J. Appl. Psychol. **60**:159-170, 1975.

Henninger, D., and Dailey, C.: Measuring nursing workload in an outpatient department, J. Nurs. Adm. **13**:20-23, September 1983.

Hoffman, F.M.: Financial management series: setting nursing hours standards. II. J. Nurs. Adm. **16**:17-19, February 1986.

Hoffman, F., Schaefer, T., and Zuraikal, N.: Financial management series: setting nursing hours standards. I. J. Nurs. Adm. **16**:13-16, January 1986.

Ignatavicius, D., and Griffith, J.: Job analysis: the basis of effective appraisal, J. Nurs. Adm. **12**:37-41, July-August 1982.

Jaques, E.: Taking time seriously in evaluating jobs, Harvard Business Rev. **57**:124-132, September-October 1979.

Kawczak, B.H., et al.: Work sampling: analyzing nursing staff productivity, J. Nurs. Adm. **15**:9-14, September 1985.

McWilliams, C.A.: Systems analysis can solve nursing management problems, J. for Nurs. Leadership and Management **7**:17-26, May 1980.

Robichaud, A.M., and Hamric, A.B.: Time documentation of clinical nurse specialist activities, J. Nurs. Adm. **16**:31-36, January 1986.

Samaras, J.S., et al.: Wage evaluation methods: a model for nurse administrators, J. Nurs. Adm. **8**:13-21, June 1978.

Sheedy, S., and Whitinger, R.: Labor-based budgeting, Nurs. Management **14**:62-64, May 1983.

Snyder, E.C.: Equitable wage and salary structuring, Personnel J. **56**:240-244, May 1977.

Watkin, B.: Management topics: job evaluation, Nurs. Mirror **138**:60, May 24, 1974.

Woods, K.: Job evaluation: more than just a management technique, Personnel Management **8**:27-39, November 1976.

Job design

Durand, C.: Employer politics in job enrichment, Int. Stud. Management Organization **5**:66-86, Fall 1975.

Frank, L.L., and Hackman, J.R.: A failure of job enrichment: the case of the change that wasn't, J. Appl. Behavioral Sci. **11**:413-436, October-November-December 1975.

Hulin, C., and Blood, M.: Job enlargement: individual differences and worker responses, Psychol. Bull. **69**:41-55, 1968.

Kaplan, H.R., Tausky, C., and Bolaria, B.S.: Job enrichment, Personnel J. **48**:791-798, October 1969.

Lawler, E.E., Hackman, J.R., and Kaufman, S.: Effects of job redesign: a field experiment, J. Appl. Social Psychol. **3**:49-62, January-March 1973.

Morse, J.J.: A contingency look at job design, California Management Rev. **16**:67-73, Fall 1973.

Salancik, G.R., and Pfeffer, J.: A social information processing approach to job attitudes and task design, Adm. Sci. Q. **23**:224-253, June 1978.

Seeborg, I.S.: The influence of employee participation in job redesign, J. Appl. Behavioral Sci. **14**:87-98, January-February-March 1978.

York, L.: Key elements in implementing job enrichment, Personnel **50**:45-52, September-October 1973.

Job descriptions

Beaman, A.L.: What do first-line nursing managers do? J. Nurs. Adm. **16**:6-9, May 1986.

Brockenshire, A., and Hattstaedt, M.J.: Revising job descriptions: a consensus approach, Supervisor Nurse **11**:16-20, March 1980.

Does your job description include "research"? Nurs. Times **68**:816-817, June 29, 1972.

Fralic, M.F., and O'Connor, A.: A management progression system for nurse administrators. I. J. Nurs. Adm. **13**:9-13, April 1983.

Fralic, M.F., and O'Connor, A.: A management progression system for nurse administrators. II. J. Nurs. Adm. **13**:32-38, May 1983.

Kaskubar, J.P.: Levels of nursing assistants, Supervisor Nurse **9**:26-34, May 1978.

Parker, J.E., and Raniere, T.M.: Job description: key to your future, Occupational Health Nurs. 9-11, August 1981.

Parker, J.K.: Job description for nursing supervisor, Supervisor Nurse **9**:37, May 1978.

Reynolds, M.L.: A classification system for RNs, Supervisor Nurse **11**:26-28, October 1980.

Steel, J.L.: What manual? getting policies and procedures on the line, Nurs. Management **13**:43-46, March 1982.

Stevens, B.J.: A second look at "new position descriptions," J. Nurs. Adm. **3**:21-23, November-December 1973.

Watkin, B.: Job descriptions, Nurs. Mirror **138**:81, April 26, 1974.

PART 3

STAFF

———————— OBJECTIVES ————————

After completing this part, the reader will be able to:

Identify at least three activities related to selection
of personnel.

Discuss affirmative action.

Compare and contrast assignment systems for staffing.

Describe different staff schedules.

Analyze variables affecting staffing.

———————— STUDY QUESTIONS ————————

1
What information should a résumé contain?

2
How does one conduct a pre-employment interview?

3
What does an affirmative action program involve?

4
What are the pros and cons of assignment systems for staffing?

5
What are the pros and cons of different staffing schedules?

6
What variables affect staffing?

NATURE AND PURPOSE OF STAFFING

Staffing is the third managerial function. Having planned and organized, the manager must now staff to accomplish the goals of the organization. Staffing involves the selection of personnel and assignment systems and the determination of staffing schedules. There are many variables to be considered when planning for staffing. The more accurate the assessment, the higher the probability of containing costs while providing high-quality care.

SELECTION OF PERSONNEL
Recruitment and retention

The acquisition of qualified people in any agency is critical for the establishment, maintenance, and growth of the organization. Therefore, active recruitment is important, and the attraction of qualified applicants is the first step in selection of personnel. Modes for active recruitment include employee recommendations and word of mouth; advertisements in local newspapers, nursing organization bulletins, and nursing journals; recruitment literature such as flyers and newsletters; career days; contacts with schools' graduating classes; placement services; open houses; and frequent, low-cost, credit-carrying, continuing education courses for outsiders as well as employees.

Word of mouth can be very effective, but it can also lead to the hiring of friends and relatives of the current work force; this practice may foster nepotism and violate equal opportunity employment requirements. The use of advertisements, employment agencies, and contacts with schools' graduating classes offers the prospective employer a broader field for selection and more opportunities to hire from minority groups. Hiring minority group members may require active recruitment to meet public policy.

Each institution needs someone responsible for recruitment. The recruiter should know nursing qualifications and the needs of the institution. She should be able to represent the institution with candor and enthusiasm. It is important that the recruiter relate well to people. Referrals from employees should be sought, and in-house applicants encouraged; however, favoritism should not be shown. To aid in the selection of the best candidate for the job, an adequate budget should be provided for necessary advertisement, and these advertisements should depict an institution that cares about employees and patients. That image should also be reflected at open houses, during conventions, and at high school and college career days.

The content is more important than the form of advertising. The recruiter should determine the needs and desires of potential applicants and demonstrate how the institution will meet those needs. New graduates are likely to be interested in thorough orientation, in-service education, staff development, and intern programs. Some nurses will be interested in tuition reimbursement and release time to work on educational degrees. Single people will be more interested in health benefits than married women whose husbands have family coverage. Older nurses will be increasingly interested in retirement plans. Refresher courses, chartered buses for people who live in suburban areas, childcare programs, part-time work, and flexible personnel policies may appeal to inactive nurses. The nurse recruiter needs to assess the interests of the nurse and show how the institution can address her concerns.

The recruiter should respond to inquiries immediately. Records of inquiries noting the origin (how the job applicant learned of the opening) and disposition (hired or not and length of tenure) should be compiled and evaluated. The most productive recruitment method should be maximized. Out-of-town or state applicants should be assisted with information about the community and housing.

The major sources of manpower are persons seeking their first jobs, dissatisfied employees, and the unemployed. These classifications are important, for the categories indicate types of information the supervisor should obtain, and they influence the selection process. The recent graduate or the nurse who has not practiced since graduation may have a limited idea about job potentials. Her choice of a first job may be strongly influenced by her education, achievement level, geographical preference, salary, mate's occupation, and peer pressure. She is likely to take several jobs before settling down. This variety of jobs, along with growing family responsibilities and maturity, helps develop the nurse's capabilities.

The dissatisfied employee is often not actively seeking other employment but is likely to be receptive to news of openings and job offers. If the supervisor attributes the dissatisfaction to the misuse of the person's talents and abilities, she may explore how to better utilize that person within her own agency. Job dissatisfaction is not uncommon, for every job has disadvantages. Agencies that require special job skills should expect applications from nurses who are looking for a better job with fewer disadvantages.

Hiring an unemployed worker who has been released from a previous job because of an infraction or a quarrel with the previous employer demands careful assessment. The supervisor may wish to hire the nurse who was fired because she refused to falsify records or perform a task for which she was not adequately prepared. She would not want to hire a nurse who was terminated because of high absenteeism and irresponsibility, unless the nurse could adequately explain the situation and assure the supervisor that the problem had been resolved. For instance, the prospective employee might explain that her child was dying at that time, or that she was having a marital crisis and has since been divorced. It is unlikely that a nurse applicant has been laid off from a previous job because of slack times. If so, the supervisor should consider the chances of the nurse's returning to her old job when the slack has ended. Seniority and other vested interests may influence the nurse's desire to return to her previous position.

Because of the costs of recruiting, selecting, and training employees, the decreased quality of care while orienting new workers, and the emotional drain of turnover on continuing employees, serious attention should be given to retention efforts. Exit interviews, particularly anonymous questionnaires, can help identify the reasons people resign. Posttermination questions mailed to the homes of former employees a month or two after their resignation may obtain more accurate information than does the exit interview. After a period of time has elapsed, a person may be less emotional and more objective with some distance from the job and may feel more anonymous with less fear of retaliation. In addition, attitude surveys can be used with current employees to identify sources of dissatisfaction and concern. Once stressors are identified, strategies to reduce them can be planned. It is important to meet personnel's psychosocial needs for advancement, responsibility, achievement, and recognition. Nurses want input into decision making and control over their own lives.

Screening of staff

Investment in well-qualified nurses can produce a high rate of return, and errors, whether they be failure to hire a promising nurse or hiring someone who fails to achieve the organization's expectations, can be expensive mistakes. In general there are three underlying philosophies in the screening process: (1) The supervisor should screen out applicants who do not fit the agency's image. Although this practice is common among some corporations, it is not a standard procedure for selecting health personnel. (2) The supervisor should try to fit the job to a promising applicant. Examples include part-time positions, split-shift hours, and opportunities for handicapped people. (3) Usually the supervisor should try to fit the applicant to the job. This philosophy assumes that both the person and the position are unique.

Application forms and résumés. Once the applicant has been attracted, she should submit biographical data. The application form is a quick way to collect demographic information. Data in the personal history—educational background, work experience, and other pertinent information—can be used to:
1. Determine whether the applicant meets minimal hiring requirements such as minimal educational level or minimal job experience requirements
2. Furnish background data useful in planning the selection interview
3. Obtain names of references that may be contacted for additional information about the applicant's work experience and general character

4. Collect information for personnel administration, that is, Social Security number, number of dependents, and so forth

Letters of reference. Letters of recommendation may be requested from references listed on the application form, from previous employers, or both. However, these letters may be inaccurate and misleading because the person writing may not have had sufficient exposure to the nurse to become familiar with her capabilities, or she may not have even known the nurse. Because of rapid turnover of nursing personnel, it is possible that few current staff members worked with the previous employee, and the current supervisor, who joined the agency after the applicant had resigned, may have to write the letter of reference based on an inadequate personnel file. The applicant may not know the current whereabouts of previous supervisors. To avoid these problems, the employee could ask that a letter of reference be sent to a placement bureau at the time of termination, but this measure does not necessarily solve the problem. She has no assurance that the letter writer can express herself well or is even willing to be accurate.

All of the above indicate that letters of reference should be used cautiously. More emphasis should be placed on comments made by previous employers and co-workers, because they tend to give more critical evaluations than do subordinates and personal acquaintances. Most emphasis should be placed on characteristics consistently cited and on the general tone of the letters.

Interview. A pre-employment interview to predict job success should be conducted with the most qualified applicants. Information obtained from the application form and letters of reference should be taken into consideration during the interview. The purposes of the interview are to obtain information, to give information, and to determine if the applicant meets the requirements for the position. The interviewer judges the applicant's dependability, willingness to assume responsibility for the job, willingness and ability to work with others, interest in the job, adaptability, consistency of goals with available opportunities, and conformance of manners and appearance to job requirements. The interviewer answers questions, explains policies and procedures, and helps acquaint the applicant with the position. Finally, the interviewer must predict whether the applicant's overall performance will be satisfactory. The value of the interview is determined by the interviewer's ability to evaluate the applicant and to predict accurately her future success.

The interview has definite purposes and should avoid social chitchat, although a brief warm-up period may help put the interviewee at ease. One of the main purposes is to learn about the prospective employee. Therefore it behooves the interviewer to concentrate on listening, as well as to provide necessary information and answer questions from the applicant. The supervisor should avoid giving clues about what pleases or displeases her, should not be argumentative, and should try to avoid premature judgment. She should also beware of the halo effect—judgment based on appearances. Although an individual wears clothing that reflects her personality, she is likely to select clothes for the interview that project the image she wishes to convey.

It is advisable to train supervisors in the art of interviewing. Training might include methods of establishing rapport with an interviewee, interviewing techniques, therapeutic communication, and predicting applicant job performance. It is helpful to construct an interview recording form designed for the needs of the agency or for a specific position. Use of the job description to define and specify job dimensions on the form increases interviewer reliability. A personal profile of what the person hired should be, including education, experience, abilities, aptitudes, and interests, is helpful. Standardization of the interview promotes nondiscriminatory hiring practices and is particularly important when more than one person does the interviewing.

The heading of the form contains the date, name of the applicant, position desired, and the interviewer's name. The body categorizes traits required for the position. This allows the interviewer to assess the applicant more systematically. One area might be work history. Does the applicant's work history indicate that she has the ability to learn and understand the requirements of the job for which she is applying? More specifically, is there any evidence of lack of ability? Has she had past experience in performing the same or similar tasks? Is she familiar with the equipment and procedures? Has she had special project or task force assignments? Has she had job progression? Education is another area to be evaluated. Has the applicant had adequate formal education? Is there evidence of on-the-job training? Has she participated in continuing education or in self-initiated skill development by reading books and journals and watching related television specials? Is the nurse active in professional organizations?

Certainly the applicant's dependability demands assessment. Is it likely that she will have a good attendance record and maintain good work habits? Or is there evidence of poor work habits or work performance? What do her past attendance and safety records indicate? Of equal concern is the nurse's sense of responsibility. Will she seek assistance when needed and take initiative when appropriate to get the job done? Will she see jobs through to the end? Is there evidence of past independent thought and action, or does she tend to blame others for problems? Finally, is the nurse capable of assuming leadership when required?

Is the applicant cooperative and able to get along with others and work well as a team member, or does she have a preference for working alone? Is there evidence of success or friction with supervisors, peers, and subordinates? Is she open to criticism, or does she react excessively? Is the nurse involved in the community? Has she been open and candid during the interview? Job interest, poise, manners, appearance, and aspirations are other areas to investigate.*

During the interview, the interviewer explains the purpose and plan of the interview. This helps create a positive climate. The interviewer learns the most by listening rather than talking, and can encourage the job candidate to talk freely by asking open-ended questions. These are nondirective questions that help reveal feelings and attitudes. Examples of nondirective questions are: What qualifies you for this job? What aspects of your last job appealed to you? How were your relations with your peers?

Closed-ended questions are directive and can often be answered yes or no. They solicit less information than open-ended questions but are appropriate for objective and factual information. Examples of closed-ended questions are: Who was your last employer? How long did you work for that agency? Did you get along with your co-workers? Do you think you are qualified for this job?

The funnel technique incorporates both open-ended and closed-ended questions. When using the funnel technique, the interviewer starts with an open-ended question such as, "What subjects did you like most in school?" This gets objective information and sets a nonthreatening tone. The scope of the discussion is then funneled by asking a self-appraisal question such as, "Why do you think you liked those courses in particular?" This elicits subjective information. The interviewer closes the discussion of a particular subject by asking direct questions to clarify the self-appraisal. A direct question might be, "What classes did you take for your nursing electives?"

A grid of topics to explore and the funnel technique can help the interviewer sequence questions in a logical order and decide what kind of questions to ask.

Topic to explore	Open-ended question	Self-appraisal question	Direct question

Initially it may be helpful to fill in the topics and potential questions. The questions may be modified during the interview.

---

*These questions are adapted and modified from Osburn, H.G., and Manese, W. R.: How to install and validate employee selection techniques, Washington, D.C., 1971, American Petroleum Institute, pp. 69-70.

Topic to Explore	Open-ended question	Self-appraisal question	Direct question
Education	Why did you choose to go to that school?	What courses were most useful to you and how were they useful?	What courses did you take as electives?
Prior employment	Where have you worked?	What did you like best about your last job? What did you like least about your last job?	How long did you work there? What was your title? On what service areas did you work?
Life experiences	What life experiences have you had that help qualify you for this job?	How will raising your own children help you in this job?	How long have you spoken Spanish? How frequently do you use sign language?
Professional	What are your professional goals?	How do you plan to accomplish your goals?	What do you plan to be doing five years from now?

After obtaining information from the candidate, it is appropriate for the interviewer to share information about the job, policies, the agency, and how the interviewee will be informed of the decision. The applicant is given an opportunity to ask questions. The interviewer closes the interview by telling the applicant when and how she can expect to hear the decision. For example, the interviewer can say, "I will be interviewing a few more applicants this week. You can expect to hear from me by the first of next week." Or, "You should receive a letter regarding our decision within two weeks."

The facts collected during the interview are used as the basis for assumptions or inferences. They should be checked throughout the interview as new information is collected. It is possible to make both positive and negative assumptions from the same information. For example, if an applicant did not work for 3 months between jobs, the negative assumption could be that the person was escaping, undirected, or lazy. A positive inference could be that the applicant was clarifying goals and fulfilling personal objectives. Inferences are often more reflective of the person making them than of the applicant, thus making it particularly important to test interpretations.

Testing. Personality and interest testing is sometimes done but does require a trained psychologist. Ability tests are rarely used when hiring nurses. However, in-basket exercises, problem analysis, mock selection interviews, oral presentations, and debates have been used to select management personnel. Testing is useful for selecting clerical help. Tests can measure knowledge and skills possessed and estimate the rate at which the applicant can acquire the knowledge and skills required for the position. They measure clerical and mechanical aptitudes, general intelligence, and mental, perceptual, and psychomotor abilities.

EQUAL OPPORTUNITY AND AFFIRMATIVE ACTION

The employer is subject to a number of legal requirements that have been enacted to provide equal opportunity and affirmative action in the work place. Requirements for providing equal opportunity are contained in Title VI and Title VII of the Civil Rights Act of 1964, Title IX of the Education Amendments of 1972, the Equal Pay Act of 1963, and the Age Discrimination in Employment Act of 1967. Affirmative action requirements are contained in Executive Order 11246, Section 503 of the Rehabilitation Act of 1973, and in Section 402 of the Vietnam Era Veterans Readjustment Assistance Act of 1974.

Title VI and Title VII of the Civil Rights Act of 1964, as amended by the Equal Employment Act of 1972, prohibit discrimination because of race, color, religion, sex, or national origin in any term, condition, or privilege of employment.

Title IX of the Education Amendments of 1972 prohibits discrimination on the basis of sex in any educational program or activity receiving federal financial assistance. The equal Pay Act, as amended by the Education Amendments of 1972, requires the same pay for men and women doing substantially equal work, requiring substantially equal skill, effort, and responsibility under similar working conditions in the same establishment.

The Age Discrimination in Employment Act of 1967, as amended, prohibits age discrimination against individuals between 40 and 70 years of age.

Executive Order 11246 (as amended by EO 11375) prohibits all government contracting agencies from discriminating against any employee or applicant for employment and requires that contractors take affirmative action to ensure that applicants are employed and that employees are treated during employment without regard to their race, color, religion, sex, or national origin.

Sections 503 and 504 of the Rehabilitation Act of 1973 prohibit discrimination because of handicap in employment and in programs and activities receiving federal funds. Section 503, in addition, requires contractors to take affirmative action to employ and advance in employment qualified handicapped individuals.

Section 402 of the Vietnam Era Veterans Readjustment Assistance Act of 1974 requires contractors to take affirmative action to employ and advance in employment qualified disabled veterans and veterans of the Vietnam era.

Affirmative action in Executive Order 11246 requires the employer to make extra efforts to recruit, employ, and promote qualified members of formerly excluded groups. It is based on the premise that unless action is taken to overcome systematic exclusion and discrimination based on national origin, race, color, sex, or religion, employment practices will perpetuate the status quo indefinitely. In addition to the elimination of all existing discriminatory practices, affirmative action requires actions beyond neutral nondiscrimination.

A major portion of an affirmative action program must recognize and remove barriers and establish affirmative measures to remedy past discriminatory practices. Such measures include additional aid to prepare disadvantaged people for jobs. It is noteworthy that recent Supreme Court rulings state that such measures are not restricted to workers who have not individually been victims of discrimination.

Development of an affirmative action program includes the addition of affirmative action intent to the agency's philosophy, development of affirmative action policies and procedures, appointment of a manager responsible for the program, inclusion of affirmative action responsibilities in appropriate job descriptions, and publication of the affirmative action commitment internally to all employees and externally to sources for recruitment, to minority and women's organizations, to organizations of handicapped individuals, to appropriate veterans' service organizations, to community agencies, and to the community in general.

The affirmative action policy is disseminated internally by including it in the policy manual, annual reports, and other media, such as the agency newsletter. It can also be posted on bulletin boards. Nondiscrimination clauses are included in union agreements. Articles about the affirmative action program, its progress, and the activities of disadvantaged workers are published in agency publications. When employees are pictured in handbooks or advertising brochures, minority and nonminority men and women should be included.

Top administration should discuss the intent of the policy and individuals' responsibilities for its implementation with management personnel. Special meetings should be scheduled with all employees and the policy discussed in orientation and management training classes.

A work-force analysis of job classifications by departments is the first step toward identifying where minorities, women, and men are currently employed and discovering areas of concentration and underutilization. The availability of minorities, women, and handicapped persons having requisite skills is considered when determining whether there is underutilization: How many minorities, women, and handicapped persons are in the geographical area from which the institution recruits? What percentage of the total work force in the area is minorities, women, and handicapped persons? How many are unemployed? How many can be recruited from the local community or the nation? Are there training programs available to prepare minorities, women, and handicapped people with skills the agency can use? Can the agency prepare minorities, women, and handicapped personnel? A hospital may be able to prepare nurse's aides or assistants but would need to rely on other institutions to prepare licensed practical or vocational nurses and registered nurses. Are there disadvantaged people already employed by the agency who are transferable or promotable? Programs to correct underutilization must be developed when there are fewer minorities, women, and handicapped persons in a job classification than would be expected by their availability.

Once management has completed its utilization and availability analysis, it establishes goals and timetables to improve utilization. To correct identifiable deficiencies, management needs goals that are measurable and attainable. Goals for minorities and women are presented separately. Those goals and the timetables for completion along with supportive data and analysis are major parts of the written affirmative action program.

Programs to achieve these goals must be developed and implemented next. This phase begins with a review of the employment process to identify barriers. Recruitment procedures and the selection process—including job requirements, job descriptions, application forms, testing, and interviewing—are examined. The upward mobility system—including training, assignments, job progressions, seniority, transfers, and promotions and disciplinary action policies—are reviewed. Wage and salary structure, benefits, conditions of employment, and union contracts are also studied. Appropriate changes are made, and an internal audit and reporting system to monitor and evaluate the affirmative action program is implemented. Records of referrals, placements, transfers, promotions, and terminations should be maintained for 3 years. Formal reports regarding attainment of goals and timetables are prepared on a regular basis. The manager of the affirmative action program reviews the reports with other managers, advises top administration of the program effectiveness, and submits recommendations for improvement of unsatisfactory performance.

Compliance status is not judged solely by whether goals have been met by the time set for achieving them. A review of the program's content and the efforts made toward realization of the goals are factors that are considered in determining its effectiveness.

It is important to keep in mind that goals are not inflexible quotas that must be met but are targets that are reasonably attainable through good faith efforts. Goals, therefore, should be realistic, measurable, and achievable by the time established.

When interviewing applicants for positions, one should remember that some employment inquiries are acceptable whereas others are not. The purpose of the question determines its propriety. Appropriate inquiries have a direct relationship to the applicant's capacity to do the job. Inappropriate questions may receive answers that will limit the person's opportunities because of ancestry, race, color, age, religion, sex, marital or parental status, or handicap. Some information needed for payroll or personnel purposes—such as age, proof of citizenship, and number of dependents—can be obtained after the person has been hired. Questions about the applicant's religious preferences, sex, marital status, credit rating, number and ages of dependents, or marital and family plans are not appropriate. Questions that would identify the person as being over forty or general questions about disabilities are not acceptable. The applicant may be asked to prove she is over eighteen and able to perform job-related functions. One can ask for an address and length of residence in a city or state but not for rental or ownership information. Questions about ability to read, write, or speak a language are acceptable, but questions about one's primary language or how one acquired the ability to use a language are unacceptable. One's legal right to remain in the United States can be questioned, but questions about naturalization of parents or spouse are unacceptable. The applicant may be asked to list membership in clubs, organizations, societies, and associations, excluding those that would indicate the national origin, race, color, or religion of the membership. Requests for all memberships are not appropriate. General questions about military service are inappropriate.

When interviewing minority candidates, the interviewer should not pretend interest in, or knowledge of, an ethnic culture or use ethnic vernacular or a foreign language she does not speak well. It is inappropriate to talk about one's minority friends or to expect the candidate to know all other minority members. Lack of eye contact should not be judged negatively, since some cultures interpret direct eye contact as disrespectful. The interviewer should be aware that body language and voice tone give messages that provoke confidence or mistrust and suggest support or indifference.

The manager should be aware that some minority applicants may not have well-defined aspirations and career goals because their opportunities may have been limited and they may feel they have little control over their careers. Minority applicants often have frequently changed jobs in search of better pay. Therefore, steady work and work progression histories may be of little use in evaluating minority applicants who have had limited opportunities.

Orientation

Having made her choice from the available applicants, the manager introduces the nurse to her new job, agency policies, facilities, and co-workers. Orientation is important, and the supervisor who does not take the time to assist a new employee is making a serious mistake. Communicating regulations and exactly what is expected of the nurse diminishes uncertainty, relieves anxiety, and prevents unnecessary misunderstandings. One's security usually increases when someone is considerate enough to help one adjust to a new situation. The manner in which the nurse is treated during her first day at a new job may be critical to her future job satisfaction and performance.

Orientation to the institution typically includes a tour of the facilities; a description of the organizational structure; a discussion of different departmental functions; a presentation of the philosophy, goals, and standards; an interpretation of administrative policies and procedures; and possibly an explanation of hospital relationships with the community. Next the nurse will need an orientation to the nursing service, including interdepartmental relationships, departmental organization, administrative controls, philosophy, goals, policies, procedures, and job descriptions.

After the general orientation, the new nurse may be assigned to another nurse for orientation to her specific job. The new nurse will need a tour of the unit so that she knows the location of supplies, equipment, and policy and procedure books. Information about how the unit is run, specific methods of practice, and communication systems is important. Introductions to other personnel can help the new person feel welcome.

Frequent visits to see that the nurse is comfortable and that the orientation is progressing satisfactorily are helpful. Documentation of the orientation process is useful. The documentation may be a simple checklist that itemizes information such as the organizational structure, specific policies, fire and disaster plans, tour of the facilities, and procedures, with space for a signature. It can be retained in the personnel file.

Nurse internship programs are common to assist newly graduated nurses in making the adjustment from the student role to a staff nurse position. The instructor and head nurse usually work together to identify teaching-learning needs, plan rotation schedules, and evaluate the intern's performance. Classes are held on a regular basis for orientation, role adjustment, problem solving, and information about pathophysiology. There is a concentration on the mastery of technical skills. Some programs also present leadership instruction. Nurse internship programs help new graduates build self-confidence, lower frustration levels, increase nursing care planning, improve patient care, improve job satisfaction, and reduce turnover.

Near the end of the probationary period, it is advisable to have a systematic evaluation. The nurse should know what characteristics will be evaluated. Two independent judgments, such as those of the supervisor and the head nurse, may be secured and used to check reliability of the evaluation. The results of the evaluation are indicative of the success of the selection process.

Staff development

Staff development goes beyond orientation. It is a continuing liberal education of the whole person to develop her potential fully. It deals with aesthetic senses as well as technical and professional education and may include activities such as orientation, internships, in-service education, courses, conferences, seminars, journal or book clubs, programmed learning, and independent study.

The nurse manager plays an important role in the support of staff development and has a responsibility to review the goals for the staff development program and to provide a budget for those activities. She participates in needs identification and analyzes how education effects change in nursing services. In addition, she must be careful to differentiate staff development needs from administrative needs. If a staff nurse knows how to do a procedure properly but does not because the necessary supplies and equipment are not available to her, the need is administrative rather than educational. The nursing manager is legally liable for the quality of nursing services. Her ability to document staff development is strong supportive evidence for the manager. Conversely, the reception of staff development will be largely related to the reward system developed. Positive reinforcement through recognition, such as oral praise on the unit or acknowledgment of accomplishments in a newsletter, is useful. Staff development can also be related to retention, pay raises, advancement to other positions, or termination.

Preceptorship. Preceptorships may be used to help recruit, retain, orient, and develop staff. They may be used before students graduate to orient them to the agency and to recruit them for hire. If students have worked at an agency before graduation and are familiar with it, they can make sounder decisions about where to work, are not as likely to be unprepared for the work situation, and, consequently, are likely to be retained longer. The preceptorship also gives agency personnel an opportunity to evaluate the student and determine if she is someone they would want to hire.

During the preceptorship, faculty facilitate, monitor, and evaluate student learning. Faculty direct students to resources, offer suggestions regarding patient care problems, and lead discussions at conferences. The faculty member is responsible for student learning and encourages students to apply class content.

The preceptor is responsible for the quality of patient care and facilitates the student's learning. Preceptors are liaisons between students and the agency. They help students learn skills and how to organize their work. They provide real-life experiences for students before graduation to help reduce the difficulties of transition from school to work.

The professional nurturance of a preceptorship can be likened to the "good old boy" network or godfathers who look after godsons. It allows students to use and increase their knowledge and skills so they can assume increasing responsibilities. They gain experience with a variety of patients and different levels of staff. They have opportunities to discuss and adjust to professional-bureaucratic conflicts. Preceptorships are a potential recruitment tool for the agency and can increase the job satisfaction of nurses. Preceptors may even learn from the students and are likely to find the preceptor role challenging and stimulating.

There are also disadvantages to preceptorships. They add to staff nurse responsibilities and require time. Sometimes busy nurses have little time to spend with students. It becomes difficult for faculty to evaluate students because they have little direct observation of the students' work. The use of preceptors requires considerable planning and coordination. Role descriptions should clarify who chooses learning experiences for the student, who supervises the student, and who evaluates the student. Practical evaluation tools of the student, preceptor, and faculty should be developed and used. Educational and service administrative support are needed.

The faculty member serves as a preceptor of preceptors. A workshop to prepare preceptors is desirable. It is appropriate to discuss and clarify role descriptions, skill inventory lists for students, and guidelines for preceptor evaluation of students. Information about teaching methods, counseling, and evaluation is useful. Finding a time and place for the workshop and getting release time for the preceptors may create problems. Awarding continuing education credits for the workshop and preceptor experience may be considered as a way to reward preceptors.

The preceptor model can also be used by the staff development department and nurses after a graduate has been hired. The staff development faculty may present formal content in orientation and development programs that is reinforced by preceptors on the units.

Mentorship. Preceptors are role models who may become mentors. Mentors give their time, energy, and material support to teach, guide, assist, counsel, and inspire a younger nurse. It is a nurturing relationship that cannot be forced. A close, trusted counselor, usually in her forties or fifties, acquaints a younger person, usually in her twenties or thirties, with the values, customs, and resources of the profession. The mentor is a confidante who personalizes role modeling and serves as a sounding board for decisions. The mentor is a resource person who supports the development of the young person through influence and promotion.

There are phases to the mentoring process. At first, during the invitational stage, a mentor must be willing to use her time and energy to nurture someone who is goal-directed, willing to learn, and respectfully trusting of the mentor. The younger professional has a career goal, a vision of what she wants to become; the mentor is someone who has reached that goal and is willing to share the secrets of her success. Then there is a period of questioning, when the young person has self-doubt and fears of being unable to meet the goals. The mentor helps clarify those goals through self-discrimination. Next the mentor shares information about power and politics, tells how she became successful, and serves as a sounding board. The transitional phase is the final phase when the mentor helps the mentee personalize learning and become aware of her own strengths and uniqueness. The younger nurse is then prepared to be a mentor and to tell others how she became what she is.

It has been difficult to establish mentorships in nursing. Many nurses have poor self-esteem, project insecurity, are dissatisfied with nursing, and show little respect for or pride in their work. Parent-child relationships with smothering, oppressive control and overdependence are too common. Envy may develop when the younger nurse matures quickly.

Mentorship should provide an opportunity to share information, review work, provide feedback, explore issues, plan strategies, and solve problems. It helps socialize novices into professional norms, values, and standards. Career advancement and success are promoted, thus increasing self-confidence, self-esteem, and greater personal satisfaction.

ASSIGNMENT SYSTEMS FOR STAFFING

Changes in assignment systems are a response to changing needs. In the 1920s, the case method and private duty nursing were popular. By 1950, functional nursing was predominant in response to the shortage of nurses. During that decade, team nursing was introduced to maximize the knowledge and skills of professional nurses and to supervise auxiliary help. The late 1960s and 1970s have witnessed a shift back to care of the patient by a professional nurse through primary nursing. Each system has advantages and disadvantages.

Case method

In the case method each patient is assigned to a nurse for total patient care while that nurse is on duty. The patient has a different nurse each shift and no guarantee of having the same nurses the next day. The head nurse, with no obligation to assign nurses to the same patient, supervises and evaluates all of the care given on her unit. Popular during the 1920s along with private duty nursing, the case method emphasized following physicians' orders.

Functional nursing

In the 1950s, with few registered and only some practical nurses available, much patient care was given by nurses' aides. In functional nursing, hierarchical structure predominates. The medication nurse, treatment nurse, and bedside nurse are all products of this system. The functional method implements classic scientific management, which emphasizes efficiency, division of labor, and rigid controls. Procedural descriptions are used to describe the standard of care, and psychological needs are slighted. Registered nurses keep busy with managerial and nonnursing duties, while nurses' aides deliver the patient care.

Although efficient, the functional assignment method does not encourage patient and staff satisfaction. Regimentation of tasks may bore the nurse who no longer has the satisfaction of seeing the effects of her total patient care. On the other hand, the functional system may work satisfactorily during critical staffing shortages. Routinized patient care for patients with similar needs may meet those needs more consistently than other systems, and some staff members may be satisfied by doing repetitious jobs well.

Team nursing

After World War II, registered nurses were still scarce, although the number of auxiliary personnel had increased. Team nursing was introduced during the 1950s to improve nursing services by utilizing the knowledge and skills of professional nurses and to supervise the increasing numbers of auxiliary nursing staff. The result was an improvement in patient and staff satisfaction. Team nursing is a philosophy that supports the achievement of goals through group action. Each team member is encouraged to make suggestions and share ideas. When a team member sees her suggestion implemented, job satisfaction is increased, and the individual is motivated to give even better care.

The team is led by a professional or technical nurse who plans, interprets, coordinates, supervises, and evaluates the nursing care. The team leader assigns team members to patients by matching patient needs with staff's knowledge and skills. She also does the work other members of the team are not qualified to perform. She sets goals and priorities for patient care; centralizes information through the use of a Kardex; directs the planning of care by directing care conferences and developing care plans; fixes responsibility for the work; provides for coverage during absences, such as breaks, meals, and conferences; and coordinates and evaluates team activities. The team members report to the team leader, who reports to the head nurse. This is a form of decentralization that frees the head nurse to manage the unit.

One of the main features of team nursing is the nursing care conference. Its primary purpose is the development and revision of nursing care plans by providing an opportunity to identify and solve problems. Precision in the identification of problems is increased through information sharing. The belief that the total group has more information about a topic than any one person enhances the staff's appreciation of group work. A resulting consensus increases the commitment to the decisions made. Identification of the problem and determination of goals early in the conference necessarily precede planning intervention. During the conference, one care plan can be developed or the care plans for a case load can be updated.

Team conferences also provide the opportunity to identify and work through staff educational needs. Nurses can review standards of care by comparing the actual patient's condition to the textbook example. They can review procedures and learn specialized nursing care and the operation of infrequently used equipment. By studying critical incidents, they may prevent problems from recurring and identify the contributing components of excellent care. Team conferences also provide an opportunity to discuss and resolve interpersonal problems and the chance to prevent future ones. Consequently, team spirit is fostered.

The team leader is responsible for planning and conducting the team conference, which should be limited in time and scope. Meeting for 15 to 30 minutes at the same time each day helps the conference become a part of the daily routine. A time that least interferes with other activities and a place away from the hub of activity are preferable. The team leader must arrange for coverage of the unit during the conference, because the relief of patient care responsibilities is essential to prevent interruptions. Staff should be informed of the time, place, and purpose of the conference, so that they can plan their other work around the conference and be well prepared on arrival. Interest can be stimulated by allowing the staff to decide whom they wish to discuss at the next conference and by having one of the team members record patient problems and solutions during the conference.

Preparation of the meeting area is also a responsibility of the team leader. Temperature, ventilation, lighting, and chair arrangements should be controlled. Refreshments may be appropriate. The team leader introduces the topic and starts the meeting on time to motivate latecomers to be more prompt. A brief review of the patient's condition is appropriate. The team leader monitors the group process, records problems and solutions on the nursing care plan or delegates that task, does appropriate teaching, and summarizes the major points. The nursing care plan is then available to the staff. The team leader serves as a role model by referring to the care plan while receiving and giving reports, making out assignments, and administering nursing care.

The nursing care plan is another main feature of team nursing. A care plan identifying present and potential problems and long- and short-term objectives should be developed for each patient. The care plan should be realistic to avoid morale problems that result from setting unattainable objectives. Care plans should be individualistic, reflecting the interrelatedness of psychosocial and physiological needs and involving patient and family participation. Problems, mutually acceptable goals, objectives, actions, and responses are identified. The care is evaluated according to how well the objectives are met.

Team nursing contributes to the satisfaction of patient and staff needs. Each patient is treated as a unique individual. Staff can identify their contributions and the correlation between their work and patient outcomes. The closer interaction of staff contributes to an esprit de corps.

Because each staff member does many tasks for a limited number of patients instead of a single task for a large number of patients, there is an increased likelihood of errors and a need to spend more time monitoring for them. It also takes time to coordinate delegated work. Although the team leader probably has the least contact with the patients, she is responsible for assessment, planning, and communicating with the physician. Continuity of care is not a given, as patients are not assigned to the same staff all of the time and large assignments make individualized patient care difficult. Changing team membership makes it difficult for the team leader to know team members well enough to match their talents with patient needs. Team nursing is similar to functional nursing when the team leader administers medications and treatments other team members are not qualified to give. Team conferences are often omitted because they are difficult to fit into busy days, and care plans (if done) usually note functional duties relative to the physician's orders. Care plans rarely depict the patient as a total person and consequently are not comprehensive. Medication precautions, fluid intake requirements, dietary and environmental adaptations, protective measures, psychological support, teaching, rehabilitation, and referrals are seldom mentioned. In reality the key features of team nursing— nursing care conferences and nursing care plans—often receive inadequate attention, and resulting care is routinized.

Modular nursing

Modular nursing is a modification of team and primary nursing. It is sometimes used when there are not enough registered nurses to practice primary nursing. Each registered nurse, assisted by paraprofessionals, delivers as much care as possible to a group of patients. The registered nurse plans the care, delivers as much of it as possible, and directs the paraprofessionals for the more technical aspects of care.

Primary nursing

During the late 1960s and early 1970s, primary nursing was instituted in some hospitals by professional nurses who were unhappy with fragmented care and lack of direct patient contact. Based on the philosophy that patients, instead of tasks, should be the focus of professional nurses, primary nursing features a registered nurse who gives total patient care to four to six patients while she is on duty. She remains responsible for the care of those patients 24 hours a day throughout the patient's hospitalization. The associate nurse cares for the patient by using the care plan developed by the primary nurse while the primary nurse is off duty. The associate nurse is to contact the primary nurse regarding changes in the care plan. The number of patients assigned to one nurse varies according to length of hospitalization, complexity of care, number of medical and para-medical personnel involved with the patient's care, availability of support systems, and the shift worked. Day-shift nurses are assigned the most patients; evening nurses have some; and night nurses are primarily auxiliary nurses because of the reduced contact with patients and families.

The primary nurse does the admission interview and develops the nursing care plan, including teaching and discharge planning, which she shares with the associate nurse. The primary nurse has autonomy and authority for the care of her patients. Consequently, accountability is placed and continuity of care is facilitated. An efficient method, primary nursing decreases the number of people in the chain of command and reduces the number of errors that can result from a relay of orders. Other advantages include mobile use of auxiliary workers and increased satisfaction by both nurse and patient. The nurse can identify the patient outcome as a result of her work. A patient has the security of knowing his nurse is available and has to cope with fewer people than in other assignment systems. Research suggests that patients have fewer complications and a shorter hospitalization when cared for by a primary nurse.

Unfortunately, primary nursing confines a nurse's talents to her own patients. Other patients cannot benefit, and if a patient has a nurse who is not capable, he may be worse off than if he were exposed to numerous people, some of whom might meet his needs. Another problem occurs when the associate nurse changes the care plan without discussing the reasons with the primary nurse. Thus it is critical that the primary nurse communicate verbal and written plans to the associate nurse. The success of primary nursing seems dependent on the quality of the nursing staff and administrative support.

Pure applications of case method, functional method, team nursing, modular nursing, and primary nursing are possible, but seldom do they exist in pristine form. Rather, it is common to find elements from more than one assignment system combined and used at the same time.

Leveling of staff

The level of staff available greatly influences the assignment systems used. When there are a few registered nurses and a few practical nurses, many aides are quickly oriented and used. This is an expensive and relatively dangerous mix, because aides do not have the educational background to do most of what needs to be done or to recognize what needs to be reported. After the aides have done all they can, there is still much work to be done. Consequently, there is considerable downtime. This staffing mix lends itself best to functional nursing.

Team nursing is appropriate when there are some registered nurses, even more practical nurses, and fewer aides. The registered nurses plan and direct the care, pass medications, and do the more complicated treatments. Although this provides better physical care, the staff is still not adequately educated to understand the pathophysiological basis of symptoms, to plan nursing intervention, and to detect changes in the status of the patient at an early stage so they may promptly report pertinent information to the physician. There is also a dearth of patient education and response to psychosocial needs.

Modular nursing is appropriate when more registered nurses are available, and primary nursing works best with a staff of all registered nurses. Research regarding all-registered nursing staffs indicates there is an increase in staff, patient, and physician satisfaction. There is an increase in professional orientation, personal liking of colleagues, and cooperation with others. Collegial relationships are more common and there is more mobility on units because nurses can cover for each other. There is greater competence in skills, creative interventions, personalized care, and continuity of care.

All-registered nurse staffing is economical. It has been found to save money because of the decreased turnover, sick leave, unpaid absences, float hours, and overtime. Registered nurses can give better care in fewer hours. Patients have fewer complications, shorter hospitalizations, and lower readmission rates. Hospitals also generate more revenue when patients have shorter stays with a concentration of treatments.

STAFFING SCHEDULES

Staffing schedules are largely influenced by staffing policies. To determine staffing policies, one must consider the following questions:

What is the best organization for staffing—centralized or decentralized to clinical areas or nursing units?

Who is responsible for the original scheduling or daily adjustments?

Where are nursing hours posted and an accurate copy kept?

For what period of time will schedules be prepared—1, 2, 4, or 6 weeks?

How far in advance will personnel know their work schedule?

Will there be an adjustment in staffing based on the identification of patient needs?

Will there be shift rotation?

If there is shift rotation, how often—daily, weekly, monthly?

How much time should elapse between rotated shifts?

What day starts a calendar week—Sunday or Monday?

Will there be 2 days off each week or an average of 2 days a week?

How often are weekends off guaranteed?

What days does a weekend comprise—Friday, Saturday, Sunday?

Will days off be split or consecutive?

What are the maximal and minimal work spans?

How many holiday and vacation days are allowed?

How far in advance of scheduling should employees request time off?

How will holiday time off be determined?

Will part-time help be used?

If so, what is the most economical ratio between full- and part-time personnel?

Will part-time help be allowed to specify when they can and cannot work?

Will part-time help be required to work weekends? If so, how often?

Centralized scheduling

Two major advantages of centralized scheduling are fairness to employees through consistent, objective, and impartial application of policies and opportunities for cost containment through better use of resources. Centralized scheduling also relieves head nurses from time-consuming duties, freeing them for other activities. Centralized scheduling is not without its critics, however. Lack of individualized treatment of employees is a chief complaint, and centralized scheduling has brought to the surface previously unrecognized organizational and managerial problems.

Organizational and managerial problems can be reduced when (1) the philosophy and goals of the agency are identified; (2) the goals, objectives, and organizational structure are defined; (3) scheduling policies are stated; (4) standards of nursing care practices are set; (5) acuity of care is determined as it relates to staffing needs; (6) patient needs, personnel privileges such as vacation and personal leave, and staff development are taken into account in personnel schedules; and (7) quality of care is measured.

Resistance to centralized scheduling may be reduced when head nurses prepare and control their own budgets, understand and approve the scheduling policies, and have open communication with the scheduler. Line and staff accountability need to be carefully defined to prevent confusion over responsibility and authority when staff personnel make decisions where line managers are accountable. Line authority is accountable for decisions, and staff provides support to help line make decisions.

The staff functions of the scheduler include scheduling employees according to staffing policies, implementing procedures for position control and reallocation of staff, maintaining records for line managers, gathering information and preparing reports to help line authority prepare personnel budgets, and maintaining communications with other appropriate departments, such as personnel and payroll.

Line responsibilities of head nurses include developing a master staffing pattern; establishing procedures for adjustment of staff; clarifying requirements for each job description and staff position; hiring, developing, promoting, disciplining, and firing employees when appropriate; and defining and controlling the personnel budget.

Computers can be used for centralized scheduling. Before implementing a computer system, an analysis of policies and procedures is done and baseline data collected. Agency policies regarding the nature of the schedule—straight, alternating, or rotating shifts; frequency of alternating or rotating shifts; work stretch; weekends-off sequence; and use of part-time help—are constants in the information process system. Variables such as census, acuity of patients, special requests, special assignments, vacations, and holidays can be fed into the computer.

Advantages of centralized computer scheduling include cost-effectiveness through the reduction of clerical staff and better utilization of professional nurses by decreasing the time spent in non-patient-care activities; unbiased, consistent scheduling; equitable application of agency policies; an easy-to-read work schedule developed in advance so employees know what their schedules are and can plan their personal lives accordingly; and availability of data for monitoring the effect of staff size and composition, quality of care, and cost.

Decentralized staffing

When head nurses are given authority and assume responsibility, they can staff their own units through decentralized staffing. Personnel feel that they get more personalized attention with decentralized staffing. Staffing is easier and less complicated when done for a small area instead of for the whole agency. Each head nurse learns the responsibility and challenges of staffing. With a philosophy of sharing and mutual trust, head nurses can work together to solve chronic staffing problems. Because of their knowledge and experience, head nurses can form a support system and offer each other informed advice. Supervisors and charge nurses are freed from staffing responsibilities and have more time for other tasks.

Unfortunately, some staff members may receive individualized treatment at the expense of others, and work schedules can be used as a punishment-reward system by the head nurse. Staffing, which is very time-consuming, takes the head nurse away from other duties or forces her to do the scheduling while off duty. Decentralized staffing may utilize resources less efficiently and consequently make cost containment more difficult.

Alternating or rotating work shifts

Although straight shifts are used by some institutions or for some personnel within institutions, rotating work shifts are common for staff nurses. The frequency of alternating between days and evenings, or days and nights, or rotating through all three shifts varies among institutions. Some nurses may work all three shifts within 7 days.

Alternating and rotating work shifts create stress for staff nurses. Environmental cues, such as sunrise and sunset, fluctuate in a predictable cycle. Instruments that designate hours, minutes, and seconds correspond to the natural daily cycle and allow knowledge of one's location in that cycle. Social and work routines synchronize with the internal circadian rhythms as the body rhythms are timed to coincide with the usual activities. Thus, when environmental conditions are changed by altering work hours, sleep time, hour for rising, meal times, and social and recreational activities, the body must make accommodations for the environmental changes. Body rhythms need time to adjust to the discrepancy between the person's activity cycle and the new demands of the environment. The ability of the body functions to adjust varies considerably among individuals. It may take 2 to 3 days to 2 weeks for a person to adjust to a different sleep-wake cycle.

Alternating or rotating work shifts affect the health of nurses and the quality of their work. The rapid shift of work schedules causes stress. Nurses complain of restlessness and nervousness while trying to sleep, wakefulness or sleepiness at inappropriate times, anorexia, digestive disturbance, disruption in bowel habits, fatigue, slower reaction time, lower job performance, and error proneness. There are changes in the patterning of temperature, blood pressure, and urine excretory cycles, and a possible lowered resistance to disease. Resultant increase in medication errors, equipment failures, and errors in problem solving are probable.

To guarantee that a nurse works her share of weekends, holidays, and unpopular evening and night hours, alternating and rotating assignments currently focus on the time patterns of an individual nurse rather than on well-integrated work groups. The rotation of personnel on an individual basis is disruptive to the development of work groups.

The Federal Aviation Agency's (FAA) rotation of teams of airport personnel may be used as a model by nursing service. The FAA rotates entire teams consisting of four or five controllers plus trainees and a leader, chosen because of their qualifications, amount of experience, and anticipated compatibility. Their schedules are planned a year in advance so that team members can plan their personal lives with confidence. Emergencies and vacations are handled within the team. Absenteeism affects the work load of the peers with whom one must continue to work; therefore, team identification reduces absenteeism because of team pressure. Controllers have a low turnover rate.

In hospitals, rotation of teams instead of individuals could contribute to team development. If a group of personnel works together consistently, they can help each other through the dependence of the orientation phase of group development and the conflict experienced during the organizational phase, when the role negotiations of who will be responsible for what occurs. The staff has a chance to become an interdependent, cohesive group with good communication and effective problem-solving abilities. Unfortunately, there is usually a high turnover of nursing personnel, which complicates team development. Perhaps more attention to team development would reduce the turnover.

Permanent shifts

Permanent shifts relieve nurses from stress and health-related problems associated with alternating and rotating shifts. They also provide social, educational, and psychological advantages. When the nurse is able to choose the shift that best suits her personal life, she can participate in social activities (such as hobbies, sports, and community, professional, or church organizations) even when they require regular attendance. She may be able to continue her education by planning courses around her work schedule. Childcare arrangements can be stable. The nurse may develop a sense of belonging to a shift and feel and work better because the shift suits her. In studies conducted with Montreal nurses, nurses working permanent shifts had higher averages on psychological scales such as mental health, job satisfaction, social involvement, and commitment to the organization. They had fewer health problems and a decrease in tardiness, absenteeism, and turnover.

Although the day shift is not always the preferred shift, it is likely to be the most popular one. Consequently, assignment to preferred shift may need to be done on a seniority-priority basis. This usually results in a predominance of new graduates staffing the evening and night shifts. The head nurse may have difficulty evaluating the evening and night shift personnel unless she does some observations during those shifts; therefore, it may be easier for evening and night supervisors to evaluate permanent staff on those shifts. One disadvantage of permanent shifts is that nurses may not develop an appreciation for the work load or problems of other shifts.

Block or cyclical scheduling

Block or cyclical scheduling uses the same schedule repeatedly. With a 6-day forward rotation, personnel are scheduled to work 6 successive days followed by at least 2 days off. The schedule repeats itself every 6 weeks.

Personnel can be scheduled with every other weekend off and 1 day during the week so that there are no more than 4 consecutive days of work. Several blocks are possible. Because nurses are not exhausted by working too many consecutive days, sick leave can be reduced. By having one team member at a time vacation and by rotating holidays among the workers, vacations and holidays can be scheduled to avoid changes in the block. However, some nurses fear that one day off at a time is not adequate to feel rested. But nurses who currently do not work more than 4 consecutive days report that 1 day is adequate to refresh themselves.

There are several advantages to established rotations. Personnel know their schedules in advance and consequently can plan their personal lives. Absences because of social events decrease because staff can plan their social activities around their work schedules. There is a decrease in preoccupation with staffing, time for scheduling, time for maintenance of schedule, and conflict over preferred days off. Staff is treated more fairly by equitable distribution of popular and unpopular days on duty. The scheduling of appropriate number and category mix of personnel is simplified. Once the appropriate mix is determined, it is repeated. This helps establish stable work groups and decreases floating, thus promoting team spirit and continuity of care. A decrease in flexibility of staffing, however, may be perceived as a disadvantage.

Variable staffing

Variable staffing is a method that uses patient needs to determine the number and mix of staff. Time measures are done for direct and indirect patient care. A patient classification system is developed, and tables are designed to determine the number of nursing hours required depending on the number of patients in each category. This provides the information to determine staff needs by skill levels. Nursing pools, floats, and part-time help can be used to supplement the regular staff to accomplish the variable staffing. With a study of previous staffing needs, redistribution of peak routine work, and slight overstaffing in some areas to create float personnel for last-moment needs, there may be little need to call in unscheduled staff.

Eight-hour shift, five-day workweek

The 5-day, 40-hour workweek became popular during the late 1940s. It was a radical change from the 10-hour day, 5-day workweek that contained split shifts and few holidays. It has been a predominant pattern since then. The shifts are usually 7 AM to 3:30 PM, 3 PM to 11:30 PM, and 11 PM to 7:30 AM, allowing for a half-hour lunch break and a half-hour overlap time between shifts to provide for continuity of care.

Ten-hour day, four-day workweek

The Intensive Coronary Care Unit at Saint Elizabeth Community Health Center in Lincoln, Nebraska, has implemented the 10-hour day, 4-day workweek with an every-other-weekend-off staffing pattern. The shifts are 7 AM to 5:30 PM, 1 PM to 11:30 PM, and 9 PM to 7:30 AM. A cyclical schedule is used that allows at least 14 hours off between shifts and a 4-day weekend every 6 weeks for those who rotate. The workweek begins on Sunday, and the weekend is Saturday and Sunday for all shifts. The main problem is fatigue, but it was not found to be as serious a problem as anticipated. The long weekends and extra days off are attractions (Bauer, 1971).

Ten-hour day plus five- or six-hour shift

Roger Williams General Hospital in Providence, Rhode Island, has implemented two 10-hour shifts and one 5-hour shift. The shifts are 7 AM to 5 PM, 5 PM to 10 PM, and 9 PM to 7 AM. A 2-week cyclical schedule posts 2 days on, 2 days off, 3 on, 2 off, 2 on, and 3 off with two teams working complementary schedules. The younger nurses seem to have a more positive attitude toward the 10-hour shift and cite the social opportunities as a major benefit. However, the 10-hour system did contribute to greater fatigue, poorer communication between physicians and nurses, and discontinuity of patient care (Colt et al., 1974).

Nursing service at Sacred Heart Hospital in Eau Claire, Wisconsin, was able to capitalize on a pool of inactive registered nurses by developing a 6-hour evening shift and a 10-hour day shift. Shifts are 7 AM to 5 PM, 5 PM to 11 PM, and 11 PM to 7 AM. Problems encountered were overtime, which may have been partially due to adjustment, and absences of ill nurses from 10-hour shifts—a difficult deficit to fill, and one that burdened other staff members and lowered morale (Minor, et al., 1971).

Ten-hour shift, seven-day workweek

Evergreen General Hospital in Kirkland, Washington, has implemented a 7-70 plan that includes a 10-hour shift 7 days a week, followed by 7 consecutive days off. Two teams alternate weeks from Tuesday through Monday. There is no rotation of shifts. Each team contains permanent day, evening, and night shifts. The shifts are 6:45 AM to 5:15 PM, 12:45 PM to 11:15 PM, and 9:15 PM to 7:45 AM. Initially there was no extra pay for holiday or vacation time, because that was compensated for in the pay for 80 hours when only 70 hours were worked. Later, vacation time was instituted, dependent on length of employment and ranging from 70 hours annually for 1 to 3 years of employment to 140 hours per year for 11 or more years of employment.

Advantages of the 10-hour day, 7-day workweek include increased continuity of care, more consistency of care between weekdays and weekends, improved communications, better understanding of the patients' needs resulting from longer time with patients, more consistent patient teaching, more flexibility for meeting patient needs instead of hospital regimens, and improved job satisfaction because of advanced knowledge of work schedule and prolonged rest periods that facilitated a more normal home life and more control over one's personal affairs. Sick leave and resignations decreased. However, nurses did get tired by the end of the 7-day workweek (Hutchins and Cleveland, 1978).

Twelve-hour shift, seven-day workweek

The 12-hour shift, starting at 7 or 7:30 AM and ending at 7 or 7:30 PM, has been adopted by some institutions. The better utilization of nursing personnel lowers staffing requirements; this consequently lowers the cost per patient day. Nurses find they get to know their patients better because they have more time to study charts and can visit patients more frequently. They have more time to get new admissions settled before the change of shift and feel that they can give better patient care because they are not so rushed. They find that there are fewer communication gaps and better continuity of care. Consequently, there are improved nurse-patient relations.

Working relations are improved. Personnel work with the same group of people, so team development is possible. There is less friction and no 3-to-11 shift to blame for problems. Less daily reporting results in less confusion about physicians' orders and changes in procedures and routines. Less time is required for staffing, thus freeing supervisors and head nurses for other duties.

Total time off is increased with an increased usefullness of time. Travel time is reduced. Nurses find they have more time to relax and enjoy their days off and are able to return to work refreshed. Flexibility for personal schedules improves staff morale.

Overtime pay has been of some concern. The 1966 Amendments to the Fair Labor Standards Act permit agencies to calculate overtime pay on a 14-consecutive-day work period. Consequently, overtime pay is only required for more than 80 hours in a 2-week period.

Some nurses complain that the extra time they have for learning and research becomes boring. Mental exhaustion and tension increase by the end of the workweek. Increases in minor accidents and medication errors have been reported. Others, however, have reported no such increases as a result of the cumulative fatigue. Nurses also complain that their home and social lives suffer the week they work.

The wide variety of staffing practices suggests there is no right or wrong staffing schedule. Rather, there is much variability to consider when designing the best staffing schedule for a given situation.

Baylor plan

Baylor University Medical Center in Dallas, Texas, started a 2-days alternative plan. Nurses have the option to work two 12-hour days on the weekends and be paid for 36 hours for day shifts, or 40 hours for night shifts, or to work five

8-hour shifts Monday through Friday. This plan requires a larger nursing staff but has filled weekend positions and reduced turnover. Some hospitals have implemented the Baylor plan indicating that the extra pay on weekends compensates for vacations, holidays, and sick time.

Some hospitals have nurses work 12-hour shifts when they work weekends. This way fewer people have to work weekends and, consequently, staff can have weekends off more frequently.

Variations

Medical College of Virginia Hospitals in Richmond has combined two 8-hour shifts and two 12-hour shifts per week for a total of 40 hours in a 4-day week (Alivizatos, 1981).

Intensive care nurses at Baptist Medical Center–Montclair in Birmingham, Alabama, have worked seven consecutive 8-hour nights from 10:30 PM to 7 AM, followed by seven nights off. They opted to be paid for 7½ hours for the 16 hours in excess of 40 per week rather than to accrue time off. The system was so popular it was expanded to other units.

When staff nurses designed their own staffing pattern at Valley Medical Center in Fresno, California, they designed a 3-day workweek with two 13-hour days, one 14-hour day, and 4 days off. It has decreased absenteeism and turnover and increased staff morale.

At Woman's Hospital of Texas in Houston, personnel can work the 5-day, 40-hour week, the two 16-hour weekend shifts for 40 hours' pay, or the three 12-hour shifts with at least one of those days on the weekend. The staff scheduling is done at the unit level. If a nurse wishes to work the three 12-hour day shift, she must have a buddy complete the 24-hour coverage.

Shared jobs where two part-time nurses fill one full-time position; half-shifts where two nurses each work 4 hours to fill one 8-hour shift; shifts at nontraditional times such as 9:00 AM to 5:00 PM or 10:00 AM to 6:00 PM; and 8 or fewer staggered hours scheduled during the busiest times are also options.

VARIABLES AFFECTING STAFFING

Although institutional and nursing service philosophy and objectives guide staffing, various patient, staff, and environmental factors also affect staffing patterns. The types of patients, their expectations, fluctuations in admissions, length of stay, and complexity of care complicate staffing. Personnel policies, educational and experiential levels of staff, job descriptions, the mix of work titles or leveling, hour and rotation policies, absenteeism, and the competitive market also affect staffing. Environmental factors, such as the floor plan of the unit and hospital, number of patient beds, availability of supplies and equipment, the organizational structure, and support services from other departments and agencies are also considered when planning staffing patterns.

Staffing studies

Three major types of staffing studies are used to predict the number, level, and mix of personnel required for staffing. Nursing care needed may be predicted from patient classification systems by assigning patients to categories according to diagnosis, acuity of care, or amount of self-sufficiency. Number, level, and mix of staff needed can be determined by noting the number of patients in each category. Then a cost-effective nursing personnel budget based on the needs of patients and the qualifications of nursing personnel can be determined. Patient classification systems can be combined with nursing care plans, and costs to individual patients can be determined. Systems that charge patients for the care they receive can be designed.

Time standards can be determined for nursing procedures by listing and analyzing the procedures required by each patient. The time required for each patient and the sum for all patients on a unit can then be calculated. Formulas deduced from statistical analysis of work sampling data can be used to predict the number of nursing care hours needed.

Patient classification systems. To develop patient classification systems, acuity definitions must be established and validated through work sampling. Warstler (1972) identifies five categories for patient classification: category I, self-care requiring from 1 to 2 hours per day; category II, minimal care requiring from 3 to 4 hours; category III, intermediate care requiring from 5 to 6 hours; category IV, modified intensive care requiring from 7 to 8 hours; and category V, intensive care requiring from 10 to 14 hours.

Regnery (1977) developed a four-level patient care classification system for public health nursing service that describes the characteristics of the family situation, psychological component, therapeutic competence, knowledge of health conditions, health attitudes, principles of general hygiene, environmental milieu, and community resources for each level. Level I is for clients who require a high degree of nursing skill, level II includes families that need regular public health nursing service, level III is for people requiring occasional service, and level IV is for clients and families requiring limited public health nursing service. Other four-level patient classification systems include category 1, minimal nursing care; category 2, moderate nursing care; category 3, considerable direct nursing care; and category 4, intensive nursing care. Another four-category system labels the levels self-, partial, complete, and intensive care.

Three-level categories have been labeled minimal, moderate, and maximal;

minimal, intermediate, and intensive; and essential, progressive, and comprehensive. Nurses at the Visiting Nurse Association of Cleveland classify therapeutic visits as essential nursing care. The progressive patient care category is for the client who is achieving independence in situations requiring continuing evaluation. Clients requiring a high degree of nursing knowledge and skill are placed in the comprehensive nursing care category.

Time standards. When figuring time standards for nursing care, one should consider both direct and indirect care. Direct care involves the patient and includes feeding, bathing, treating, and giving medications. Indirect care involves all activities that are not direct care, such as preparation of and cleaning up after medications and treatments, clinical work, reporting, communications, and coffee and lunch breaks.

Once the number and kind of care activities required by each patient are identified and the length of time it takes to do the activities calculated, one can add up the time required by all patients on a unit and divide by the number of productive work hours on a shift to determine the number of personnel needed. The mix of nursing personnel can be predicted by categorizing the care needed by the qualifications needed to give it, adding the time in each category, dividing by productive hours on a shift, and obtaining the number of specific types of personnel required to meet the patients' needs. Once this is accomplished, patients can be charged by the level of care required.

Staffing formulas. When determining the number of staff to hire, one must consider hours needing coverage, vacations, holidays, absenteeism, and staff development time. If nurses work 5 days a week and coverage is needed for 7 days, it takes 1.4 nurses to have one nurse on duty 7 days and 2.8 to have two nurses on duty for 7 days. This is calculated by multiplying the number needed on duty by days of the week needing coverage and dividing by the number of days each employee works per week to determine the number of personnel needed for coverage. For example:

Number needed		Days of week		Number of days each workweek		Number of people required
1	×	7	÷	5	=	1.4
2	×	7	÷	5	=	2.8
3	×	7	÷	5	=	4.2
4	×	7	÷	5	=	5.6
5	×	7	÷	5	=	7.0

This figure does not allow for vacations, holidays, absenteeism, or staff development time.

To calculate vacation coverage, multiply the number of vacation days per year by the number of people at that skill level. Dividing the total number of vacation days per skill level by the total days worked per year per person determines the number of people needed for vacation coverage. For example:

$$\begin{matrix}\text{Number of} \\ \text{vacation days per year}\end{matrix} \times \begin{matrix}\text{Number of} \\ \text{full-time people at} \\ \text{that skill level}\end{matrix} = \begin{matrix}\text{Total vacation days} \\ \text{by skill level}\end{matrix}$$

$$\begin{matrix}\text{Total vacation days} \\ \text{by skill level}\end{matrix} \div \begin{matrix}\text{Total days worked} \\ \text{per person per year}\end{matrix} = \begin{matrix}\text{Number of} \\ \text{full-time people needed for} \\ \text{vacation relief coverage}\end{matrix}$$

To determine holiday coverage, multiply total number of personnel required (7-day coverage per skill level) by the number of holidays to determine the number of holiday days to be staffed. Then divide the total holiday relief days by the total days worked per year per person to obtain the number of personnel required per skill level for holiday coverage per year.

$$\begin{matrix}\text{Number of} \\ \text{personnel}\end{matrix} \times \begin{matrix}\text{Number of} \\ \text{holidays}\end{matrix} = \begin{matrix}\text{Number of} \\ \text{holidays needing coverage}\end{matrix}$$

$$\begin{matrix}\text{Number of} \\ \text{holiday relief days}\end{matrix} \div \begin{matrix}\text{Number of} \\ \text{days worked per year} \\ \text{per person}\end{matrix} = \begin{matrix}\text{Number of} \\ \text{personnel required for} \\ \text{holiday coverage per year}\end{matrix}$$

The percentage of absenteeism is used to calculate absentee relief coverage.

Weeks/year × Days worked/week
× % of absenteeism   = Absentee days/person/year
Personnel requirements (7 days/week)
× Absenteeism days/person/year   = Absentee coverage for staffing
Absentee coverage required ÷ Total
days worked/person/year   = Full-time personnel required for absentee coverage per year

Personnel required for staff development relief per year can also be calculated.

$$\begin{matrix}\text{Number of} \\ \text{hours required or recommended} \\ \text{for staff development} \\ \text{per year per person}\end{matrix} \times \begin{matrix}\text{Number of} \\ \text{staff}\end{matrix} = \begin{matrix}\text{Number of} \\ \text{hours per year for} \\ \text{staff development} \\ \text{needing relief coverage}\end{matrix}$$

$$\begin{matrix}\text{Number of} \\ \text{staff development} \\ \text{hours needing} \\ \text{coverage}\end{matrix} \div \begin{matrix}\text{Hours worked} \\ \text{/day}\end{matrix} \div \begin{matrix}\text{Total days worked} \\ \text{/person}\end{matrix} = \begin{matrix}\text{Full-time personnel} \\ \text{required for staff} \\ \text{development coverage}\end{matrix}$$

A staffing slide rule can be developed to save time when computing the number of budgeted positions needed to meet staffing standards by preparing a table that identifies the number of persons needed on duty, number of persons needed to cover days off, and number of persons needed to cover additional days off for vacation, holiday, sick, and personal leaves. For example:

Number needed on duty	Number needed to cover days off	15.6 extra days + 6%	18.2 extra days + 7%	20.8 extra days + 8%	23.4 extra days + 9%
1	1.4	1.46	1.47	1.48	1.49
2	2.8	2.92	2.94	2.96	2.98
3	4.2	4.38	4.41	4.44	4.47
4	5.6	5.84	5.88	5.92	5.96
5	7.0	7.30	7.35	7.40	7.45

Staffing to meet fluctuating needs

Full-time staff. Full-time staff may be hired to meet the average staffing needs of an institution. The most common adjustment for an increased work load is to transfer staff from a less busy area to the overloaded area. This is economical for the agency but disrupts the unity of work groups, causes the transferred nurse to feel insecure, and contributes to job dissatisfaction and turnover. Some units require specialized knowledge and skill that not every nurse has.

In the companion floor system, two units relieve each other. Staff nurses are oriented to the second unit and know that if they are transferred it will be to the companion unit. Thus staff aggravation is minimized, flexibility is possible, and quality of care is maintained.

A complementary or float staff is at best full-time staff nurses who are oriented to many areas and like the challenge of different types of patients and settings. Unfortunately, most nurses prefer stability. Consequently, the float staff is likely to be part-time staff or new personnel waiting for a permanent assignment.

Having full-time staff work double shifts and overtime is another option. The nurse is already oriented to the area and continuity of care is facilitated. There are also disadvantages, however. Institutional costs increase. The nurses may become tired, errors are likely to increase with fatigue, and overtime may interfere with the nurses' personal lives.

Part-time staff. Flexible working hours can be an incentive for inactive nurses to start part-time employment and can thus reduce staffing shortage. Most nurses are women who have to combine their nursing role with many others, such as wife, mother, and homemaker. A part-time job can broaden the woman's horizons beyond her home, increase her income, give her ego satisfaction, and help her maintain her nursing skills. It is not uncommon for nurses to want to work part-time while continuing their education. Part-time nurses tend to work more than their share of unpopular hours, and some prefer evening and night duty exclusively. When the part-time nurse's other responsibilities decrease, she is a likely candidate for full-time work.

There are, of course, disadvantages to the use of part-time nurses. Educational and administrative expenses are higher proportionately for part-time than for full-time help. For example, it is likely to cost as much to orient a part-time as a full-time nurse, thus costing more per hours worked. Maintaining continuity of care is complicated, because two or more part-time people may fill budgeted full-time positions. There are also disadvantages for the employee. The part-time nurse may not receive benefits such as paid sick or vacation days and is not likely to be considered for promotion. Sometimes benefits are prorated for part-time workers.

Temporary help is another option. Some institutions hire temporary help for the summer to give relief for vacations. The University of Virginia Hospital in Charlottesville has used temporary bed and bath teams to reduce weekend staffing shortages (Rinker et al., 1975). Rochester Methodist Hospital in Rochester, Minnesota, has used a "premium day" approach to reduce the weekend staffing shortage. A staff nurse gets an extra day off (a premium day) if she works one additional weekend within a 4-week schedule (Fisher et al., 1974). Some nurses may be willing to work on an on-call basis the year around.

External temporary help agencies are available in some areas. The use of such agencies can greatly reduce the amount of time middle management must spend on staffing. The supervisor merely calls the external agency and requests so many nurses, and the agency makes the necessary contacts. The agency has a registry of available nurses who are allowed to have highly flexible, self-determined schedules. This allows some nurses to work who could not otherwise and consequently helps those nurses maintain their skills. It is then more likely for those nurses to return to nursing practice on a full-time basis than if they had remained inactive. Their availability may boost morale, and they may introduce new ideas and stimulate creativity among the regular staff.

Unfortunately, there are also disadvantages to temporary help agencies. The matching of the nurses' credentials and qualifications with assignments and orientation to assignments are severe problems. Although some temporary help agencies do keep orientation information and procedure manuals for their client institutions on file, their use may still be optional. It is likely to take considerable time for the regular staff to orient the temporary help, errors are likely to increase, and continuity of care is jeopardized. The temporary nurses get preferred schedules, leaving the regular staff with more of the less-attractive hours. Consequently, morale may be lowered.

A central placement service run by the state board of nursing or the state nurses' association could be useful for matching nurses' qualifications and interests with vacancies and anticipated vacancies throughout the state.

There are many variables to be considered when planning staffing schedules. The more accurately those variables are assessed, the better one is able to contain costs while providing high-quality care.

Using the case study in the appendix:

Write one advertisement for the local newspaper and one for a national nursing journal to recruit staff for one of the new units.

Develop your résumé. Write a letter of reference for a classmate. Interview a classmate for one of the new positions and be interviewed by a classmate for one of the new positions.

Determine what assignment system will be used on one of the new units. Determine how the scheduling will be done and how shifts and workweeks will be defined (8-, 10-, or 12-hour days on a permanent or rotating basis). Determine the number and level of staff to hire for the new ward. Discuss the rationale for and advantages and disadvantages of your decisions with your classmates.

BIBLIOGRAPHY

Books

Alexander, E.L.: Nursing administration in the hospital health care system, ed. 2, St. Louis, 1978, The C. V. Mosby Co.

Althaus, J.N., et al.: Nursing decentralization: the El Camino experience, Wakefield, Mass., 1981, Aspen Publishing Co.

Berger, M.S., et al., editors: Management for nurses, ed. 2, St. Louis, 1980, The C. V. Mosby Co.

Blum, M.L., and Naylor, J.C.: Industrial psychology: its theoretical and social foundations, New York, 1956, Harper & Row, Publishers.

Bradford, L.P.: Making meetings work: a guide for leaders and group members, La Jolla, Calif., 1976, University Associates, Inc.

Cooper, S.S., and Byrns, H.H.: A plan for continuing education in nursing in five North Central states, Bethesda, Md., 1973, Department of Health, Education and Welfare, Public Health Service (no. NIH 71-4151).

Curtis, F.S., et al.: Continuing education in nursing, Boulder, Colo., 1969, Western Interstate Commission for Higher Education.

Deines, E.: Staffing for DRGs: a unit-specific approach for nurse managers, Chapel Hill, N.C., 1983, W.L. Ganong Co.

DiVincenti, M.: Administering nursing service, ed. 2, Boston, 1977, Little, Brown & Co.

Douglas, L.M.: Review of leadership in nursing, St. Louis, 1977, The C. V. Mosby Co.

Eckles, R.W., Carmichael, R.L., and Sarchet, B.R.: Essentials of management for first-line supervision, New York, 1974, John Wiley & Sons, Inc.

Feldman, D.C., and Arnold, H.J.: Managing individual and group behavior in organizations, New York, 1983, McGraw-Hill Book Co.

Fraser, L.P.: Contemporary staffing techniques in nursing, Norwalk, Conn., 1983, Appleton & Lange.

French, W.L.: The personnel management process, ed. 5, Boston, 1982, Houghton Mifflin Co.

Ganong, J.M., and Ganong, W.L.: Nursing management, Rockville, Md., 1980, Aspen Publishing Co.

Gillies, D.A.: Nursing management: a systems approach, Philadelphia, 1982, W.B. Saunders Co.

Hilliard, M.: Orientation and evaluation of the professional nurse, St. Louis, 1974, The C. V. Mosby Co.

Jelinek, R.C., Munson, F., and Smith, R.L.: SUM (Service Unit Management): an organizational approach to improved patient care, Battle Creek, Mich., 1971, W.K. Kellogg Foundation.

Kirk, R.K.: Nursing management tools, Boston, 1981, Little, Brown & Co.

Kron, T.: The management of patient care: putting leadership skills to work, Philadelphia, 1981, W.B. Saunders Co.

Laliberty, R., and Christopher, W.I.: Enhancing productivity in health care facilities, Owings Mills, Md., 1984, National Health Publishing.

MacVicar, J., and Boroch, R.: Approaches to staff development for departments of nursing: an annotated bibliography, New York, 1977, National League for Nursing (pub. no. 20-1658).

Marram, G., et al.: Cost-effectiveness of primary and team nursing, Wakefield, Mass., 1976, Aspen Publishing Co.

Marram, G.D., Schlegel, M.W., and Bevis, E.O.: Primary nursing: a model for individualized care, St. Louis, 1974, The C. V. Mosby Co.

Marriner, A.: Contemporary nursing management: issues and practice, St. Louis, 1982, The C. V. Mosby Co.

Mayer, G.G., and Bailey, K.: The middle manager in primary nursing, New York, 1982, Springer Publishing Co.

Meyer, D.: GRASP: a patient information and workload management system, Morgantown, N.C., 1978, MCS.

Newcomb, D.P., and Swansburg, R.C.: The team plan, New York, 1971, G.P. Putnam's Sons.

Osburn, H.G., and Manese, W.R.: How to install and validate employee selection techniques, Washington, D.C., 1971, American Petroleum Institute.

Popiel, E.S.: Nursing and the process of continuing education, ed. 2, St. Louis, 1977, The C. V. Mosby Co.

Price, E.M.: Staffing for patient care, New York, 1970, Springer Publishing Co.

Robbins, S.P.: Organizational behavior: concepts, controversies, and applications, ed. 3, Englewood Cliffs, N.J., 1986, Prentice-Hall, Inc.

Rowland, H.S., and Rowland, B.L.: Nursing administration handbook, ed. 2, Germantown, Md., 1985, Aspen Systems Corp.

Schindler-Rainman, E., Lippitt, R., and Cole, J.: Taking your meetings out of the doldrums, La Jolla, Calif., 1977, University Associates, Inc.

Schweiger, J.L.: The nurse as manager, New York, 1980, John Wiley & Sons, Inc.

Sheridan, R.S., Bronstein, J.E., and Walker, D.D.: The new nurse manager: a guide to management development, Rockville, Md., 1984, Aspen Systems Corp.

Simms, L.M., Price, S.A., and Ervin, N.E.: The professional practice of nursing administration, New York, 1985, John Wiley & Sons, Inc.

Staffing 2, Wakefield, Mass., 1975, Aspen Publishing Co.

Stevens, B.J.: The nurse as executive, ed. 2, Wakefield, Mass., 1980, Aspen Publishing Co.

Stewart, C.J., and Cash, W.B.: Interviewing: principles and practices, ed. 4, Dubuque, Iowa, 1985, W.C. Brown Co., Publishers.

Sullivan, E.J., and Decker, P.J.: Effective management in nursing, Reading, Mass., 1985, Addison-Wesley Publishing Co.

Swansburg, R.C.: A programed instruction book: in-service education, New York, 1968, G.P. Putnam's Sons.

Swansburg, R.C.: Team nursing: a programed learning experience, New York, 1968, G.P. Putnam's Sons.

Tobin, H.M., et al.: The process of staff development, ed. 2, St. Louis, 1979, The C. V. Mosby Co.

Veninga, R.L.: The human side of health administration, Englewood Cliffs, N.J., 1982, Prentice-Hall, Inc.

Vogt, J.F., et al.: Retaining professional nurses: a planned process, St. Louis, 1983, The C. V. Mosby Co.

Warstler, M.E., editor: Staffing: a journal of nursing administration reader, Wakefield, Mass., 1974, Contemporary Publishing, Inc.

Zurlage, C., editor: The nurse as personnel manager, Chicago, 1982, S-N Publications.

Journals

Selection of personnel

Carr, A.J.: Checklist for appointment of nursing staff, Nurs. Times **68**:85-87, June 1, 1972.

Ertl, N.: Choosing successful managers: participative selection can help, J. Nurs. Adm. **14**:(4)27–33, April 1984.

Esler, R.O.: Getting a new job, Am. J. Nurs. **81**:758-760, April 1981.

Filoromo, T.: Changing jobs? A look at employment agencies and executive search firms, Nurs. Econ. **1**:202–205, November-December 1983.

Fredericks, C.D.: Selection and placement of professional nurse applicants, Supervisor Nurse **10**:16-21, December 1979.

Hanger, T.I.: The employee process, Supervisor Nurse **5**:40-46, August 1974.

Johnson, E.P., Wagner, D.H., and Sweeney, J.P.: Identifying the right nurse manager: An objective selection process, J. Nurs. Adm. **14**:(11)24–30, November 1984.

Marriner, A.: The selection of personnel, Supervisor Nurse **7**:18-22, January 1976.

Mondy, R.W., and Mills, H.N.: Choice not chance in nurse selection, Supervisor Nurse **9**:35-38, November 1978.

Niederbaumer, L.: What the nursing service director expects, Nurs. Clin. North Am. **3**:99-110, March 1968.

Plaszczynski, L.: A systematic approach to leadership selection, J. Nurs. Adm. **9**:6-15, March 1979.

Roter, B.: Personnel selection: an update, Personnel J. **55**:23-37, January 1976.

Spurr, D.O., Maierle, M.A., and Haywood, L.J.: The anatomy of peer selection, J. Nurs. Adm. **10**:25-28, July 1980.

Sullivan, E.J., Decker, P.J., and Hailstone, S.: Assessment center technology: selecting head nurses, J. Nurs. Adm. **15**:(5)13–18, May 1985.

Recruitment and retention

Aiken, L.H.: The nurse labor market, J. Nurs. Adm. **14**:18-23, January 1984.

Bayley, E.W.: Breaking a turnover cycle—a successful approach, J. Nurs. Leadership Management **12**:19-21, March 1981.

Beauchamp, S.P.: Use supervisory personnel to recruit nurses! Supervisor Nurse **11**:36, December 1980.

Beyers, M., Mullner, R., Byre, C.S., and Whitehead, S.F.: Results of the nursing personnel survey. I. RN recruitment and orientation, J. Nurs. Adm. **13**:34-37, April 1983.

Beyers, M., Mullner, R., Byre, C.S., and Whitehead, S.F.: Results of the nursing personnel survey. II. RN vacancies and turnover, J. Nurs. Adm. **13**:26-31, May 1983.

Brief, A.P.: Turnover among hospital nurses: a suggested model, J. Nurs. Adm. **7**:55-58, October 1976.

Brief, A.P., Aldag, R.J., and Jacox, A.: A study: the impact of task characteristics on employee response in hospital nursing, Nurs. Adm. Q. 2:107-114, Summer 1978.

Brown, L.E., and Lewin B.A.: Supplemental staffing agencies: friend . . . or foe? Nurs. Management 13:37-47, September 1982.

Campbell, J.P., and Williams, T.: Marketing to nurses through an incentive program, J. Nurs. Adm. 13:9-12, October 1983.

Connelly, J.A., and Strauser, K.S.: Managing recruitment and retention problems: an application of the marketing process, J. Nurs. Adm. 13:17-22, October 1983.

Crout, T.K., and Crout, J.C.: Care plan for retaining the new nurse, Nurs. Management, 15:30-33, December 1984.

Deets, C., and Froebe, D.J.: Incentives for nurse employment, Nurs. Res. 33:242-246, July-August 1984.

Duxbury, M.L., and Armstrong, G.D.: Calculating nurse turnover indices, J. Nurs. Adm. 12:18-24, March 1982.

Felt, B.L.: Absenteeism in nursing, Nurs. Management 13:35-38, January 1982.

Fredericks, C.: Reversing the turnover trend, Nurs. Management 12:42-44, December 1981.

Ginzberg, E., et al.: Nurse discontent: the search for realistic solutions, J. Nurs. Adm. 12:7-11, November 1982.

Hill, B.S.: Retention crisis: staff development can help, Nurs. Management 13:20-21, January 1982.

Hofmann, P.B.: Accurate measurement of nursing turnover: the first step in its reduction, J. Nurs. Adm. 11:37-39, November-December 1981.

Johnston, P.F.: Head nurses as middle managers, J. Nurs. Adm. 13:22-26, November 1983.

Jones, B.M.: Focus: on the AHA's commission on nursing: nursing shortage, Nurs. Management 12:63-64, November 1981.

Kasprisin, C.A., and Young, W.B.: Nurse internship program reduces turnover, raises commitment, Nurs. Health Care 6:137-140, March 1985.

Massemino, L., Kilgallon, J., and Trelease, J.: Nurse day, Nurs. Management 12:32-33, December 1981.

McCloskey, J.: Influence of rewards and incentives on staff nurse turnover rate, Nurs. Res. 23:239-247, May-June 1974.

Mullner, R., Byre, C.S., and Whitehead, S.: Hospital vacancies, Am. J. Nurs. 82:592-594, April 1982.

Munro, B.H.: Young graduate nurses: who are they and what do they want? J. Nurs. Adm. 13:21-26, June 1983.

Murphy, E.C.: Practical management course, module 7: the bookends of management: hiring and firing, Nurs. Management 14:21-24, December 1983.

Nursing service problem: absenteeism and coverage, Regan Rep. Nurs. Law 16:4, January 1976.

The nursing shortage: current trends in recruitment and retention, Nurs. Careers 1:7-10, September 1980.

Rose, M.A.: Factors affecting nurse supply and demand: an exploration, J. Nurs. Adm. 12:31-34, February 1982.

Rotkovitch, R.: Employment opportunities: hiring a nurse. III. Am. J. Nurs. 74:680-681, April 1974.

Rozell, V.: The head nurse as a staff nurse satisfaction factor, Nurs. Adm. Q. 2:65-69, Fall 1977.

Seybolt, J.W.: Dealing with premature employee turnover, J. Nurs. Adm. 16:26-32, February 1986.

Seybolt, J.W., Pavett, C., and Walker, D.D.: Turnover among nurses: it can be managed, J. Nurs. Adm. 8:4-9, September 1978.

Smith, D.R.: Nursing shortage: some practical response please! Nurs. Management 14:38-40, November 1983.

Sredl, D.R.: Administrative turnover: total nursing turnover (tnt) = dynamite, Nurs. Management 13:24-30, November 1982.

Strilaeff, F.: Supervision and turnover of general staff nurses, Dimensions Health Service 53:36-39, November 1976.

Taylor, G.: How to use a headhunter, J. Nurs. Adm. 14:28-31, July-August 1984.

Wandelt, M.A., Pierce, P.M., and Widdowson, R.R.: Why nurses leave nursing and what can be done about it, Am. J. Nurs. 81:72-77, January 1981.

Watson, L.A.: Keeping qualified nurses, Supervisor Nurse 10:29-34, October 1979.

Weisman, C.S.: Recruit from within: hospital nurse retention in the 1980s, J. Nurs. Adm. 1:24-31, May 1982.

West, M.E.: Keeping talented RNs in hospital

practice, Nurs. Management **14**:38-44, August 1983.

Whitis, R., and Whitis, G.: The exit interview: a nursing management tool, J. Nurs. Adm. **13**:13-16, October 1983.

Wolf, G.A.: Nursing turnover: some causes and solutions, Nurs. Outlook **29**:233-236, April 1981.

Applications and résumés

Longest, B.B.: The application blank: a tool for reducing turnover, Hosp. Prog. **52**:71-96, July 1971.

Parker, M.C.: How to write your resume, Am. J. Nurs. **79**:1739-1741, October 1979.

Letters of reference

Creighton, H.: Law: for the nurse supervisor, Supervisor Nurse **10**:68-69, January 1979.

Cuthbert, B.L.: Please list three names . . . , Am. J. Nurs. **77**:1596-1599, October 1977.

Employment interview

Battle, E.H., et al.: Developing a rating interview guide, J. Nurs. Adm. **15**:39-45, October 1985.

Bowden, M.S., and Carbiener, A.O.: A team approach to interviewing, Supervisor Nurse **9**:14-26, November 1978.

Brydon, P.C., and Myli, A.R.: After the interview who gets the job? Am. J. Nurs. **84**:736-738, June 1984.

Dale, R., and Buley, K.E.: The group interview, Supervisor Nurse **9**:40-44, November 1978.

Goodale, J.G.: Tailoring the selection interview to the job, Personnel J. **53**:62-83, February 1976.

Hakel, M.D.: Similarity of post-interview trait rating intercorrelations as a contributor to interrater agreement in a structured employment interview, J. Appl. Psychol. **55**:443-448, 1971.

Kaiser, P.: Ten steps to interviewing job applicants, Am. J. Nurs. **78**:627-630, April 1978.

Kowalski, K.E.: Job interviewing: an effective tool for hiring staff nurses, Nurs. Digest **5**::58-62, Fall 1977.

LaRocco, S.: Interviewing and selecting staff, Nurs. Management **13**:22-24, September 1982.

Manfredi, C.: The interviewing and selection process, Supervisor Nurse **5**:22-27, May 1974.

Mondy, R.W., and Mills, H.N.: Choice not chance in nurse selection, Supervisor Nurse **9**:35-38, November 1978.

Parker, T.: How to develop skills in the use of interviewing techniques, Hosp. Top. **52**:10-15, November-December 1974.

Poteet, G.W.: The employment interview: avoiding discriminatory questioning, J. Nurs. Adm. **14**:38-42, April 1984.

Tebbit, B.V.: Preparing the interviewer, Supervisor Nurse **8**:44-48, April 1977.

Thomson, W.: Conducting an interview, Nurs. Times **68**:484-485, April 20, 1972.

Wagner, R.: The employment interview: a critical summary, Personnel Psychol. **11**:17-46, 1949.

Watkin, B.: Management topics: employment interviewing, Nurs. Mirror **138**:51, April 19, 1974.

Wright, O.R.: Summary of research on the selection interview since 1964, Personnel Psychol. **22**:391-413, 1969.

Job testing

Gerschefske, L.: Assessment and development for head nurse positions, Supervisor Nurse **11**:21-25, February 1980.

Orientation

Barnes, D.J., Harmon, P., and Kish, J.P.: A displacement orientation program: effects on transferred nurses, J. Nurs. Adm. **16**:45-50, July-August 1986.

Schofield, V.M.: Orientation of nurse executives, J. Nurs. Adm. **16**:13-17, November 1986.

Staff development

Charron, D.C.: Save the new graduate, Nurs. Management **13**:45-46, November 1982.

Dear, M.R., et al.: Evaluating a hospital nursing internship, J. Nurs. Adm. **12**:16-20, November 1982.

Sovie, M.D.: Fostering professional nursing careers in hospitals: the role of staff development. I. J. Nurs. Adm. **12**:5-10, December 1982.

Preceptorship

Chickerella, B.G., and Lutz, W.J.: Professional nurturance: preceptorships for undergraduate nursing students, Am. J. Nurs. **81**:107-109, January 1981.

Dell, M.S., and Griffith, E.: A preceptor program

for nurses' clinical orientation, J. Nurs. Adm. 7:37-38, January 1977.

Limón, S., Bargagliotti, L.A., and Spencer, J.B.: Who precepts the preceptor? Nurs. Health Care 2:433-436, October 1981.

Limón, S., Bargagliotti, L.A.,and Spencer, J.B.: Providing preceptors for nursing students: what questions should you ask? J. Nurs. Adm. 12:16-19, June 1982.

Limón, S., Spencer, J.B., and Waters, V.: A clinical preceptorship to prepare reality-based ADN graduates, Nurs. Health Care, 2:267-269, May 1981.

May, L.: Clinical preceptors for new nurses, Am. J. Nurs. 80:1824-1826, October 1980.

McGrath, B.J., and Koewing, J.R.: A clinical preceptorship for new graduate nurses, J. Nurs. Adm. 8:12-18, March 1978.

Mentorship

Atwood, A.H.: The mentor in clinical practice, Nurs. Outlook 27:714-717, November 1979.

Bolton, E.B.: A conceptual analysis of the mentor relationship in the career development of women, Adult Educ. 30:195-207, Summer 1980.

Cole, J.R.: Women in science, Am. Sci. 69:385-391, July-August 1981.

Darling, L.A.W.: Becoming a mentoring manager, J. Nurs. Adm. 15:43-44, June 1985.

Darling, L.A.W.: Can a non-bonder be an effective mentor? J. Nurs. Adm. 15:30-31, February 1985.

Darling, L.A.W.: The case for mentor moderation, J. Nurs. Adm. 15:42-43, July-August 1985.

Darling, L.A.W.: Cultivating minor mentors, J. Nurs. Adm. 15:41-42, September 1985.

Darling, L.A.W.: Endings in mentor relationships, J. Nurs. Adm. 15:40-41, November 1985.

Darling, L.A.W.: Mentors and mentoring, J. Nurs. Adm. 15:42-43, March 1985.

Darling, L.A.W.: Mentor matching, J. Nurs. Adm. 15:45-46, January 1985.

Darling, L.A.W.: Mentor types and life cycles, J. Nurs. Adm. 14:43-44, November 1984.

Darling, L.A.W.: Self-mentoring strategies, J. Nurs. Adm. 15:42-43, April 1985.

Darling L.A.W.: So you've never had a mentor . . . not to worry, J. Nurs. Adm. 14:38-39, December 1984.

Darling, L.A.W.: What do nurses want in a mentor? J. Nurs. Adm. 14:42-44, October 1984.

Darling, L.A.W.: What to do about toxic mentors, J. Nurs. Adm. 15:43-44, May 1985.

Hagerty, B.: A second look at mentors, Nurs. Outlook 34:16-19, 24, January-February 1986.

Hamilton, M.S.: Mentorhood: a key to nursing leadership, Nurs. Leadership 4:4-13, March 1981.

Heider (Campbell), N.: Do nurses need mentors? Image 18:110-113, Fall 1986.

Kelly, L.Y.: End paper: power guide—the mentor relationship, Nurs. Outlook 26:339, May 1978.

May, K.M., Meleis, A.I., and Winstead-Fry, P.: Mentorship for scholarliness: opportunities and dilemmas, Nurs. Outlook 30:22-28, January 1982.

Pilette, P.C.: Mentoring: an encounter of the leadership kind, Nurs. Leadership 3:22-26, June 1980.

Reskin, B.F.: Academic sponsorship and scientists' careers, Sociol. Educ. 52:129-146, July 1979.

Roche, G.R.: Much ado about mentors, Harvard Business Rev. 58:14-28, January-February 1979.

Schoor, T.: The lost art of mentorship, Am. J. Nurs. 78:1873, November 1978.

Vance, C.N.: The mentor connection, J. Nurs. Adm. 12:7-13, April 1982.

Team nursing

Allen, R.: Turning staff into a team, Nurs. 75 5:91-92, March 1975.

Brooks, E.: First seven years are the hardest, Am. J. Nurs. 49:276-280, May 1949.

Brooks, E.: Team nursing—1961, Am. J. Nurs. 61:88-91, April 1961.

Dolora, Sister M.: A team leader development program, Hosp. Prog. 48:104-108, October 1967.

Elizabeth, Sister R.: Team nursing, revised, Hosp. Prog. 45:112-120, July 1964.

Elizabeth, Sister R.: The team assignment plan, Hosp. Prog. 46:76-104, February 1975.

Fogt, J.: Team nursing: concepts and procedures, Hosp. Prog. 45:65-67, February 1964.

Fogt, J.: Team nursing: the team leader, Hosp. Prog. 45:104-106, March 1964.

Fosberg, G.C.: Teaching management skills in a team nursing setting, Nurs. Outlook 15:67-68, April 1967.

Germaine, A.: What makes team nursing tick? J. Nurs. Adm. **1**:46-49, 1971.

Kelly, P.A., and Lambert, K.L.: The effect of a modified team approach on nurse-patient interaction and job satisfaction, J. Nurs. Adm. **8**:3-9, April 1978.

Kramer, M.: Team nursing: a means or an end? Nurs. Outlook **19**:648-652, October 1971.

Kron, T.: Team nursing: how valid is it today? J. Nurs. Adm. **1**:19-22, 1971.

Lio, A.M.: Leadership and responsibility in team nursing, Nurs. Clin. North Am. **8**:267-281, June 1973.

O'Brien, M.: Team nursing in school health, Nurs. Outlook **17**:28-30, July 1969.

Parramore, B., and Yeager, W.: Team nursing in public health, Nurs. Outlook **16**:54-56, June 1968.

Radthe, M.,and Wilson, A.: Team conferences that work, Am. J. Nurs. **73**:506-508, March 1973.

Williams, M.: Myths and assumptions about team nursing, Nurs. Forum **3**:61-84, 1964.

Wyatt, L.J., and Hannah, H.D.: Does team nursing work in a psychiatric hospital? Am. J. Nurs. **64**:132-135, June 1964.

Primary nursing

Ahmed, M.C.: Professionalizing assignments, Nurs. Management **12**:45-48, October 1981.

Anderson, M.: Primary nursing in day-by-day practice, Am. J. Nurs. **76**:802-805, May 1976.

Anderson, M., and Choi, T.: Primary nursing in an organizational context, J. Nurs. Adm. **10**:26-31, March 1980.

Bailey, K., et al.: A tool for implementing primary nursing: a color-coded bulletin board, Supervisor Nurse **12**:56-58, August 1981.

Bakke, K.: Primary nursing: perceptions of a staff nurse, Am. J. Nurs. **74**:1432-1434, August 1974.

Beltran, H., et al.: An adaptation of primary nursing, Supervisor Nurse **10**:16-19, July 1979.

Betrus, A., et al.: Organizing for primary care in obstetrics, Nurs. Management **16**:31-33, November 1985.

Betz, M., Dickerson, T., and Wyatt, D.: Cost and quality: primary and team nursing compared, Nurs. Health Care **1**:150-157, October 1980.

Brown, B., editor: Primary nursing, Nurs. Adm. Q. **1**:79-85, Winter 1977.

Carey, R.G.: Evaluation of a primary nursing unit, Am. J. Nurs. **79**:1253-1255, July 1979.

Ciske, K.: Primary nursing: an organization that promotes professional practice, J. Nurs. Adm. **4**:28-31, 1974.

Ciske, K.: Primary nursing: evaluation, Am. J. Nurs. **74**:1436-1438, August 1974.

Ciske, K.: Misconceptions about staffing and patient assignment in primary nursing. IV. Nurs. Adm. Q. **1**:61-68, Winter 1977.

Ciske, K.L., Verhey, C.A., and Egan, E.C.: Improving peer relationships through contracting in primary nursing, J. Nurs. Adm. **13**:5-9, February 1983.

Corpuz, T.: Primary nursing meets needs, expectations of patients and staff, Hospitals **51**:95-96 + , June 1, 1977.

Culpepper, R.C., et al.: The effect of primary nursing on nursing quality assurance, J. Nurs. Adm. **16**:24-31, November 1986.

Daeffler, R.J.: Patients' perceptions of care under team and primary nursing, J. Nurs. Adm. **5**:20-26, 1975.

Dahlen, A.L.: With primary nursing we have it all together, Am. J. Nurs. **78**:426-428, March 1978.

Deiman, P.A., Noble, E., and Russell, M.E.: Achieving a professional practice model: how primary nursing can help, J. Nurs. Adm. **14**:16-21, July-August 1984.

Demers, P.M.: Developing a primary nurse, Nurs. Management **12**:28-30, December 1981.

Elpern, E.: Structural and organizational supports for primary nursing . . . Rush-Presbyterian–St. Luke's Medical Center, Nurs. Clin. North Am. **12**:205-219, June 1977.

Fairbanks, J.N.: Staffing a primary nursing unit, Nurs. Adm. Q. **1**:79-85, Summer 1977.

Felton, G.: Increasing the quality of nursing care by introducing the concept of primary nursing: a model project, Nurs. Res. **24**:27-32, 1975.

Fogleson, D.H.: Evaluating conversion to primary nursing, Nurs. Management **14**:25-26, August 1983.

Ingersoll, G.L.: Implementing primary nursing in a surgical outpatient department, Nurs. Management **15**:32-38, May 1984.

Jones, K.: Study documents effect of primary nursing on renal transplant patients, Hospitals **49**:85-89, 1975.

Kent, L.A., and Larson, E.: Evaluating the effectiveness of primary nursing practice, J. Nurs. Adm. **13**:34-41, January 1983.

Knecht, A.A.: Innovation on Four Tower West: why? Am. J. Nurs. **73**:809-810, May 1973.

Logsdon, A.: Why primary nursing? Nurs. Clin. North Am. **8**:283-291, 1973.

Manthey, M.: Primary nursing is alive and well in the hospital, Am. J. Nurs. **73**:83-87, January 1973.

Manthey, M., and Kramer, M.: A dialogue on primary nursing between Marie Manthey and Marlene Kramer, Nurs. Forum **9**:356-379, 1971.

Manthey, M., et al.: Primary nursing: a return to the concept of "my nurse" and "my patient," Nurs. Forum **9**:65-83, 1970.

Marram, G.D.: Innovation on Four Tower West: what happened? Am. J. Nurs. **73**:814-816, May 1973.

Marram, G.D.: The comparative costs of operating a team and primary nursing unit, J. Nurs. Adm. **6**:21-24, May 1976.

McAdam, E.: Primary nursing demands change, Nurs. Management **13**:50-53, May 1982.

McCarthy, D., and Schifalacqua, M.M.: Primary nursing: its implementation and six month outcome, J. Nurs. Adm. **8**:29-32, May 1978.

McGreevy, M.E., and Coates, M.R.: Primary nursing implementation using the project nurse and the nursing process framework, J. Nurs. Adm. **10**:9-15, February 1980.

Molke, T., and Schreiber, R.: A common-sense approach to primary nursing, Nurs. Management **13**:32-35, April 1982.

Mundinger, M.: Primary nurse: role evolution, Nurs. Outlook **21**:642-645, October 1973.

Mutchner, L.L.: How well are we practicing primary nursing? J. Nurs. Adm. **16**:8-13, September 1986.

O'Leary, J., and Hill, E.: Viewpoints: staffing a primary nursing unit, Nurs. Adm. Q. **1**:69-78, Summer 1977.

Osinski, E.G., and Morrison, W.H.: The all-RN staff, Supervisor Nurse **9**:66-74, September 1978.

Osinski, E., and Powals, J.G.: The all-RN staff three years later, Supervisor Nurse **9**:25-27, October 1978.

Page, M.: Primary nursing: perceptions of a head nurse, Am. J. Nurs. **74**:1435-1436, August 1974.

Paradise, R.L., and Kendall, V.M.: Ambulatory care: primary nursing brings continuity, Nurs. Management **16**:27-30, December 1985.

Reinkemeyer, Sister A.N.: It won't be hospital nursing, Am. J. Nurs. **68**:1936-1940, September 1968.

Robinson, M.A.: Primary nurse: specialist in total care, RN **37**:31-33, 1974.

Romero, M., et al.: Symposium on primary nursing: patient and staff perceptions as a basis for change . . . Rush-Presbyterian–St. Luke's Medical Center, Nurs. Clin. North Am. **12**:197-203, June 1977.

Schlegel, M.: Innovation on Four Tower West: how? Am. J. Nurs. **73**:811-813, May 1973.

Servellen, G.M.: Primary nursing: variations in practice, J. Nurs. Adm. **11**:40-46, September 1981.

Shukla, R.K.: Primary or team nursing? Two conditions determine the choice, J. Nurs. Adm. **12**:12-15, November 1982.

Spitzer, R.: Making primary nursing work, Supervisor Nurse **10**:12-14, January 1979.

Spoth, J.: Primary nursing: the agony and the ecstasy . . . Rush-Presbyterian–St. Luke's Medical Center, Nurs. Clin. North Am. **12**: 221-234, June 1977.

Steckel, S.B.: Introduction to the study of primary nursing, Nurs. Dimensions **7**:74-77, Winter 1980.

Steckel, S.B., Barnfather, J., and Owens, M.: Implementing primary nursing within a research design, Nurs. Dimensions **7**:78-81, Winter 1980.

Stegman, C.B., and Dison, C.C.: Changing service-education relationships: the impact of primary nursing, J. Nurs. Adm. **13**:26-29, March 1984.

van Servellen, G.M.: Primary nursing: variations in practice, J. Nurs. Adm. **11**:40-46, September 1981.

Weeks, L.C., Barrett, M., and Snead, C.: Primary nursing: teamwork is the answer, J. Nurs. Adm. **15**:21-26, September 1985.

Werner, J., et al.: Primary nursing: the Evanston story—primary nursing comes alive . . . the Evanston Hospital, Nurs. Adm. Q. **1**:9-50, Winter 1977.

Williams, L.: Evaluation of nursing care: a primary nursing project. I. Report of the controlled study, Supervisor Nurse **6**:32-39, January 1975.

Wobbe, R.: Primary versus team nursing, Supervisor Nurse **9**:34-37, March 1978.

Wolff, K.G.: Change: implementation of primary nursing through adhocracy, J. Nurs. Adm. **12**:24-27, December 1977.

Zander, K.S.: Primary nursing won't work . . . unless the head nurse lets it, J. Nurs. Adm. **12**:19-23, October 1977.

Zander, K.S.: Second generation primary nursing: a new agenda, J. Nurs. Adm. **15**:18-24, March 1985.

Leveling of staff

The composition of the nursing staff, Hospitals **43**:30, August 16, 1969.

Halloran, E.J.: RN staffing: more care—less cost, Nurs. Management **14**:18-22, September 1983.

Halloran, E.J., and Kiley, M.: Case mix management, Nurs. Management **15**:39-45, February 1984.

Hallstrom, B.J.: Utilization of nursing personnel: a task-specific approach, Nurs. Outlook **19**:664-667, October 1971.

Hinshaw A.S., Scofield, R., and Atwood, J.R.: Staff, patient, and cost outcomes of all-registered nurse staffing, J. Nurs. Adm. **11**:30-36, November-December 1981.

Lombard, H.: As I see it . . . what can nursing do to control costs? Am. Nurse **12**:11-13, June 1980.

Minetti, R., and Hutchinson, J.: System achieves optimal staffing, Hospitals **49**:61-64, May 1, 1975.

Minyard, K., Wall, J., and Turner, R.: Financial management series: RNs may cost less than you think, J. Nurs. Adm. **16**:28-35, May 1986.

Nicolaou, P.: The first professional degree: invest wisely (editorial), Michigan Nurse **55**:3, January 1982.

Norby, R.B., Freund, L.E., and Wagner, B.: A nurse staffing system based upon assignment difficulty, J. Nurs. Adm. **7**:2-24, November 1977.

Nursing service problem: utilization of nurses aides, Regan Rep. Nurs. Law **17**:4, October 1976.

Nursing service problem: volunteer nurses, Regan Rep. Nurs. Law **13**:4, September 1972.

Osinski, E.G., and Powals, J.G.: The all-RN staff three years later, Supervisor Nurse **9**:25-27, October 1978.

Osinski, E.G., and Powals, J.G.: The cost of all-RN staffed primary nursing, Supervisor Nurse **11**:16-21, January 1980.

Salkever, D.S., et al.: Episode-based efficiency comparisons for physicians and nurse practitioners, Med. Care **20**:143-153, February 1982.

Staffing

Aydelotte, M.K.: Staffing for high-quality care, Hospitals **47**:58-65, January 16, 1973.

Aydelotte, M.K.: Joint commission on accreditation of hospitals on nursing services: standard 1—staffing for quality care, J. Nurs. Adm. **3**:33-36, March-April 1973.

Charter, D.: How the Friesen concept affects nurse staffing, Can. Hosp. **47**:52-58, September 1970.

Christie, L.S.: Research staffing needs in psychiatric hospitals, Nurs. Times **70**:1870-1871, November 28, 1974.

Clark, E.L.: A model of nurse staffing, J. Nurs. Adm. **7**:22-27, February 1977.

Coulton, M.R.: Labor disputes: a challenge to nurse staffing, J. Nurs. Adm. **6**:15-20, May 1976.

Del Bueno, D.J.: Adapting staffing plans and standards to suit budgets, JOGN Nurs. **3**:26-29, September-October 1974.

Del Bueno, D.J., McLuckey, P., and Altano, R.: Staffing and patient care, Supervisor Nurse **4**:22-29, May 1973.

Dias, K., Dziekan, N.C., and Willis, B.: Work designs: extended shifts balance workloads—and budgets, too! Nurs. Management **17**:36-38, November 1986.

Eliopoulos, C.: Nurse staffing in long-term care facilities: the case against a high ratio of RNs, J. Nurs. Adm. **13**:29-31, October 1983.

Flynn, R.: Reflections on the midnight shift, Nurs. Management **14**:30-31, November 1983.

Froebe, D.: Scheduling: by team or individually, J. Nurs. Adm. **4**:34-36, May-June 1974.

Gale, D., and Roark, T.: Adaptability: a mobile nursing unit in-house, Nurs. Management **16**:48-50, November 1985.

Gates, N.: Planning and staffing an ENT unit, Nurs. Mirror **140**:52-57, May 1, 1975.

Hoffman, F.M.: Cost per RN hired, J. Nurs. Adm. **15**:27-29, February 1985.

Holdt, S.H.: Schedule yourself on all three shifts, Nurs. Management **14**:43-44, March 1983.

Holle, M.L.: Staffing: what the books don't tell you! Nurs. Management **13**:14-16, March 1982.

Hubbard, E.D., et al.: A proposed system for

scheduling nurses, Hosp. Adm. **20**:44-61, Fall 1975.

Kaye, G.H., and Krol, S.: This time . . . traditional responses won't work, Supervisor Nurse **12**:13-17, July 1981.

Keene, A.: On staffing advice for the new head nurse, Nurs. Management **14**:53-54, January 1983.

Latham, J., and Fagan, J.: Control of Christmas holiday census and staffing, J. Nurs. Adm. **9**:19-23, October 1979.

Lillesand, K., and Mathews, L.L.: The staffing function and management techniques, Nurs. Adm. Q. **1**:27-30, Summer 1977.

Miller, C.: Is staffing "realignment" just another word for "layoff"? RN **43**:113-124, September 1980.

Miller, M.L.: Implementing self-scheduling, J. Nurs. Adm. **14**:33-36, March 1984.

Monaghan, J.J., Perro, K.B., and Haran, M.L.: Critical care staff shortages, Nurs. Management **14**:38-39, January 1983.

Naber, M., Seizyk, J., and Wilde, N.: Standards + nursing care needs = staffing methodology, Nurs. Adm. Q. **2**:1-11, Fall 1977.

Norby, R.B., and Freund, L.E.: A model for nurse staffing and organizational analysis, Nurs. Adm. Q. **1**:1-13, Summer 1977.

Nursing service problem: summer vacation replacements, Regan Rep. Nurs. Law **13**:4, June 1972.

Nursing service problem: staffing shortages, Regan Rep. Nurs. Law **14**:4, December 1973.

Nursing service problem: chronic understaffing, Regan Rep. Nurs. Law **16**:4, July 1975.

On the scene: a family-centered approach to staffing, Nurs. Adm. Q. **2**:13-29, Fall 1977.

Panwar, S.: Introducing family-centered care for mothers and newborns, Nurs. Management **17**:45-47, November 1986.

Poole, P.: How nursing service can relieve staffing problems, Can. Hosp. **47**:42-43, July 1970.

Price, E.M.: Innovations in scheduling for the operating room, AORN J. **18**:983-996, November 1973.

Rustia, J., Wilson, C., and Quinn, J.: Use of physician-hired nurses: a survey, J. Nurs. Adm. **15**:35-40, September 1985.

Schmid, M., and Gerlach, C.: LDRP: staffing a single care maternity system, Nurs. Management **17**:36-40, August 1986.

Schmied, E.A.: Nurse staffing after hospitals merge, Nurs. Adm. Q. **2**:71-77, Fall 1977.

Segall, M., and Sauer, K.: Nurse staffing in the context of institutional and state level planning, Nurs. Adm. Q. **2**:39-50, Fall 1977.

Serdensky, S.M., Collins, K., and Hanrahan, S.: Evaluating staff nurse floating, Nurs. Success Today **3**:20-23, August 1986.

Shaheen, P.P.: Staffing and scheduling: reconcile practical means with the real goal, Nurs. Management **16**:64-72, October 1985.

Simendinger, E.A., and Gilbert, V.: Flexible staffing, Supervisor Nurse **10**:43-46, March 1979.

Smith, M.L.: Resource team: a staffing solution, Nurs. Management **12**:39-40, November 1981.

Somers, J.B.: Purpose and performance: a system analysis of nurse staffing, J. Nurs. Adm. **7**:4-9, February 1977.

Stanton, M.P., Laughlin, J.A., and Wheeler, C.E.: Do extended shifts satisfy nurses more? Nurs. Management **14**:49-52, October 1983.

Thorpe, R.: Cross-training program for nurses: a solution to a staffing problem, Supervisor Nurse **11**:65-67, October 1980.

Tomsky, C.N.: Acuity-based staffing controls costs, Nurs. Management **14**:36-37, October 1983.

Torrez, Sister M.R.: Systems approach to staffing, Nurs. Management **14**:54-58, May 1983.

Trofino, J.: Reducing work loads for staff nurses, Nurs. Management **13**:37-38, March 1982.

Vestal, K.W., and Dean, D.: Pulling staff: problem or solution? Supervisor Nurse **12**:44-46, September 1981.

Warner, D.M.: Nurse staffing, scheduling, and reallocation in the hospital, Hosp. Health Services Adm. **21**:77-90, Summer 1976.

Williams, A.: Student learning: team vs. primary nursing, Supervisor Nurse **12**:48-51, September 1981.

Williams, M.A., and Murphy, L.N.: Subjective and objective measures of staffing adequacy, J. Nurs. Adm. **9**:21-29, November 1979.

Wimpsett, J.: When the patient census climbs too high . . . , Nurs. Management **14**:28-31, June 1983.

Centralized scheduling

Ballantyne, D.J.: A computerized scheduling system with centralized staffing, J. Nurs. Adm. **9**:38-45, March 1979.

Duraiswamy, N., Welton, R., and Reisman, A.: Using computer simulation to predict ICU staffing needs, J. Nurs. Adm. **11**:39-44, February 1981.

Durham R.C.: How to schedule the nursing staff by computer, Hosp. Management **112**:16, September 1971.

Jackson, R.M., and Kortge, C.: Automated proficiency reports, Hospitals **45**:76-78, January 1, 1971.

Jacmen, C., and Stuerke, N.M.: Computerization helps solve staff scheduling problems, Nurs. Econ. **1**:209-211, November-December 1983.

Jelinek, R.C., Zinn, T.K., and Brya, J.R.: Tell the computer how sick the patients are and it will tell how many nurses they need, Mod. Hosp. **121**:81-85, December 1973.

Murray, D.J.: Computer makes the schedules for nurses, Mod. Hosp. **119**:104-105, December 1971.

Ross, B.T.: Computerized system aids staffing in strikes, Hospitals **49**:50-52, September 16, 1975.

Swanburg, G., and Smith, E.L.: Centralized scheduling: is it worth the effort? Nurs. Adm. Q. **1**:51-57, Summer 1977.

Tillock, E.E., Abendroth, W.W., and Clapp, G.D.: Central scheduling smooths the work flow, Mod. Hosp. **109**:123-166, September 1967.

Trout, F.: Central staffing office smooths personnel problems, Dimens. Health Serv. **52**:15-17, August 1975.

Decentralized scheduling

Althaus, J.N., et al.: Nurse staffing in a decentralized organization. I. J. Nurs. Adm. **12**:34-39, March 1982.

Althaus, J.N., et al.: Nurse staffing in a decentralized organization. II. J. Nurs. Adm. **12**:18-22, April 1982.

Burkhalter, P.: Staffing by complexes, Supervisor Nurse **4**:20-28, March 1973.

Fine, R.B.: Decentralization and staffing, Nurs. Adm. Q. **1**:59-66, Summer 1977.

Alternating or rotating work shifts

Felton, G.: Body rhythm effects on rotating work shifts, J. Nurs. Adm. **5**:16-19, March-April 1975.

Felton, G., and Patterson, M.G.: Shift rotation is against nature, Am. J. Nurs. **71**:760-763, April 1971.

Gibson, V.J.: Rotation of critical care nursing personnel, Supervisor Nurse **9**:15-17, May 1978.

Levenstein, A.: Art and science of management: shift rotation—a nursing challenge, Nurs. Management **13**:16-17, February 1982.

Patterson, M., and Felton, G.: Those nurses who won't rotate shifts may know what's good for them—and their patients, Mod. Hosp. **116**:123-128, April 1971.

Tonges, M.C., and Jones, E.N.: Interunit rotation: a chance to choose, Nurs. Management **16**:31-33, February 1985.

Permanent shifts

Rose, M.: Shift work: how does it affect you? Am. J. Nurs. **84**:442-447, April 1984.

Saunders, H.: Let's have permanent shifts, Can. Nurse **66**:21-22, June 1970.

Weaver, C.G.: A permanent day shift for staff, Nurs. Management **13**:30-32, February 1982.

Block or cyclical scheduling

Ellis, T.: If cyclical staffing pattern is too rigid, you may lose face—and some good employees, Mod. Hosp. **119**:109, August 1972.

Eusanio, P.L.: Effective scheduling—the foundation for quality care, J. Nurs. Adm. **13**:12-17, January 1978.

Gahan, K., and Talley, R.: A block scheduling system, J. Nurs. Adm. **5**:39-41, November-December 1975.

Morrish, A.R., and O'Connor, A.R.: Cyclic scheduling, Hospitals **44**:66-71, February 16, 1970.

Morrish, A.R., and O'Connor, A.R.: Cyclic scheduling, J. Nurs. Adm. **1**:49-54, September-October 1971.

Price, E.M.: Techniques to improve staffing, Am. J. Nurs. **70**:2112-2115, October 1970.

Price, E.M.: A study of innovative staffing, Hosp. Prog. **53**:67-72, January 1972.

Price, E.M.: Staffing: the most basic nursing service problem, Supervisor Nurse **6**:26-31, July 1975.

Warstler, M.E.: Cyclic work schedules and a nonnurse coordinator of staffing, J. Nurs. Adm. **3**:45-51, November-December 1973.

Ten-hour day, four-day workweek

Bauer, J.: Clinical staffing with a 10-hour day, 4-day workweek, J. Nurs. Adm. **1**:12-14, November-December 1971.

Four-day workweek? Oh, those long weekends! RN **35**:42-45, January 1972.

Shaw, P.: The 10-hour day in the 4-day week, Supervisor Nurse **9**:47-56, October 1978.

Ten-hour day plus five- or six-hour shift

Colt, A.M., and Corley, T.F.: What nurses think of the 10-hour shift, Hospitals **48**:134-142, February 1, 1974.

Minor, M.A.: Ten- and 6-hour nursing shifts solve staffing problem, Hosp. Prog. **52**:62-66, July 1971.

Ricci, J.A.: Ten-hour night shift: cost vs. cost savings, Nurs. Management **15**:34-42, January 1984.

Ten-hour shift, seven-day workweek

Aft, L.S., Watt, J.R., and Thomason, C.Y.: Scheduling 7-day weeks poses equity problems, Hospitals **49**:93-96, September 1, 1975.

Boyarski, R.P.: Nursing workweek equalizes shifts, time off, Hosp. Prog. **57**:36-45, July 1976.

Cleveland, R.T., and Hutchins, C.L.: Seven days' vacation every other week, Hospitals **48**:81-85, August 1, 1974.

Deans, J.H., and McSwain, G.: Nurses have more time on, more time off, with seven-day week scheduling, Mod. Hosp. **118**:107-108, June 1972.

DeMarsh, K.G., and McLellan, E.I.: Nurses sold on shortened workweek, Can. Hosp. **48**:64-65, November 1971.

Hutchins, C., and Cleveland, R.: For staff nurses and patients—the 7-70 plan, Am. J. Nurs. **78**:230-233, February 1978.

Price, E.M.: Seven days on and seven days off, Am. J. Nurs. **81**:1142-1143, June 1981.

Stinson, S.M., and Hazlett, C.B.: Nurse and physician opinion of a modified workweek trial, J. Nurs. Adm. **5**:21-26, September 1975.

Twelve-hour shift

Cales, A.D.: A twelve-hour schedule experiment, Supervisor Nurse **7**:71-76, June 1976.

Ganong, W.L., Ganong, J.M., and Harrison, E.T.: The 12-hour shift: better quality, lower cost, J. Nurs. Adm. **6**:17-29, February 1976.

The good and bad of twelve-hour shifts, RN **38**:47-52, September 1975.

Hoffman, T., and Fischer, S.: Weekend sched-uling: the 12-hour shift, Dimensions Crit. Care Nurs. **2**:171-173, May-June 1983.

Mech, A., Mills, M.E., and Arnold, B.: Wage and hour laws: their impact on 12-hour scheduling, J. Nurs. Adm. **14**:24-25, March 1984.

Ryan, S.M.: The modified workweek for nursing staff on two pediatric units, J. Nurs. Adm. **5**:31-34, July-August 1975.

Ryan, S.M.: The modified workweek for nursing staff on two pediatric units, Nurs. Digest **4**:29-31, November-December 1976.

Underwood, A.B.: What a 12-hour shift offers, Am. J. Nurs. **75**:1176-1178, July 1975.

Vik, A.G., and MacKay, R.C.: How does the 12-hour shift affect patient care? J. Nurs. Adm. **12**:11-14, January 1982.

Baylor plan

Alivizatos, M.S.: A new concept in scheduling for nurses, Supervisor Nurse **12**:20-22, February 1981.

Dison, C.C., Carter, N., and Bromley, P.: Making the change to flex time, Am. J. Nurs. **81**:2162-2164, December 1981.

Henson, L.: Baylor's two days alternative—today, Am. J. Nurs. **84**:936-938, July 1984.

Variations

Arnold, B., and Mills, M.E.: Core-12: Implementation of flexible scheduling, J. Nurs. Adm. **13**:9-14, July-August 1983.

Braun, A.E., and Schweiger, J.L.: Proper staffing schedules: a must for coronary care, **14**:27-28, October 1983.

The demise of the traditional 5-40 workweek? Am. J. Nurs. **81**:1138-1141, June 1981.

Imig, S.I., Powell, J.A., and Thorman, K.: Primary nursing and flexi-staffing: do they mix? Nurs. Management **15**:39-42, August 1984.

McGillick, K.: Modifying schedules makes jobs more satisfying, Nurs. Management **14**:53-55, December 1983.

Ross, M.: Shift: how does it affect you? Am. J. Nurs. **8**:442-447, April 1984.

Roy, M.J., and Runge, E.: Flexi-hour nurses, Nurs. Management **14**:54-56, September 1983.

Patient classification systems

Alward, R.R.: Patient classification systems: the ideal vs. reality, J. Nurs. Adm. **13**:14-19, February 1983.

Anderson, B.: The numbers game: personnel

staffing, Supervisor Nurse 5:13-19, February 1974.

Auger, J.A., and Dee, V.: A patient classification system based on the behavioral system model of nursing. I. J. Nurs. Adm. 13:38-43, April 1983.

Barham, V.Z., and Schneider, W.R.: Matrix: a unique patient classification system, J. Nurs. Adm. 10:25-31, December 1980.

Barr, A., Moores, B., and Rhys-Hearn, C.: A review of the various methods of measuring the dependency of patients on nursing staff, Int. J. Nurs. Stud. 10:195-208, August 1973.

Billings, D.M.: Patient classification in critical care, Dimensions Crit. Care Nurs. 2:36-43, January-February 1983.

Chagnon, M., et al.: Validation of patient classification through evaluation of the nursing staff degree of occupation, Med. Care 16:465-475, June 1978.

Clayton, A., and St. Germain, D.: A four-year experience with GRASP. I, Dimensions, 8-11, November 1981.

Clayton, A., and St. Germain, D.: A four-year experience with GRASP. II, Dimensions, 24-26, December 1981.

Cochran, Sister J.: Refining a patient-acuity system over four years, Hosp. Prog. 60:56-60, February 1979.

Cochran, Sister J., and Derr, D.: Patient acuity system for nurse staffing, Hosp. Prog. 56:51-54, November 1975.

Costello, S., and Summers, B.Y.: Documenting patient care: getting it all together, Nurs. Management 16:31-34, June 1985.

Dale, R.L., and Mable, R.J.: Nursing classification system: foundation for personnel planning and control, J. Nurs. Adm. 13:10-13, February 1983.

Daubert, E.A.: Patient classification system and outcome criteria, Nurs. Outlook 27:450-454, July 1979.

Davis, A.: Classifying rehabilitation patients, Nurs. Management 14:47-51, February 1983.

Dee, V., and Auger, J.A.: A patient classification system based on the behavioral system model of nursing. II. J. Nurs. Adm. 13:18-23, May 1983.

Des Ormeaux, S.P.: Implementation of the C.A.S.H. patient classification system for staffing determination, Supervisor Nurse 8:29-35, April 1977.

Dijkers, M., and Paradise, T.: PCS: one system for both staffing and costing, Nurs. Management 17:25-34, January 1986.

Donnelly, L.J.: Patient classification: an effective management tool, Nurs. Management 12:42-43, November 1981.

Ebener, M.K.: Reliability and validity basics for evaluating classification systems, Nurs. Econ. 3:324-327, November-December 1985.

Eklof, M., and Qu, W.: Validating a psychiatric patient classification system, J. Nurs. Adm. 16:10-17, May 1986.

Evans, C.L.S.: A practical staffing calculator, Nurs. Management 15:68-69, April 1984.

Evans, S.K., Laundon, T., and Yamamoto, W.G.: Projecting staffing requirements for intensive care units, J. Nurs. Adm. 10:34-42, July 1980.

Fine, R.B.: Controlling nurses' workloads, Am. J. Nurs. 74:2206-2207, December 1974.

Fray, C.P.: An accountability—classification instrument for orthopaedic patients, J. Nurs. Adm. 14:32-39, July-August 1984.

Giovannetti, P., and Mayer, G.M.: Building confidence in patient classification systems, Nurs. Management 15:31-34, August 1984.

Grohar, M.E., Myers, J., and McSweeney, M.: A comparison of patient acuity and nursing resource use, J. Nurs. Adm. 16:19-23, June 1986.

Hearn, C.R.: Evaluation of patients' nursing needs: prediction of staffing. III, Nurs. Times 77-80, October 3, 1974.

Hearn, C.R.: Evaluation of patients' nursing needs: prediction of staffing. IV, Nurs. Times 81-84, October 10, 1974.

Hoffman, F., and Wakefield, D.S.: Ambulatory care patient classification, J. Nurs. Adm. 16:23-30, April 1986.

Jackson, B.S., and Resnich, J.: Comparing classification systems, Nurs. Management 13:13-19, November 1982.

Jelinek, R.C., Zinn, T.K., and Brya, J.R.: Tell the computer how sick the patients are and it will tell how many nurses they need, Mod. Hosp. 121:81-85, December 1973.

Johnson, K.: A practical approach to patient classification, Nurs. Management 15:39-46, June 1984.

Martin, K.: A client classification system adaptable for computerization, Nurs. Outlook 30:515-517, November-December 1982.

Matthews, A.: Patient allocation: a review, Nurs. Times **71**:65-68, July 10, 1975.

Matthews, A.: Patient allocation. II, Nurs. Times **71**:69-72, July 17, 1975.

Matthews, A.: Patient allocation. III, Nurs. Times **71**:73-76, July 24, 1975.

Matthews, A.: Patient allocation. IV, Nurs. Times **71**:77-79, July 31, 1975.

McWhirt, F.D.: Staffing in a psychiatric unit, Supervisor Nurse **8**:27-33, December 1977.

Meijers, A.: Nursing: using workload measurement systems, Dimensions 49, September 1983.

Meyer, D.: Workload management system ensures stable nurse-patient ratio, Hospitals **52**:81-85, March 1978.

Mills, R.: A simple method for predicting days of increased patient census, J. Nurs. Adm. **7**:15-20, February 1977.

Mina, E.S.: P.R.N.: the choice of Toronto General, Dimensions 22-24, November 1981.

Nyberg, J., and Simler, M.: Developing a framework for an integrated nursing department, J. Nurs. Adm. **9**:9-15, November 1979.

O'Connor, T.J., and Efurd, N.: System predicts patient census, forecasts staffing needs, costs, Hospitals **52**:95-101, March 16, 1978.

O'Donnovan, T.R.: A penetration coefficient approach to nursing staffing, Nurs. Adm. Q. **2**:31-38, Fall 1977.

Pardee, G.: Classifying patients to predict staff requirements, Am. J. Nurs. **68**:517-520, March 1968.

Plummer, J.: Patient classification proves staffing needs, Dimens. Health Serv. **53**:36-38, May 1976.

Price, J.: Patient care classification system, Nurs. Outlook **20**:445-448, July 1972.

Rahr, V.: Rationale for determining staffing patterns: what's missing, Supervisor Nurse **4**:60-66, May 1973.

Ramey, I.G.: Eleven steps to proper staffing, Hospitals **27**:98-104, March 16, 1973.

Regnery, G.: Patient care needs: an index for community health staffing, Nurs. Adm. Q. **2**:79-89, Fall 1977.

Reinert, P., and Grant, D.R.: A classification system to meet today's needs, J. Nurs. Adm. **11**:21-25, January 1981.

Reitz, J.A.: Toward a comprehensive nursing intensity index. I. Development, Nurs. Management **16**:21-30, August 1985.

Reitz, J.A.: Toward a comprehensive nursing intensity index. II. Testing, Nurs. Management **16**:31-42, September 1985.

Roehrl, P.K.: Patient classification: a pilot test, Supervisor Nurse **9**:21-25, February 1979.

Ryan, T., Barker, B.L., and Marciante, F.A.: A system for determining appropriate nurse staffing, J. Nurs. Adm. **5**:30-38, June 1975.

Sawyer, J., Levy, J., Harris, C., and Dixon, B.: Indirect hours of care per patient per day in a Midwest extended care facility, Nurs. Management **17**:52-60, October 1986.

Schroder, P.J., et al.: Testing validity and reliability in a psychiatric patient classification system, Nurs. Management **17**:49-54, January 1986.

Smith, C.A.: Adequate staffing: it's more than a game of numbers, Nurs. Adm. Q. **1**:15-25, Summer 1977.

Tarcinale, M.A.: Patient classification: cutting the margin of human error, Nurs. Management **17**:49-51, October 1986.

Thornton, L.M.R.: Nursing algorithms, J. Nurs. Adm. **15**:11-15, January 1985.

Unger, J.: Building a classification system that works, J. Nurs. Adm. **15**:18-24, July-August 1985.

Vanputte, A.W., et al.: Accounting for patient acuity: the nursing time dimension, Nurs. Management **16**:27-36, October 1985.

Vaughan, R.G., and MacLeod, V.: Comparing acuity among hospitals: who has the sickest patients? J. Nurs. Adm. **15**:25-28, May 1985.

Vaughan, R.G., and MacLeod, V.: Nurse staffing studies: no need to reinvent the wheel, J. Nurs. Adm. **10**:9-15, March 1980.

Warstler, M.E.: Some management techniques for nursing service administrators, J. Nurs. Adm. **2**:25-34, November-December 1972.

Williams, M.A.: Quantification of direct nursing care activities: J. Nurs. Adm. **7**:15-18, October 1977.

Wolf, G.A., Lesic, L.K., and Leak, A.G.: Primary nursing: the impact on nursing costs within DRGs, J. Nurs. Adm. **16**:9-11, March 1986.

Staffing formulas

Carr, A.J.: Workload and staffing on night duty, Nurs. Times **72**:105-108, July 29, 1976.

Cleland, V.: Relating nursing staff quality to patients' needs, J. Nurs. Adm. **12**:32-37, April 1982.

Duckett, S.: Nurse rostering with game theory, J. Nurs. Adm. **7**:58-59, January 1977.

Finlayson, H.: The numbers approach to nursing management, Dimensions **53**:39-44, May 1976.

Fraser, L.P.: The reconstructed worksheet: one

answer to the scheduling dilemma, J. Nurs. Adm. **2**:12-16, September-October 1972.

Hanson, R.L.: Staffing statistics: their use and usefulness, J. Nurs. Adm. **12**:29-35, November 1982.

Hanson, R.L., and Cleland, V.: Dialogue in print: relating nursing staff quality to patients' needs, J. Nurs. Adm. **12**:29-31, September 1982.

Harman, R.J.: Nursing services information system, J. Nurs. Adm. **7**:14-20, March 1977.

Harris, D.H.: Nursing staffing requirements, Hospitals **44**:64-70, April 16, 1970.

Kaplan, R.S.: Approaches and techniques: analysis and control of nurse staffing, Health Services Res. **10**:278-296, Fall 1975.

McNally, J.K.: SCANS analyzes daily staffing patterns, Mod. Hosp. **116**:115-116, May 1971.

Miller, E.A.: Staffing with the aid of dependency indices, Nurs. Times **72**:113-115, August 12, 1976.

Nield, M.: Developing a projected nurse staffing program, Supervisor Nurse **6**:17-24, July 1975.

O'Donovan, T.R.: A penetration coefficient approach to nursing staffing, Nurs. Adm. Q. **2**:31-38, Fall 1977.

Spruill, M.L., Wallace, M.J., and Glasberg, A.: Staffing cost analysis technique (SCAT), Managerial Planning **26**:32-38, May-June 1978.

Part-time staff

Amenta, M.M.: Staffing through temporary help agencies, Supervisor Nurse **8**:19-25, December 1977.

Boyer, C.M.: The use of supplemental nurses: why, where, how? J. Nurs. Adm. **9**:56-60, March 1979.

Chaska, N.L., et al.: A joint effort to mediate the "outside source" staffing dilemma, J. Nurs. Adm. **10**:13-18, December 1980.

DiPaolo, V.: Predicting contracts to increase by one-third, Mod. Health Care **8**:50-52, July 1977.

Duffus, A.J., and Smith, N.: Temporary staffing service: an answer to fluctuating needs in hospital staffing, Hosp. Top. **54**:43-48, November-December 1976.

Fisher, D.W., and Thomas, E.: A "premium day" approach to weekend nurse staffing, J. Nurs. Adm. **4**:59-60, September-October 1974.

Jett, M.: Use of temporary nursing personnel as cost-control measure, Hosp. Top. **55**:48-50, July-August 1977.

Johnson, P.D., and Marcella, M.J.: Part-time nursing employment: worry or worth? Supervisor Nurse **8**:34-36, January 1977.

Kehrer, B.H., Deiman, P.A., and Szapiro, N.: The temporary nursing service RN, Nurs. Outlook **32**:212-217, July-August 1984.

Langford, T., and Prescott, P.A.: Hospitals and supplemental nursing agencies: an uneasy balance, J. Nurs. Adm. **9**:16-20, November 1979.

Letter to the editor, J. Nurs. Adm. **11**:4 + , October 1977.

Lewin, B.A., and Brown, L.E.: Monitoring supplemental staffing agencies, Supervisor Nurse **12**:56-63, September 1981.

Luneski, I.D.: Temporary nursing: is it for you? RN **36**:46-50, September 1973.

Marriner, A.: Variables affecting staffing, Supervisor Nurse **10**:62-65, September 1979.

Prescott, P.A.: Supplemental nursing services: how much do hospitals really pay? Am. J. Nurs. **82**:1208-1213, August 1982.

Prescott, P.A., and Langford, T.L.: Supplemental nursing service: boon or bane? Am. J. Nurs. **79**:2140-2144, December 1979.

Prescott, P.A., et al.: Supplemental nursing service: who uses them, who does not? Am. J. Nurs. **82**:1714-1717, November 1982.

Rinker, K.L., Norris, C.L., and Jordan, M.F.: "Bed and bath teams": one solution to the weekend staffing shortage, J. Nurs. Adm. **5**:34-35, May 1975.

Shanks, K., and Potempa, K.: A system for using supplemental staff, J. Nurs. Adm. **11**:41-46, October 1981.

Stover, W.R.: Temporary nurse service, Am. J. Nurs. **75**:1998-1999, November 1975.

Thompson, D.D.: Supplemental staffing: can it be cost-effective? Hospitals **55**:74-77, March 16, 1981.

Trivedi, V.M., and Warner, D.M.: A branch and bound algorithm for optimum allocation of float nurses, Management Sci. **22**:972-981, May 1976.

Trout, F.: Placement service would cure staffing ills, Dimens. Health Serv. **52**:13-14, July 1975.

Wakefield, D.S., and Mathis, S.: Formulating a managerial strategy for parttime nurses, J. Nurs. Adm. **15**:35-39, January 1985.

Wiley, L.: Career guide: should you join a rent-a-nurse for temporary service? Nursing 76 **6**:81-88, September 1976.

PART
4

DIRECT

────────────── **OBJECTIVES** ──────────────

After completing this part, the reader will be able to:

Name at least five theories of leadership.

Discuss the development of management thought.

Identify at least five sources of power.

Discuss the political process.

Compare conflict resolution strategies.

Assess motivational factors.

Assist with communication processes.

Do transactional analysis.

Behave assertively.

────────────── **STUDY QUESTIONS** ──────────────

1
What are five theories of leadership?
2
How has management thought evolved?
3
What are sources of power?
4
How can one get involved in politics?
5
What strategies help resolve conflict?
6
How can personnel be motivated?
7
What are pros and cons of various communication channels?
8
What is transactional analysis?
9
What are assertiveness techniques?

NATURE AND PURPOSE OF DIRECTING

After the manager has planned, organized, and staffed, she must direct personnel and activities to accomplish the goals of the organization. Knowledge of one's leadership style, managerial philosophy, sources of power and authority, and political strategies is important. To get the work done by others, the manager must deal with conflict and motivate and discipline staff; all of these tasks require good communication skills and assertive behavior.

THEORIES OF LEADERSHIP

Nursing is not recognized for the leaders it produces. Rather, leadership—the ability to lead, guide, direct, or show the way—is a quality often lacking in the nursing profession. The reasons are several. Nursing seems to attract people who rank lower in self-esteem and initiative and higher in submissiveness and need for structure than people in other occupations. Schools of nursing have placed little emphasis on teaching leadership, and what education has been offered has often been taught in an apprenticeship manner. Moreover, the autocratic leadership style, so prevalent in nursing, does not foster leadership in others. Instead, it contributes to the belief that nurses are paid to follow orders rather than to think.

Most nurses are female, and role conflicts are common. A woman must maintain heavy responsibilities to run a household, raise a family, and pursue a leadership role in nursing. Leadership is associated with aggressiveness, which traditionally has been considered a masculine characteristic, whereas passivity has been thought to be a feminine trait. When a nurse does accept a position of leadership, she may find it less than rewarding. More than likely, her primary reason for choosing a career in nursing was to work directly with patients, but her new role blocks fulfillment of her initial goal. The high attrition rate in nursing is directly related to this conflict. For many, the frustrations over role contradictions and the stifling atmosphere of an autocratic system are too much to endure. Unable to tolerate the barriers to service and self-fulfillment, many potential nursing leaders leave the field.

The problem of role conflicts in an autocratic system can be reduced by a greater emphasis on leadership in nursing education and service. Theories of leadership are numerous. The following survey covers the alternatives, beginning with the oldest notion and advancing to ideas currently in vogue. By familiarizing herself with them, the nurse can select and adapt the most suitable approach for dealing with different situations. As a role model herself, the nursing leader can reduce the autocratic atmosphere and, hence, some of the role conflicts.

Great man theory

The great man theory argues that few people are born with the necessary characteristics to be great. Leaders are well rounded and simultaneously display both instrumental and supportive leadership behavior. Instrumental activities include planning, organizing, and controlling the activities of subordinates to accomplish the organization's goals. Obtaining and allocating resources such as people, equipment, materials, funds, and space are particularly important. Supportive leadership is socially oriented and allows for participation and consultation from subordinates for decisions that affect them. People who use both instrumental and supportive leadership behaviors are considered "great men" and supposedly are effective leaders in any situation. Many find this theory unattractive because of its premise that leaders are born and not made, which suggests that leadership cannot be developed.

Charismatic theory

A person may be a leader because she is charismatic, but relatively little is known about this intangible characteristic. What constitutes charisma? Most agree that it is an inspirational quality possessed by some people that makes others feel better in their presence. The charismatic leader inspires others by obtaining emotional commitment from followers and by arousing strong feelings of loyalty and enthusiasm. Under charismatic leadership, one may overcome obstacles not thought possible. However, because charisma is so elusive, some may sense it while others do not.

Trait theory

Until the mid-1940s, the trait theory was the basis for most leadership research. Early work in this area maintained that traits are inherited, but later theories suggested that traits could be obtained through learning and experience. Researchers identified the leadership traits as energy, drive, enthusiasm, ambition, aggressiveness, decisiveness, self-assurance, self-confidence, friendliness, affection, honesty, fairness, loyalty, dependability, technical mastery, and teaching skill. Asking themselves what traits leaders possessed, various researchers arrived at different conclusions, but identified some common leadership traits:

1. Leaders need to be more intelligent than the group they lead. However, a highly intelligent person may not find leadership responsibilities challenging enough, may prefer to work with abstract ideas and research, and may have difficulty relating to the group.
2. Leaders must possess initiative, the ability to perceive and start courses of action not considered by others.

3. Creativity is an asset. Having originality, the ability to think of new so-lutions to problems and ideas of new ways to be productive, is helpful.

4. Emotional maturity with integrity, a sense of purpose and direction, per-sistence, dependability, and objectivity, is another important trait. Mature leaders do what they say they will and are consistent in their actions. They often work long hours, apply themselves intensely, and spread enthusi-asm to followers. Energy, drive, and good health are necessary to endure the long hours, overcome obstacles, and sustain continuous achievement. Self-assurance is self-confidence. It is hoped that the leader perceives her-self as an effective problem solver who can successfully handle the diffi-culties that confront her.

5. Communication skills are important. The leader needs to perceive the meaning of messages from others and to speak and write clearly.

6. Persuasion often is used by leaders to gain the consent of followers. The leader may make suggestions, supply supportive data, ask penetrating questions, make compromises, and request action to persuade others.

7. Leaders need to be perceptive enough to distinguish their allies from their opponents and to place their subordinates in suitable positions.

8. Leaders participate in social activities. They can socialize with all kinds of people and adapt to various groups. Approachable, friendly, and helpful, they gain the confidence and loyalty of others in such a way that makes people willing to cooperate.

The trait theory expanded knowledge about leadership, but it was not with-out its flaws. Few, if any, traits are identified in all trait theory research. They are not mutually exclusive, and there is considerable overlap between categories or definitions of the characteristics. It is not clear which traits are most important, which traits are needed to acquire leadership, and which traits are needed to maintain it. Trait theory does not view personality as an integrated whole, does not deal with subordinates, and avoids environmental influences and situational factors.

Situational theories

Situational theories became popular during the 1950s. These theories suggest that the traits required of a leader differ according to varying situations. Among the variables that determine the effectiveness of leadership style are factors such as the personality of the leader; the performance requirements of both the leader and followers; the attitudes, needs, and expectations of the leader and followers; the degree of interpersonal contact possible; time pressures; physical environ-ment; organizational structure; the nature of the organization; the state of the organization's development; and the influence of the leader outside of the group. A person may be a leader in one situation and a follower in another or

---

Table 2.   Group-atmosphere scale

Describe the atmosphere of your group by checking the following items:

	8	7	6	5	4	3	2	1	
1. Friendly	:___:___:___:___:___:___:___:								Unfriendly
2. Accepting	:___:___:___:___:___:___:___:								Rejecting
3. Satisfying	:___:___:___:___:___:___:___:								Frustrating
4. Enthusiastic	:___:___:___:___:___:___:___:								Unenthusiastic
5. Productive	:___:___:___:___:___:___:___:								Nonproductive
6. Warm	:___:___:___:___:___:___:___:								Cold
7. Cooperative	:___:___:___:___:___:___:___:								Uncooperative
8. Supportive	:___:___:___:___:___:___:___:								Hostile
9. Interesting	:___:___:___:___:___:___:___:								Boring
10. Successful	:___:___:___:___:___:___:___:								Unsuccessful

From Fiedler, F.E.: A theory of leadership effectiveness, New York, 1967, McGraw-Hill Book Co., p. 269.

---

a leader at one time and a follower at others, because the type of leadership needed depends on the situation.

Contingency theory

During the 1960s, Fred Fiedler (1922-   ) introduced the contingency model of leadership. Refuting the ideal leadership style theory, he argued that a leadership style will be effective or ineffective, dependent on the situation. He identified three aspects of a situation that structure the leader's role: (1) leader-member relations, (2) task structure, and (3) position power.

Leader-member relations involve the amount of confidence and loyalty the followers have in their leader. Leadership is assessed by a group-atmosphere scale. Fiedler also used a sociometric index of the least-preferred co-worker (LPC) score (Table 2). Followers were asked to think of everyone they have ever worked with and to rate the least-preferred co-worker on an eight-point bipolar adjective scale, which includes adjectives such as friendly and cooperative. A high score describes the person in favorable terms, and a low score is a negative rating. Although the LPC scores are difficult to interpret and it is hard to say what they measure, Fiedler suggests that high scorers are relationship oriented and low scorers are mostly task oriented.

Task structure is high if it is easy to define and measure a task. The structure is low if it is difficult to define the task and to measure progress toward its completion. Fiedler used four criteria to determine the degree of task structure: (1) goal clarity— goal understood by followers; (2) the extent to which a decision can be verified—know who is responsible for what; (3) multiplicity of goal paths—number of solutions; and (4) specificity of solution—number of correct

Table 3. Summary of Fiedler investigations of leadership

	Group situation			Leadership style correlating with productivity
Condition	Leader-member relations	Task structure	Position power	
1	Good	Structured	Strong	Directive
2	Good	Structured	Weak	Directive
3	Good	Unstructured	Strong	Directive
4	Good	Unstructured	Weak	Permissive
5	Moderately poor	Structured	Strong	Permissive
6	Moderately poor	Structured	Weak	No data
7	Moderately poor	Unstructured	Strong	No relationship found
8	Moderately poor	Unstructured	Weak	Directive

From Donnelly, J.H., Jr.: Gibson, J.L., and Ivancevich, J.M.: Fundamentals of management: functions, behavior, models Dallas, Tex.: Business Publications, 1981. © 1981 by Business Publications, Inc.

answers. Technical nursing, which focuses on procedures, may have a high task structure, but situations involving human relations and value judgments may have numerous solutions with no specific correct answer and consequently have low task structure.

Position power refers to the authority inherent in a position, the power to use rewards and punishment, and the organization's support of one's decisions. Directors of nursing, supervisors, and sometimes head nurses have high position power with the right to hire and fire, promote, and adjust salaries. People with low position power may be elected, function in an acting position, or be subject to removal by peers or subordinates. Elected committee chairpersons have low position power. Team leaders and staff nurses usually have low position power. Given the critical conditions, Fiedler argues that one can predict the most productive leadership style (Table 3).

If a task is structured but the leader is disliked and therefore needs to be diplomatic, or if the task is ambiguous and the leader is liked and therefore seeks the cooperation of the workers, the considerate, accepting leadership style probably will be most productive. When a disliked leader faces ambiguous tasks, a directive style is more productive. The most productive leadership style is contingent on the situational variables.

Empirical evidence does not supply conclusive evidence for the contingency model. It is difficult to say what the psychologically distant manager and psychologically closer manager measures are really recording. Correlations were used for predicted direction even when they were not statistically significant. The model is primarily academic in that it has not been used in management development for improving group performance and organizational effectiveness, and Fiedler's complex, three-dimensional contingency model has contributed to leadership theories.

Path-goal theory

Robert J. House derived the path-goal theory from the expectancy theory. The expectancy theory argues that a person acts as she does because she expects her behavior to produce satisfactory results. In the path-goal relationship, the leader facilitates task accomplishment by minimizing obstructions to the goals and by rewarding followers for completing their tasks. The leader helps subordinates assess needs, explores alternatives, helps subordinates make the most beneficial decisions, rewards personnel for task achievement, and provides additional opportunities for satisfying goal accomplishment.

House noted that studies done during the 1950s revealed that leaders who structured activities for subordinates generally had more productive work groups and got higher performance evaluations from superiors. Structure includes planning, organizing, directing, and controlling through activities such as clarifying expectations of subordinates, scheduling work, making assignments, determining procedures, and setting standards. Structured activity can increase motivation by reducing role ambiguity and allowing for externally imposed controls. In contrast, considerate leaders had more satisfied workers. They created an atmosphere of friendliness, warmth, and support by tending to the personal welfare of their subordinates. Leader consideration seems particularly important for routine jobs. People who do a variety of tasks may find their jobs more satisfying and have less need for social support.

House recognized that individual differences will affect the subordinates' perception of leader behavior. For instance, experienced subordinates may prefer a task-oriented style, whereas less mature, less experienced, and consequently less secure subordinates may prefer a considerate leader. Subordinates with a high need for achievement probably will prefer a task-oriented leader, but people with a high need for affiliation will prefer a considerate leader. The path-goal theory introduced subordinates as a variable.

Life-cycle theory

The life-cycle theory predicts the most appropriate leadership style from the level of maturity of the followers. Paul Hersey and Kenneth H. Blanchard illustrate this theory in a four-quadrant model (Fig. 4-1). A horizontal continuum registers low emphasis on the accomplishment of tasks on the left side of the model to a high emphasis on task behavior on the right side. The vertical continuum depicts low emphasis on interpersonal relationships at the bottom of the model to high emphasis on relationships at the top. The lower left quadrant, therefore, represents a laissez-faire type of leadership style with little concern

Fig. 4-1. Life cycle theory of leadership. (From Paul Hersey and Kenneth H. Blanchard, Management of organizational behavior: utilizing human resources, 3rd ed., © 1977, p. 194. Reprinted by permission of Prentice-Hall, Inc., Englewood Cliffs, New Jersey.)

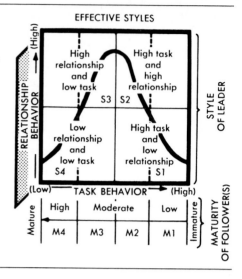

for production or relationships. The lower right quadrant represents an autocratic leadership style with considerable concern for production but little concern for relationships. The upper right quadrant designates a high concern for both tasks and relationships. The left upper quadrant represents a leadership style that stresses relationships but shows little concern for tasks.

The maturity level of the group or individual is depicted on a continuum from high maturity on the left to low maturity on the right under the four quadrants. The maturity levels are superimposed on the quadrants with dashed lines. The best leadership style for given levels of maturity is shown by a curvilinear line in the four quadrants. To determine the most appropriate leadership style, one must assess the maturity level of the individual or group, plot it on the maturity continuum, and project a line at a right angle from that point until it intersects with the curvilinear line. The quadrant in which the intersection occurs depicts the most appropriate leadership style. With increased maturity, less structure and emotional support are needed. In contrast, high-task and low-relationship style is considered best for below-average maturity. The leadership styles in quadrants 2 and 3 are recommended for the average group or individual.

This model is consistent with Argyris's immaturity-maturity continuum, which indicates that as a person matures, she progresses from a passive to an active state and from dependence to independence. With maturity she passes from a need for structure and little relationship through a decreasing need for structure and increasing need for relationship to little need for either. The progression is not always smooth. Stress may cause members of the group to regress, and the leader must adjust her behavior accordingly. The life-cycle theory therefore emphasizes the importance of the maturity level of the group, and the leader needs to adapt leadership styles accordingly.

Integrative leadership model

From a review of leadership theories, obviously there is no one best leadership style. Leaders are rarely totally people- or task-oriented. Leader, followers, situation—all influence leadership effectiveness. Consequently, an integration of leadership theories seems appropriate. The leader needs to be aware of her own behavior and influence on others, individual differences of followers, group characteristics, motivation, task structures, environmental factors, and situational variables, and adjust her leadership style accordingly. Leadership behavior needs to be adaptive.

DEVELOPMENT OF MANAGEMENT THOUGHT

A familiarity with the development of management thought can be useful to nursing leaders in creating their own management styles. No single management theory is sufficient in itself to guide the nursing leader's every action. But through an eclectic approach, drawing from the best and most applicable theories in each situation, nurse administrators can create individual management styles to meet their particular needs.

Scientific management

Theories of management do not remain static. Since the introduction of the earliest principles of scientific management nearly a century ago, management thought has been marked by constant change. Frederick W. Taylor (1856-1915) is generally recognized as the father of scientific management. Through the use of stopwatch studies, he applied the principles of observation, measurement, and scientific comparison to determine the most efficient way to accomplish a task. Taylor conducted time-and-motion studies to time workers, analyze their movements, and set work standards. He usually found that the same result could be obtained in less time with fewer or shorter motions. When the most efficient way to complete a task was determined, workers were trained to follow that method. The most productive workers were hired, and even when they were paid an incentive wage, labor costs per unit were reduced.

Taylor, an engineer in steel manufacture, brought his pioneering experience in scientific management to the service of Bethlehem Steel in 1898 and later became an independent business consultant. Identifying the responsibilities of management and separating them from the functions of the workers, Taylor threw aside rule-of-thumb judgments and developed a systematic approach to determine the most efficient means of production. He considered management's function to be planning. Working conditions and methods had to be standardized to maximize production. It was management's responsibility to select and train workers rather than allow them to choose their own jobs and methods and train themselves. An incentive plan whereby workers were paid according to their rates of production was introduced to minimize worker dissent and reduce resistance to improved methods, increase production, and produce higher profits. Taylor's scientific management reduced wasted efforts, set standards for performance, encouraged specialization, and stressed the selection of qualified workers who could be developed for a particular job. His *Shop Management* (1911) and *The Principles of Scientific Method* (1912) spread his ideas throughout Europe and America.

Frank B. Gilbreth (1868-1924) and Lillian M. Gilbreth (1878-1972) also did pioneering work in time-and-motion studies. They emphasized the benefits of job simplification and the establishment of work standards as well as the effects of the incentive wage plans and fatigue on work performance. As an apprentice bricklayer, Frank Gilbreth was instructed differently by each workman on how to lay bricks. To add to his confusion, the men used one set of motions to teach him, another for a slow pace, and still another for a fast pace. Wondering what methods would be most efficient, the young bricklayer started studying the workers' motions. Gilbreth reduced the number of motions required to lay a brick from eighteen to four by developing a new way to stack bricks; developed an adjustable stand to eliminate excessive stooping, bending, and walking back and forth; and prescribed a mortar consistency that prevented excessive tapping on the brick with a trowel. His system of "speed work" eliminated haste and also increased work output by cutting out unnecessary motions. Workers could be paid higher wages because they accomplished more in a shorter time.

The Gilbreths were among the first to use motion-picture films to analyze workers' motions. Because early cameras did not work at a steady speed, Gilbreth developed a microchronometer, a clock with a large hand measuring $\frac{1}{2000}$ of a minute. The clock was photographed with the task and used to study motion patterns. A small, blinking electric bulb was attached to the worker's hand so speed and direction of movement could be studied. For his study of hand motions, Gilbreth developed seventeen classifications for hand movements, such as "find," "select," "grasp," "position," and "rest," which he labeled "therbligs" (Gilbreth spelled backward with the 'th' transposed). They also developed the flow diagram and the process chart to record their observations. The work process was diagramed to indicate operations, delays, inspection, transportation, and storage, and the process was then studied to shorten, combine, or eliminate steps. The Gilbreths recommended written instructions to avoid misunderstandings and started a merit-rating system for workers.

Lillian Gilbreth is known as the first lady of management. Her doctoral dissertation, *The Psychology of Management* (1914), was published with the author listed as L.M. Gilbreth, thus obscuring the fact that she was a woman. It was one of the first contributions toward understanding human factors in industry. Her work on the effects of fatigue complemented her husband's efforts. The Gilbreths and their twelve children are the subjects of the popular book *Cheaper by the Dozen*.

Henry L. Gantt (1861-1919), a disciple of Taylor, also was concerned with problems of efficiency. He contributed to scientific management by refining previous work rather than introducing new concepts. The Gantt chart, a forerunner of the PERT chart, depicts the relationship of the work planned or completed on one axis to the amount of time needed or used on the other. Gantt also developed a task and bonus remuneration plan whereby workers received a guaranteed day's wage plus a bonus for production above the standard to stimulate higher performance. Gantt recommended that workers be selected scientifically and provided with detailed instructions for their tasks. He argued for a more humanitarian approach by management, placing emphasis on service rather than profit objectives, recognizing useful nonmonetary incentives such as job security, and encouraging staff development.

Appearing before the Interstate Commerce Commission in 1910, Harrington Emerson (1853-1936) testified that the railroads could save $1 million a day by using principles of scientific management. Emerson, one of the first management consultants, originated the term "efficiency engineering." With emphasis on conservation and the organization's goals and objectives, he defined twelve principles of efficiency. Five are related to interpersonal relations and seven to systems in management: (1) goals and ideas should be clear and well defined, the primary objective being to produce the best product as quickly as possible at minimal expense; (2) changes should be evaluated—management should not ignore "common sense" by assuming that bigness is necessarily better; (3) "competent counsel" is essential; (4) management can strengthen "discipline," or adherence to the rules, by (5) justice, or equal enforcement on all; (6) records, including adequate, reliable, and immediate information about the expenses of equipment and manpower, should be available as a basis for decisions; (7) dispatching or production scheduling is recommended; (8) standardized schedules, (9) standardized conditions, and (10) standardized operations can be facilitated through the use of (11) written instructions; (12) "efficiency rewards" should be given for successful completion of tasks. Emerson moved beyond scientific management toward classic organizational theory.

Morris Cook (1872-1960) applied scientific management to university settings and municipal management. Studying the cost of input efforts and the resulting outputs of teaching and research, he found that management practices in education were lacking. Committee management was inefficient, inbreeding was common, and departmental autonomy undermined university coordination. Cook recommended a student hour as the standard by which to measure the efficiency of professional time. He also recommended extensive use of assistants so that more expensive faculty time could be used for more sophisticated tasks. Cook felt that professors should spend their time teaching and conducting research rather than being on committees and should leave administration to specialists. He advocated establishment of professional salaries on the basis of merit rather than longevity, discontinuance of tenure, and retirement of unfit teachers.

As director of public works in Philadelphia, Cook initiated efficient methods for personnel selection, inventory recording, equipment replacement, financial planning, subcontracting, standardization, public relations, and complaint handling. After his work there, he founded his own consulting firm.

Classic organization

Classic administration-organization thinking began to receive attention in 1930. Deductive rather than inductive, it viewed the organization as a whole rather than focus solely on production. Managerial activities were classified as planning, organizing, and controlling. The concepts of scalar levels, span of control, authority, responsibility, accountability, line-staff relationships, decentralization, and departmentalization became prevalent.

Henri Fayol (1841-1925), known as the "father of the management process school," was a French industrialist concerned with the management of production shops. Fayol studied the functions of managers and concluded that management is universal. All managers, regardless of the type of organization or their level in the organization, have essentially the same tasks: planning, organizing, issuing orders, coordinating, and controlling.

Fayol derived some general principles of administration from his observations. A believer in the division of work, he argued that specialization increases efficiency. Fayol recommended centralization through the use of a scalar chain or levels of authority, responsibility accompanied by authority, and unity of command and direction so that each employee receives orders from only one superior. He believed that although individual interests should be subordinated to agency interest, workers should be allowed to think through and implement plans and should be adequately remunerated for their services. Fayol encouraged development of group harmony through equal treatment and stability of tenure of personnel. A firm believer in order, he advocated "a place for everything and everything in its place." He also urged that management be taught in the colleges.

Max Weber (1864-1920), a German sociologist, earned the title of "father of organization theory" by his conceptualization of bureaucracy with emphasis on rules instead of men and on competence over favoritism as the most efficient basis for organization. He conceptualized a structure of authority that would facilitate the accomplishment of the organizational objectives. The three bases of authority, according to Weber, are (1) traditional authority, which is accepted because it seems things have always been that way, such as the rule of a king in a monarchy; (2) charisma, typified by Abraham Lincoln and Otto von Bismarck; and (3) rational legal authority, which is considered rational in formal organizations because the person has demonstrated the knowledge, skill, and ability to fulfill her position. Weber recognized that if subordinates do not believe a person qualified for the position, they may not accept her authority.

Favoring a rational, legal basis for authority, he suggested the avoidance of traditional and charismatic leadership through systematic selection of personnel. Administrators are chosen for their competence; their authority is clearly defined; they are given legal means for exercising their authority; and continuity of administration is provided. In Weber's bureaucracy, administrators are appointed, not elected. They are career officials who work for fixed salaries and do not own what they administer. Like other personnel, they are subject to strict rules that are applied impersonally and uniformly. All personnel are selected for competence; the division of labor, authority, and responsibility is clearly defined; and positions are organized into a hierarchy.

Working independently of Fayol and Weber, James Mooney (1884-1957) formed similar ideas. Mooney believed management to be the technique of directing people and organization the technique of relating functions. Organization is management's responsibility. Mooney enumerated four universal principles of organization: (1) coordination and synchronization of activities for the accomplishment of a goal can be accomplished in part through (2) functional effects, the performance of one's job description, and (3) scalar process organizes (4) authority into a hierarchy. Consequently, people get their right to command from their position in the organization.

Lyndall Urwick (1891-   ) integrated the ideas of Henri Fayol and James Mooney with those of Frederick Taylor. His conceptual framework blended scientific management and classic organization theory into the beginnings of classic management theory. He described the managerial process as planning, coordinating, and controlling, and he popularized such concepts as the balance of authority with responsibility, span of control, unity of command, use of general and special staffs, the proper utilization of personnel, delegation, and departmentalization.

Human relations

The human relations movement began in the 1940s with attention focused on the effect individuals have on the success or failure of an organization. Classic organization and management theory concentrates on the physical environment and fails to analyze the human element; human relations theory stresses the social environment. The chief concerns of the human relations movement are individuals, group process, interpersonal relations, leadership, and communication. Instead of concentrating on the organization's structure, managers encourage workers to develop their potential and help them meet their needs for recognition, accomplishment, and sense of belonging.

Chester Barnard (1886-1961) studied the functions of the executive while he was a manager for the New Jersey Bell Telephone System. Barnard saw the manager's responsibility as defining objectives, acquiring resources, and coordinating activities. Stressing the importance of cooperation between management and labor, he noted that the degree of cooperation is dependent on nonfinancial inducements, which informal organization can help provide. Formal channels of communication must be known and should be as short as possible. Barnard said authority depends on acceptance by the followers, and he stressed the role of informal organizations for aiding communication, meeting individuals' needs, and maintaining cohesiveness. Because small units are the building blocks for complex organizations, the worker contributes to the large organization as well as the basic work unit. Barnard's work, which was done at the end of the classic period before human relations were emphasized, influenced the development of a behavioral focus.

In the 1920s, Mary Parker Follett (1868-1933) stressed the importance of coordinating the psychological and sociological aspects of management. Perceiving the organization as a social system and management as a social process, she considered subordination offensive. Follett distinguished between power with others and power over others and indicated that legitimate power is produced by a circular behavior whereby superiors and subordinates mutually influence one another. The law of the situation dictates that a person does not take orders from another person but from the situation. For instance, nurses will work through their lunch break during an emergency. The problem with this idea is that it is difficult for workers to know the total situation. Follett advocated that managers study the total situation to achieve unity, because she believed that control would be obtained through cooperation among all of the elements, people, and materials. Her work was a link between the classic and human relations eras.

The Hawthorne studies, though criticized for poor research methods, stimulated considerable interest in human problems on the job. Conducted at the Chicago Hawthorne plant of Western Electric by researchers from Harvard University under the direction of psychologist Elton Mayo (1880-1949) and reported by sociologist Fritz Rothlesberger, the study investigated the effects of changes in illumination on productivity. Lighting was changed for the experimental group but remained constant for the control group. As the illumination was increased for the experimental group, the production of both groups increased. When it was decreased for the experimental group, production continued to increase for both groups until the level of illumination reached moonlight, at which point there was a significant decrease in output. The researchers concluded that lighting had little effect on production. The effects of the number and length of work breaks, refreshments, length of work days and workweeks, temperature, and humidity were observed on five volunteers with little or no effects shown. A group piecework incentive plan was studied. The researchers anticipated that fast workers would pressure slow workers to increase their output. However, they found that group norms were set and workers were pressured not to be rate-busters by overproducing or chiselers by underproducing. Workers slacked off when it became apparent that they could meet the rate for the day. Work norms obviously had more influence than wage incentive plans. The Hawthorne studies gave the human relations movement its thrust.

In the early 1930s, Kurt Lewin (1890-1947), a Jewish psychologist, fled from Germany to the United States, where he revived the study of group dynamics. Lewin maintained that groups have personalities of their own—composites of the members' personalities. He showed that group forces can overcome individual interests. He confirmed the importance of group control over output and coined the terms "life space," "space of free movement," and "field forces" to describe group pressures on individuals.

Lewin advocated democratic supervision. His research indicated that democratic groups in which participants solve their own problems and have the opportunity to consult with the leader are most effective. Autocratic leadership, on the other hand, tends to promote hostility and aggression or apathy and to decrease initiative. Conducting experiments during World War II to change people's eating habits to consumption of more organ meats, he found that only 3% of the women who attended lectures (autocratic method) changed their behavior, but 32% of the women who participated in a discussion after the lecture (democratic method) started eating more organ meats. Lewin was one of the first to apply Gestalt psychology to the study of individual personality.

Jacob L. Moreno (1892-1974) developed sociometry to analyze group behavior. Claiming that people are either attracted, repulsed, or feel indifferent toward others, he developed the sociogram to chart pairings and rankings of preferences for others. This process of classification can be used to calculate which workers are capable of harmonious interpersonal relationships. With this knowledge, work groups can be organized with a predicted minimum of disruptive tendencies, for maximal efficiency, and for promotion of high morale. Moreno also contributed to psychodrama (individual therapy), sociodrama (related to social and cultural roles), and role-playing techniques for the analysis of interpersonal relations.

Behavioral science

During the 1950s, advocates of the behavioral sciences became concerned that much scientific, classic, and neoclassic or human relations management had been accepted without scientific validation. Behavioral science emphasized the use of scientific procedures to study the psychological, sociological, and anthropological aspects of human behavior in organizations. Behavioral scientists indicated that management is not strictly a technical process, that it cannot be haphazard, and that it should not be executed through authority. Rather, they stressed the importance of maintaining a positive attitude toward people, training managers, fitting supervisory action to the situation, meeting employees' needs, promoting employees' sense of achievement, and obtaining commitment through participation in planning and decision making.

Abraham Maslow (1908-1970) initiated the human behavioral school in 1943 with his development of a hierarchy-of-needs theory. He outlined a hierarchical structure for human needs classified into five categories: (1) physiological, (2) safety, (3) love, (4) esteem, and (5) self-actualization. The physiological needs are the most important and the most necessary for survival. They include the need for oxygen, water, food, sleep, sex, and activity. Safety includes freedom from danger, threat, and deprivation, such as physical harm, economic distress, ill health, and unnecessary, unexpected occurrences. Love needs are composed of affectionate relations with others, acceptance by one's peers, recognition as a group member, and companionship. Esteem comprises self-respect, positive self-evaluation, and regard by others. Self-actualization is composed of self-fulfillment and achievement of one's full capacity. In Maslow's hierarchy, physical needs must be met before other needs become prepotent and so on, with the satisfaction of self-actualization needs being possible only after all other needs are met. Once a need is satisfied it is no longer a motivator, and the next need becomes prepotent. As a need begins to be satisfied, it decreases in importance as a motivator in relation to other needs, some of which are never completely satisfied and never cease completely to motivate.

Maslow's work has been very influential in management and has stimulated subsequent research. Although Maslow's outline is correct in general, human needs are more complex than a simple listing would indicate. Because no two people are alike, needs vary in type and intensity from one person to another. People differ in the amount of gratification needed before the next goal becomes prepotent. For example, some people do well with 6 hours of sleep a day, but others need 10 hours to function. Varying degrees of importance may be placed on the needs dependent on cultural and individual differences. One person may desire recognition, whereas a sense of belonging to a group may be more important to someone else. People do tend to attach importance to what they do not have. It is socially more acceptable to request that physical needs be met than that social or psychological goals receive attention. The process of motivation is complicated by the fact that one's needs change. When one accepts a job, the pay, work hours, and geographical location may be prepotent. Soon after, the social needs and need for achievement and recognition may become prepotent. People also meet their needs in different ways. One person may get recognition for the quantity and quality of work she produces, whereas someone else may get even more attention through negative behavior such as inferior work and tardiness. There are some situations that seem to defy Maslow's theory. Although most of us will eat if we are hungry, some people fast to achieve higher-level needs. Maslow's work marked the beginning of behavioral science. Much subsequent work has been based on his theory.

Frederick Herzberg (1923-   ) and his colleagues used the critical-incident method in 1959 to interview 200 Pittsburgh area engineers and accountants about job situations that they had found satisfying or dissatisfying. The stories were analyzed according to content and classified according to the job factors each contained. The researchers found that job factors in situations associated with satisfaction were different from job factors in situations associated with dissatisfaction. The motivators or satisfiers identified were achievement, recognition, work itself, responsibility, advancement, and the possibility for growth. These job-content factors (factors in the job) can raise the level of performance and meet the higher-order needs. In Maslow's hierarchy-of-needs model, the hygiene factors or dissatisfiers identified were supervision, company policy, working conditions, interpersonal relations with superiors, peers, and subordinates, status, job security, and the job's effect on one's personal life. These job-context factors (surrounding environmental factors) cannot motivate but can lower performance and cause job dissatisfaction. They meet lower-order needs in Maslow's model. Fig. 4-2 illustrates Herzberg's two-factor–motivation-hygiene theory.

Herzberg's theory is very controversial and has stimulated considerable research, some of which supports the theory and some of which does not. Herzberg's work has been the subject of much criticism. He studied only two jobs, and only one measure of job attitude was used. No validity or reliability data were reported. Statements of critical incidents were subject to memory loss and selective perception. The mere fact that one is more likely to blame others than himself when asked about an unpleasant experience but is willing to assume the responsibility when something good happens could explain Herzberg's findings. No observations or measurement of job behavior were taken. Wrong cate-

Fig. 4-2. Herzberg's two-factor motivation-hygiene theory of needs motivation. (From Claus, K.E., and Bailey, J.T.: Power and influence in health care, St. Louis, 1977, The C. V. Mosby Co., p. 145; diagram conceptualized by K.E. Claus from data in Herzberg, F., Mausner, B., and Snyderman, B.B.: The motivation to work, ed. 2, New York, 1959, John Wiley & Sons, Inc.)

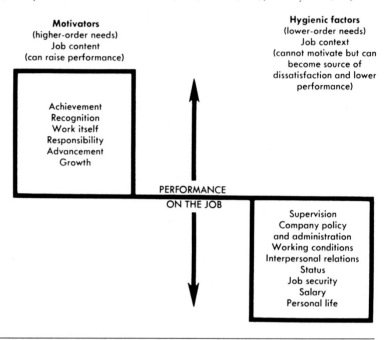

gories could be identified, and the highly subjective stories could be misclassified. Herzberg did, however, develop a taxonomy of job situations based on research that has contributed to a better understanding of human motivation. His work complements Maslow's (Fig. 4-3).

Douglas McGregor (1932-   ) developed the managerial implications of Maslow's theory. He noted that one's style of management is dependent on one's philosophy of humans and categorized those assumptions as Theory X and Theory Y. In Theory X, the manager's emphasis is on the goal of the organization. The theory assumes that people dislike work and will avoid it; consequently, workers must be directed, controlled, coerced, and threatened so that organizational goals can be met. According to Theory X, the average person wants to be directed and to avoid responsibility because she has little ambition. She desires security. The manager who accepts the assumptions of Theory X will do the thinking and planning with little input from subordinates. She will delegate little, supervise closely, and motivate workers through fear and threats, failing to make use of their potentials.

In Theory Y the emphasis is on the goal of the individual. It is the manager's

Fig. 4-3. Comparison of the Maslow and Herzberg models. (From James H. Donnelly, Jr., James L. Gibson, and John M. Ivancevich, Fundamentals of management: functions, behavior, models, ed. 4 [Dallas, Tex: Business Publications, 1981]. © 1981 by Business Publications, Inc.)

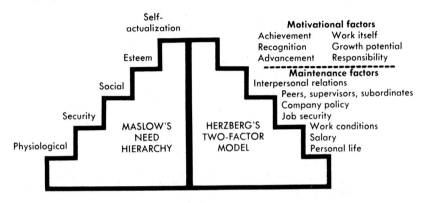

assumption that people do not inherently dislike work and that work can be a source of satisfaction. The Theory Y manager assumes that workers have the self-direction and self-control necessary for meeting their objectives and will respond to rewards for the accomplishment of those goals. She believes that under favorable conditions, people seek responsibility and display imagination, ingenuity, and creativity. According to Theory Y, human potentials are only partially utilized. The manager who believes the assumptions of Theory Y will allow participation. She will delegate, give general rather than close supervision, support job enlargement, and use positive incentives such as praise and recognition.

McGregor suggests that when people are unable to satisfy their higher-level needs, they experience personal frustrations resulting in negative behaviors. Some managers have responded to the consequences of the personal frustration with punitive measures without determining the cause. Managers with a human relations orientation have made working conditions pleasant and have provided rewards unrelated to job performance. McGregor believes that both approaches are ineffective and recommends that the work situation be structured so that the worker can meet her personal goals while working toward the goals of the organization. He suggests collaboration between the manager and the worker for integration of goals. Table 4 shows the relationship between the Maslow, Herzberg, and McGregor theories.

Chris Argyris (1923-   ), focusing his research on the coexistence of personal and organizational needs, found that individuals give priority to meeting their own needs. He found that the greater the disparity between individual and organizational needs, the more tension, conflict, dissatisfaction, and subversion

Table 4. Relationships between the Maslow, Herzberg, and McGregor theories

Maslow	Herzberg	McGregor
Physiological needs Safety needs	Hygiene factors	Theory X
The need to belong Esteem needs The need for self-actualization	Motivators	Theory Y

From Joe Kelly, *Organizational Behaviour*, rev. ed. (Homewood, Ill.: Richard D. Irwin, 1974), p. 276. © by Richard D. Irwin, Inc.

result. Argyris recommends that leaders help workers achieve self-actualization by implementing a Theory Y philosophy and maintains that this will help one's personality to grow from passivity and dependence to activity and independence. Incongruency between the mature personality and management based on classic principles makes workers subordinate, dependent, and passive, thereby causing psychological failure and job dissatisfaction. Managers can make jobs more meaningful by taking advantage of people's talents and letting them participate in planning, goal setting, and problem solving.

Rensis Likert's (1903-1981) theory of management is based on his work at the University of Michigan's Institute for Social Research. He identifies three variables in organizations: (1) causal, (2) intervening, and (3) end result. The causal variables include leadership behavior, organizational structure, policies, and controls. Intervening variables are perceptions, attitudes, and motivations. The end-result variables are measures of profits, costs, and productivity. Likert believes that managers may act in ways harmful to the organization because they evaluate end results to the exclusion of intervening variables. Consequently, he developed a Likert Scale questionnaire that includes measures of causal and intervening variables. The Likert Scale measures several factors related to leadership behavior process, motivation, managerial influence, communication, decision-making processes, goal setting, and staff development.

Likert also identifies four types of management systems: (1) exploitive-authoritative, (2) benevolent-authoritative, (3) consultative, and (4) participative group. He associates the first system with the least effective performance. Superiors show little confidence in subordinates and ignore their ideas. Consequently, subordinates do not feel free to discuss their jobs with their superiors. Responsibility for the organization's goals is at the top; goals are established through orders. What little communication is used is directed downward, is often inaccurate, and is accepted with suspicion. Although superiors do not know about their subordinates' problems, they make decisions without input from below. Policing and punishment are used as control functions by top administration. Allowed no input, the workers strongly resist the organization's goals and develop an informal organization of their own.

In the benevolent-authoritative system, the superior is condescending to subordinates. Subordinates' ideas are sometimes sought, but they do not feel very free to discuss their jobs with their superior. Top and middle management are responsible for setting goals. There is little communication, and it is mostly directed downward after being censored by the superior and is received with some suspicion. Decisions are made at the top with some delegation. Superiors do have some knowledge of the subordinates' situation, and subordinates are occasionally consulted for problem solving. Goals are established through orders with some comment invited and moderate resistance received. Rewards and punishment are used as control functions by top administration. There is usually an informal organization resisting the formal one.

In the third system, the consultative system, the superior has substantial confidence in subordinates. Their ideas are usually sought, and they feel free to discuss their work with the superior. Responsibility for setting goals is fairly general. Although there is considerable communication, both upward and downward, it has limited accuracy and is accepted with some caution. Superiors are quite familiar with the problems faced by their subordinates. Broad policy is set at the top with delegation; goals are set after discussion; and there is decision making throughout the organization. Control functions are delegated to lower levels where reward and self-guidance are used. Sometimes an informal organization resists the formal goals.

Participative management, the fourth system, is associated with the most effective performance. Superiors have complete confidence in their subordinates. Subordinates' ideas are always sought, and they feel completely free to discuss their jobs with the superior. Goals are set at all levels. There is a great deal of communication—upward, downward, and sideways—that is accurate and received with an open mind. Superiors are very well informed about the problems faced by their subordinates, and the decision making is well integrated throughout the organization with full involvement of subordinates. Because goals are established through group action, there is little or no resistance to them. There is not an informal organization resisting the goals of the formal organization, as the goals of both are the same. Control is quite widely shared through the use of self-guidance and problem solving.

Likert is a strong proponent of participative management and supportive relationships. His linking-pin concept is based on studies about the differences between good and poor supervisors as measured by their level of productivity. Good supervisors were found to have more influence on their own superiors than did poor supervisors, and their supervisory procedures were better received

Fig. 4-4. Linking-pin concept. Arrows indicate linking-pin function. (From Likert, R., and Likert, J.G.: New ways of managing conflict, New York, 1976, McGraw-Hill Book Co., p. 184.)

by their subordinates. Consequently, Likert suggests that managers form groups for supportive relationships and that those groups be linked by overlapping groups of supervisors. This facilitates three-way communications—upward, downward, and sideways. When the middle manager has the opportunity for interaction with her superior, workers can have input, and there is a chance for the individual's and the organization's goals to become similar (Fig. 4-4).

Robert Blake (1918-   ) and Jane Mouton (1930-   ) maintain that the two critical dimensions of leadership are (1) concern for people and (2) concern for production, which they depict on a 9 × 9 or 81-square managerial Grid® (Fig. 4-5). The two dimensions are independent, so a manager can be high on both, low on both, or high on one and low on the other. The vertical axis represents the manager's concern for people, and the horizontal axis represents concern for production. Each axis is on a 1-to-9 scale from a minimal concern for people or production to a maximal concern. The five basic styles are located at each corner and in the middle.

The task manager at 9,1 has the highest regard for production and the lowest concern for people. This manager stresses operating efficiency through controls and views people as tools of production. Workers are paid to do what they are told without questioning.

As reflected on the Grid, 1,1 management is impoverished. The manager has a lack of concern for both production and people. This style may be found in some managers who feel they have been repeatedly denied promotion or otherwise mistreated and who have consequently compensated through a low level of involvement with their jobs. The organization-man management at 5,5 represents a moderate concern for both people and production but not necessarily at the same time. The manager's emphasis shifts. The country club manager, 1,9, is thoughtful and friendly but has little concern for production.

Blake and Mouton consider team management, 9,9, the optimal managerial style. This manager integrates her concern for people and production. Problems

Fig. 4-5. Managerial Grid. (From Robert R. Blake and Jane Srygley Mouton, *The New Managerial Grid* [Houston: Gulf Publishing Company, 1978], p. 11. Reproduced by permission.)

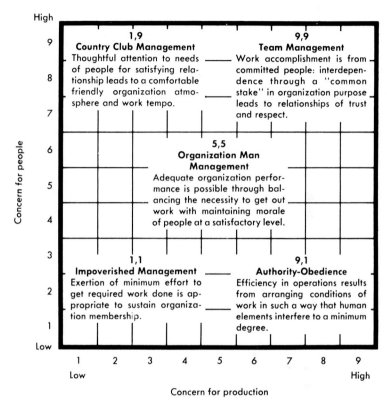

are confronted directly, and mutual trust, respect, and interdependence are fostered.

During the 1960s, Fred Fiedler (1922-   ) introduced the contingency model of leadership effectiveness. He identified three important dimensions of a situation for his contingency model: (1) leader-member relations, (2) task structure, and (3) position power. Leader-member relations refers to the amount of confidence and loyalty followers have in their leader. Task structure is related to the number of correct solutions to a problem. Position power is dependent on the amount of organizational support available to the leader.

Paul Hersey and Kenneth H. Blanchard (1939-   ) extended the work of Blake, Mouton, and Fiedler by considering the maturity of the followers in more detail. As the maturity of one's followers increases, the leadership style requires less structure and emotional support. Groups with below-average maturity function best under leaders with high task–low relationship orientations. Groups with average maturity function best under leaders with high task–high relationship or high relationship–low task orientations. The most effective leadership style is dependent on the maturity of the group.

In his prolific writings about management, Peter Drucker (1909-   ) maintains that the only way for management to justify its existence is through economic results. However, he recognizes noneconomic consequences of managerial decisions, such as job satisfaction, as by-products of the focus on economic performance. He identifies three areas of management: managing (1) a business, (2) managers, and (3) workers. Activity, decision, and relations analyses are recommended to determine the structure and organization needed. Drucker has studied the advantages and disadvantages of decentralization, supports decentralization, and says managers should create markets and products rather than being passive.

Drucker introduced management by objectives as a way to manage managers. Relying on self-control instead of control from above, the manager is directed by objectives of performance rather than by his superior. For management by objectives, the superior develops the framework, and the subordinate supplies the goals, which are agreed on by both. The subordinate gives progress reports to the superior. Objectives are developed for every level of management in the hierarchy and each unit in the organization. The superior checks objectives for compatibility with other units and contribution to the objectives at the next level of the hierarchy. Drucker maintains that it is more productive to have workers set their own norms and measure their own performance than to set minimal standards.

For managing the worker, Drucker recommends that jobs be designed to fit the worker, that the worker be given more control over her job, and that the worker be considered the most vital resource in the agency.

George S. Odiorne, Director of the Bureau of Industrial Relations of the University of Michigan, was previously Assistant Director of Personnel for General Mills, Inc., where he pioneered the installation of a management-by-objectives system. He advocates effective management through personal and agency goals and has written about the executive's responsibilities for implementing a management-by-objectives system. He also recommends training by objectives as an economic strategy for management training.

Implications for nursing administration

Surveying the development of management thought, one can see that there has been a trend from autocratic to democratic management and from a focus on efficiency to a greater regard for the well-being of personnel. Although the focus has changed, elements from each era maintain their validity and can be used by the nurse administrator. For example, Taylor's time studies and the Gilbreths' motion studies in the scientific era are illustrations of how the nurse can study complexity of care to predict staffing needs and study efficiency of nursing care. An adaption of Gantt's chart can be used to visualize the time element of planning and controlling, and the nurse administrator is well advised to heed Emerson's early notion of the importance of objectives in agencies. Nursing education could become more efficient by implementing some of Cook's recommendations.

The nurse administrator should be aware of her managerial tasks as defined by Fayol: planning, organizing, directing, coordinating, and controlling. His definition of management can help clarify the manager's role, and his principles of management can help direct one's actions. Assistance with the organizing function can be obtained from Weber's conceptualization of bureaucracy and authority and Urwick's popularization of such concepts as balancing authority with responsibility, unity of direction, unity of command, and span of control.

To a large extent the social environment results from organization and management. The work of Barnard, Follett, Mayo, and Lewin during the human relations era should remind the nurse administrator of the importance of developing her workers to their potential and meeting their needs for recognition, accomplishment, and a sense of belonging. It is hoped that the nurse administrator will consider the results of Kurt Lewin's research about autocratic and democratic leadership when determining her own style. She can use Moreno's sociometry to study the group behavior of her workers.

Much has been learned about management from the behavioral science studies. The nurse can apply Maslow's hierarchy-of-needs theory to the care of individual patients, to functions of individual workers, or to groups of people. The importance of achievement, recognition, responsibility, and advancement as motivators and satisfiers is stressed in Herzberg's two-factor theory. McGregor, Argyris, Likert, Blake, and Mouton's research all support the benefits of positive attitudes toward people, development of workers, satisfaction of their needs, and commitment through participation. Fiedler indicates that a leadership style may or may not be effective depending on the situation. The nurse administrator can use his work to assess her work situation to determine the most effective style or choose her work situation according to what fits her style best. She can also incorporate Drucker's and Odiorne's work on management by objectives for the planning, directing, and controlling phases of the management process.

By studying the development of management thought, the nurse administrator can define her management role, develop her philosophy of management, learn tools and techniques for implementation of her responsibilities, and gain an increased understanding of how to work with others to accomplish goals.

POWER AND AUTHORITY

Power and authority are closely related and often confused. Power is one's capacity to influence others, whereas authority is the right to direct others. One's power may be greater or less than the authority of her position. Authority is obtained through position power, but several other sources of power exist.

Sources of power

Reward. Much of a manager's power comes from her ability to reward others for complying. When the subordinate perceives that the superior has the ability to provide something she values, the superior has reward power. Sources of reward power include money, desired assignments, provision of personal space, or the acknowledgment of accomplishments. Rewards contribute to an independent system.

Coercive power. Coercive power is the opposite of reward power and is based on fear of punishment if one fails to conform. Undesired assignments, embarrassment in front of others, withheld pay increases, and termination are sources of coercive power that contribute to a dependent system.

Legitimate power. Their official positions in the organizational hierarchy give managers legitimate power. Legitimate power gives the superior the right to influence and the subordinate an obligation to accept that influence. The director of nursing has more legitimate power than the supervisor, who in turn has more legitimate power than the head nurse. Cultural values that give a person the right to prescribe appropriate behavior for another (such as parents for children), social structures involving a hierarchy of authority, and election processes to legitimize a person's right to an office are bases for legitimate power.

Referent power. Referent power is based on identification with a leader and what that leader symbolizes. The leader is admired and exerts influence because the followers desire to be like the leader.

Expert power. A person gains expert power through knowledge, skills, and information. Her expertise gains her respect and compliance. Knowledge of the organization and its rules, regulations, and work flow helps one to acquire power over others who need the knowledge to meet their responsibilities.

Informal sources of power. Informal sources of power are related to one's personal power rather than position power. Some people have situational power because they happen to be in the right place at the right time. Others have personal power because of their unique characteristics.

Education, experience, drive, and decisiveness are viewed positively and help establish credibility. The person with these qualities may be viewed as reliable, and therefore others are willing to cooperate. Attractiveness gains an individual access to people who will help promote her cause, because people enjoy being around others who have a happy temperament, generate a sense of well-being, and foster goodwill in others. Location also influences others, as individuals communicate more with people who are located near them in the organization, which increases their opportunities to influence. For instance, full voting membership on powerful committees places one in close proximity for persuading others and provides the opportunity to confront, negotiate, and solve problems. In general, people are most comfortable with others who share similar values, beliefs, and customs. Social pressure from people who share social norms encourages others to conform to those norms. Coalitions strengthen one's power base. Consequently, friendships and associations with people can be a source of power.

Interpersonal relationships also provide access to the informal communication network. Doing a favor for another so that she owes you a favor creates an obligation-based power. One may gain power by default when there is no one else available or by autonomy when the decision is hers to make. Control of resources, such as information, procedures, equipment, and personnel, also strengthens one's power base. Religion, politics, race, or national origin are bases for establishing power in some situations but interfere with power bases in other situations. For example, a nurse of a certain faith may be given priority for a job on the staff of an institute run by that faith, but her religion may be held against her if she seeks a position at a hospital affiliated with another religion or denomination.

Power relations

Power is interpersonal. It is a dependence relationship. Person x has power over person y to the extent that y is dependent on x for goal attainment. The power varies inversely to the availability of goals outside the particular interpersonal relationship. If a nurse wants to work for the hospital but does not care if she works for one head nurse or another, she reduces the head nurses' power. Motivational investment in the goals being mediated is a variable. The nurse who wants to work in intensive coronary care is far more dependent on one head nurse than the nurse who is willing to work on several units. Cost of goal achievement is also a factor. The nurse may not be willing to work straight nights to work on the unit of her choice. A staff nurse may not be willing to hassle with a grievance procedure to get what she thinks she deserves. Sources of dependence are numerous: knowledge, skills, interpersonal relations, and organizational authority.

Predictable behaviors occur when there is a conflict of interest among people with power. Coalition is a technique to strengthen one's power. It involves uniting to gain a sense of strength. Whether coalition occurs or not, there will probably be bargaining in an attempt to negotiate the conflict. One may leave the situation if bargaining is ineffective or adjust to lessened power if alternative positions are not readily available.

It is useful to assess one's power in a relationship before engaging in conflict. Although there is no magic formula to assess one's power, there are considerations that help identify one's power in relation to that of others. Who is the most powerful? The person who appears the most powerful may not be. Communication patterns help assess who actually has the power. The person who structures the options has more power, whereas the person who does more accommodating probably has less power. The person with the least interest in maintaining the relationship has more power. Those who gain the most from ritualized patterns have the most power, because institutionalized norms reinforce the existing power structure, and people who try to maintain the status quo are likely protecting their own power. People who are aware of their sources of power can use that knowledge, but people are often unaware of their sources of power and consequently are unable to use those sources effectively.

Kinds of power

In *Power and Innocence* Rollo May has identified five kinds of power. Exploitative power is the most destructive type. It subjects people to whatever use the power holder chooses. Slavery is an example. Manipulative power is influence over another person that may have been invited because of the person's desperation and anxiety. Operant conditioning is an example of manipulative power. Competitive power is energy used against another. One person wins and another loses, although neither the gain nor the loss is necessarily related to merit. An example is the competition of several people for one position. One person wins, the others lose—even if they were well qualified for the job. Nutrient power, such as parents caring for their children, teachers caring for students, and politicians caring for their constituents, is influence used for others. Integrative power is cooperative power with others. A person can possess the five types of power at different times.

Authority

Authority is legitimate power. It is determined by structure, which involves rules, roles, and relations. Rules legitimize authority and tend to suspend the subordinate's critical faculties. Subordinates tend to do unquestioningly what the superior with legitimate authority tells them to do. Role is position or office. Authority is inherent in the position, not in the person. Relations are related to credibility, which is obtained through knowledge and expertise.

Authority is traditionally structured as line or staff. Line authority refers to levels of authority and superior-subordinate relationships, and it therefore provides the framework for the organization. Staff authority has no command privileges. It has only the right to advise or assist managers in the performance of their duties. The staff member provides assistance when requested, must sell her idea to the manager over whom she has no authority, and must sell her idea up the line to managers who have the line authority to implement the ideas. More recently, functional authority or authority of the specialist has emerged. Functional authority is normally limited to the performance of defined duties for a limited period of time.

It is preferable for a manager's power to be equitable to the authority of her position. Her knowledge, experience, drive, and decisiveness help her achieve power. Being attractive, visible, and available are sources of informal power. More formal sources of power available to nurse managers are control of resources, reward and coercive power, association with other powerful people, and the legitimate power from her managerial position. The nurse manager's knowledge of her sources of power can help her assess and use them.

Politics

Politics is the authoritative allocation of scarce resources. It requires legitimate power to distribute goods, services, and other resources that are not as abundant as desired. A political system is a social system that gets people to do what they would not ordinarily want to do. There are several theories that help explain the dynamics of political systems. According to *game theory*, politics is a fascinating game with rules, referees, and players on opposing sides. *Elite theory* purports that political power is concentrated with people who hold top positions in large centralized institutions. These people tend to have a unified purpose because of similar social backgrounds and interests and consequently have stable power. *Pluralist theory* explains that political life is based on competition between interest groups. The influence of political groups is determined by their political organization, strategies, and leadership. These competitive relationships are unstable because interest groups and related alliances are short-lived and new coalitions and interest groups develop as old ones decline. The power of interest groups is limited by dependence on other groups and the need for compromises. *Exchange theory* states that political behavior is based on the exchange of resources. People decide what they want, what it will cost, and if they have the resources to exchange for it.

There are levels of political participation ranging from apathetic inactivists who engage in no political activity to complete activists who engage in numerous activities. As a nurse becomes involved in politics, she can expand her influence beyond a single vote. Spectator political activities include gathering political information, displaying bumper stickers or wearing buttons, initiating political discussions, trying to persuade others, and voting. As one becomes increasingly involved, she can make financial contributions, attend political meetings, and contact political leaders. Activists become active members in political parties, attend caucus meetings, contribute time to political campaigns, solicit funds, and run for offices.

Nurse managers can encourage others to become more politically active by educating them in issues, posting and circulating information, and encouraging staff discussion of political topics. She can educate and encourage others to work with legislators by providing formal classes on the legislative process, a list of key contacts, and information about voting records. The nurse manager can encourage participation in professional organizations, consumer groups, boards, legislative committee meetings and hearings, and political functions. Staff members can be sent to testify at hearings and be assigned to attend political activities. The manager can generally support political activities, exemplify political involvement, encourage others to vote, and give release time for political participation.

Nurse administrators have found that communicating with legislators, building coalitions, being knowledgeable about current issues, providing testimony, problem solving, educating and involving other nurses, and knowing the legislator before needing help are most successful political strategies. Less effective political strategies include mass mailings, petitions, demonstrating, and relying on others to protect nurses' interests. Factors that have contributed to unsuccessful political outcomes include emotionalism, lack of preparation, lack of unity among nurses, failure to build an adequate power base, failure to attend political meetings, contacting policymakers too late, lack of publicity, and lack of feedback from politicians, other nurses, and community members.*

Legislators spend so much time in sessions and at committee meetings that it can be difficult to reach them by telephone. A letter is a written record that requires a written reply and is more likely to reach the legislator. Letters should be kept brief, preferably one and not more than two pages. A personal letter is more effective than a form letter or a petition. The title and number of the bill one is addressing and a brief interpretation of it should be included. One's position should be stated succinctly. The name and address of the writer need to be legible, and when possible the writer should identify herself as a nurse and a voter in the legislator's district. One must use discretion in selecting a time to discuss an interest with a legislator. It is preferable not to talk to a legislator when he is engrossed in activities related to another bill but to wait until he can give his full attention to one's concerns. Appointments are set up

---

*Political strategies are reported in Archer, S.E., and Goehner, P.A.: Acquiring political clout: guidelines for nurse administrators, J. Nurs. Adm. **11:**49-55, November-December 1981.

ahead of time. The nurse should prepare a short, well-written statement of what legislative action is preferred and why, specifying the direct impact it will have on the legislator's constituents. The points should be concise and accompanied with news clippings, research reports, and other supportive documentation. It is preferable to deal with one issue at a time.

One should know the party of which the legislator is a member and address him as a representative or senator, as appropriate, to show respect. One should be specific and reasonable about what is wanted and should ask a legislator to do only what is within his power. A dialogue can be continued by writing to express gratitude for the meeting and by sending new information as it becomes available.

Nurse managers can take the initiative to organize political meetings. It is best to start with a small group with political and organizing experience. The group should include all organizations and important people willing to be involved. One should compile lists of members of organizations, agency directories, officers, names from newspaper articles, and so on. Personal time and money will be needed to type, copy, and mail invitations as well as for refreshments, room rental, supplies such as name tags and agendas, and follow-up correspondence.

The meeting should be held at a neutral meeting site. A map should be included with the invitation. A self-addressed, stamped response postcard and request for correction of address and telephone number should also be enclosed. Brief handouts and name tags should be prepared in advance of the meeting. A minimum of food should be served. The atmosphere of the political meeting should be kept comfortable and professional.*

Because the legislative process is complex and technical, nurses need to know the process to determine when to intervene. The state legislative process is similar to the national process that follows. First, legislation is introduced. These legislative proposals originate in a number of ways, but most originate in the executive branch. However, either individuals such as members of Congress or groups such as interest groups may introduce legislation.

Next, there is committee referral. A bill is considered read for the first time when it is referred to a committee. Only a member of Congress can introduce legislation. There is no limit to the number of bills a member may introduce. In the House of Representatives and the Senate, a bill is numbered according to its place in the order of introduction, referred to committee, labeled with the sponsor's name, and printed by the Government Printing Office. Bills are prefixed with HR when introduced in the House of Representatives and S when

---

*Davis, C.K., Oakley, D., and Sochalski, J.A.: Leadership for expanding nursing influence on health policy, J. Nurse. Adm. **12**:15-21, January 1982.

introduced in the Senate. After referral to a standing committee, most legislation is referred to a subcommittee. Most bills go no further. Each bill introduced must pass the House of Representatives and the Senate in identical form within 2 years to become a law.

After referral to a standing committee and a subcommittee, hearings are held by the subcommittee. Often only a few members of the subcommittee who have a special interest in the subject will participate in the hearings. The chairperson uses the agenda, funds, and staff to expedite, delay, or modify legislation. The subcommittee usually schedules public hearings and invites testimony from private and public witnesses. Interested individuals submit written requests to testify. Once they are informed of when to testify, rescheduling is not allowed. If a person cannot be present at the designated time, she may file a written statement for the record of the hearing. Witnesses who share common positions are urged to consolidate testimony and designate a single spokesperson. Groups with similar concerns that are unwilling to have a single spokesperson may form panels. Panelists are allowed a 6-minute presentation of the key points in their written documents and are urged to avoid repeating other presentations. All witnesses are required to file a written statement with the committee at least a day before the scheduled appearance or the preceding Friday if the testimony is to be on Monday or Tuesday. The statement should be typed on letter-sized paper and include a summary of the principal points. Witnesses should not read their written statements but should summarize the key points in no more than 6 minutes. Once the testimony has been given, each subcommittee member may ask questions.

If, after the hearing, the subcommittee members decide the legislation should go further, they consider the language line by line and section by section to determine the language of the final bill, which is then recommended to the full committee.

When presenting the bill to the floor of the House or Senate, the full committee justifies its actions in a written report that accompanies the bill. Bills that are unanimously voted out of committee have a good chance on the floor. However, dispute is likely to occur on the floor if there has been a divided committee.

After a bill has passed one house, it is sent to the other where the same process takes place. If the second house approves the bill as it was passed by the first, it is sent to the president for his signature. However, if the bill was revised or amendments added, the bill must be returned to the originating chamber for approval of the changes. If that body refuses to approve the revised bill, both versions are sent to a conference committee. The bill is sent to the president for signature or veto after the differences are reconciled and there is a final vote of acceptance by the conference committee. In the case of a presidential veto, both houses can override the veto to make the bill law.*

CONFLICT
Conflict theory

Conflict, which is closely related to power and political issues, is inevitable and can be constructive or destructive. It may offer an individual personal gain, provide prestige to the winner, be an incentive for creativity, and serve as a powerful motivator. Indeed, there seems to be an optimal level of conflict or anxiety necessary for effective functioning. Conflict that is managed instead of avoided, ignored, or suppressed can be used effectively. If conflict goes beyond the invigorating stage, it becomes debilitating. Conflict is a warning to management that something is amiss, and it should stimulate a search for new solutions through problem solving, the clarification of objectives, the establishment of group norms, and the determination of group boundaries. However, eliminating conflict is not necessary. If the manager learns the sources and types of conflicts and how to manage them, she can minimize stress on individuals and the organization and maximize effectiveness.

Sources of conflict. Conflict can arise because the individuals involved do not have the same facts. They define the problem differently, have different pieces of information, place more or less importance on various aspects, or have divergent views of their own power and authority. Varying goals and objectives or contrasting procedural strategies for accomplishing mutually acceptable goals produce conflict. Variations in personal value systems or in perceptions of ethical responsibilities can lead to divergence in choices of both goals and methods, thus producing conflict.

When people work together in a complex organization, there are numerous sources of conflict. Conflict increases with both the number of organizational levels and the number of specialties. It is greater as the degree of association increases and when some parties are dependent on others. Competition for scarce resources, ambiguous jurisdictions, and the need for consensus all contribute to conflict. Communication barriers impede understanding, and separations in time and space foster factionalism rather than mutual cooperation. Although standardized policies, rules, and procedures regulate behavior, make relationships more predictable, and decrease the number of arbitrary decisions, they impose added controls over the individual. Men and women who value

---

*The legislative process is discussed in more detail in Kalisch, B.J., and Kalisch, P.A.: Politics of nursing, Philadelphia, 1982, J.B. Lippincott.

autonomy are likely to resist such control. Clearly, the sources of conflict are endless, and the number of conflicts increases as the number of unresolved differences accumulate.

Types of conflict. Structurally based conflict is either vertical or horizontal. Differences between superiors and subordinates (vertical conflict) are often related to inadequate communication, opposing interests, and the lack of shared perceptions and attitudes. In vertical situations, the supervisor often attempts to control the subordinate's behavior, and the subordinate resists, often causing the superior to apply her position power through impersonal bureaucratic rules. Line-staff conflict, usually horizontal, is commonly a struggle between domains related to activities, expertise, and authority and is often related to interdepartmental strife.

Interdepartmental differences are related to the degree of interdependence between departments. Interdependence demands collaboration, and the latter provides the occasion for conflict. The need for consensus, the work sequence, and common use of shared facilities or services are areas of interdependence aggravated by differing departmental goals. Both the personalities and the status of the individuals involved affect attitudes such as trust and cooperation and are just as important as the communication and interaction structures.

There are several types of role conflict. *Intrasender* conflict originates in the sender who gives conflicting instructions or expects conflicting or mutually exclusive behavioral responses. For example, the same supervisor may demand a higher quality of nursing care, refuse to allow the head nurse to fire incompetent help, and, in an effort to cut costs, refuse to increase an inadequate staff or to permit overtime.

Intersender conflict arises when an individual receives conflicting messages from two or more sources. For example, management may implement an incentive plan to stimulate production while peer pressures discourage rate busting. In university settings, the dean may expect department chairpersons to function as administrators, while the faculty may expect them to act as their advocates. The matrix organization that imposes project management on a functional structure creates intersender role conflict. Any time a person is responsible to more than one supervisor, she can anticipate intersender role conflict.

Interrole conflict can occur when an individual belongs to more than one group. Simultaneous, multiple roles within the same organization or the conflicting expectations that result from being a member of more than one organization are sources of such conflict. For example, a person may be expected to attend two different committee meetings at the same time. Job expectations can easily interfere with one's family life. The individual has to develop a system of trade-offs to determine how she should behave at certain times.

Person-role conflict is the result of disparity between internal and external roles. An individual has perceived roles and expectations based on her values and perceptions of herself. When one's values, needs, or capabilities are incompatible with the role requirement, person-role conflict is created. Behavioral expectations that exceed one's current level of knowledge and skill are also stressful. If the nurse believes that people are important but must process patients through a large clinic in a relatively impersonal manner, she is bound to suffer person-role conflict.

Interperson conflict is common between people whose positions require interaction with other persons who fill various roles in the same organization or other organizations. Interperson conflict is usually not personal but rather the result of each person's acting as a protagonist for her department. For example, the director of nursing competes with other department heads for resources. Occasionally, the conflict arising from the nature of the roles involved is complicated by personal animosity.

Intragroup conflict occurs when the group faces a new problem, when new values are imposed on the group from outside, or when an individual's extra-group role conflicts with her intragroup role. In an academic setting, pressures to have baccalaureate nursing students prepared by faculty with master's degrees and graduate students prepared by faculty with doctoral degrees produces intragroup conflict. Faculty members are caught in a conflict over their teaching responsibilities, continuation of their own education, and fulfillment of expectations for community service and scholarly work. A group facing a new problem may require a change in role relationships that requires role negotiations. When intragroup conflict becomes intense, two new groups may form and give rise to intergroup conflict.

Intergroup conflict is common where two groups have different goals and can only achieve their goals at the other's expense. The conflict may be between groups on the same level or between groups on different levels within an organization. Competition between groups also produces conflict. Resolution may be reached by the dominance of one group over the other, by a compromise that rarely satisfies either group, or by an integration of goals attained when each group recognizes the role of the other group in the system. Intergroup conflict need not be dysfunctional. It can stimulate creativity, innovation, and progress. A conflict-free organization suggests stasis, a situation that offers little challenge for group members.

Role ambiguity, a condition in which the individual does not know what is expected of her, frequently occurs in organizations. Inadequate job descriptions, incomplete explanations of assigned tasks, rapid technological change, and the increasing complexity of organizations contribute to role ambiguity and produce uncertainty and frustration.

If the individual cannot meet the expectations placed on her, she will experience *role overload*. This does not involve a questioning of the legitimacy of the request or of what is expected. Rather, the person is simply unable to accomplish so much within a limited time period. As a result, quality is sacrificed for quantity, the ego is threatened, and frustration develops.

Reactions to conflict. Numerous psychological mechanisms exist for coping with one's own behavioral reactions to conflict, but such stress contributes to somatic reactions, for example, cardiovascular diseases and gastric disorders. Sublimation is one of the most constructive psychological mechanisms whereby unacceptable feelings are repressed and channeled into socially acceptable activities. Energy from hostility and anger that would be destructive if expressed directly is diverted with positive results into other activities such as jogging, tennis, or community service. Vigorous physical activity often reduces interpersonal aggression.

Someone who is displeased with the results of her behavior may increase her efforts. Working longer and harder is likely to increase one's productivity. Flight into activity, a defense mechanism whereby a person keeps busy to avoid thinking about problems, provides some temporary relief but does not solve the problems.

Identification is the practice of enhancing one's self-esteem by imitating another's behavior. The values and beliefs of the other person are internalized, and both achievements and suffering are experienced vicariously. This illustrates the adage, "If you can't beat them, join them." An individual may compensate for a real or imagined inadequacy in one area by substituting a high degree of proficiency in another area. For example, one who lacks social skills may excel academically.

Goals may be reinterpreted to attain an unmet goal, or the goal may be lowered or another goal substituted. A person promoted to vice-president with little hope of becoming president may decide that the vice-presidency is a satisfactory position. A rejected job applicant may find another job she enjoys more.

Rationalization provides acceptable explanations for undesirable beliefs or behaviors. A superior may find reasons to fire someone she does not like or pad her expense account because "everyone does it."

Attention getting may involve seeking highly visible jobs, engaging in loud or excessive talking, wearing bright or sexy clothing and unusual hair styles, or driving flashy cars. These displays are destructive only if they divert attention from problem solving.

When an individual represses unacceptable behaviors and values and substitutes the opposite attitudes and behaviors, she is using a coping mechanism called reaction formation. For example, an employee who was denied a merit pay increase may defend her supervisor and vigorously support the related policies.

216

Another mechanism people use to cope with stress is flight into fantasy. Flight into fantasy allows one to think about something else. For example, the nurse's aide may daydream about being the charge nurse. Although daydreaming, watching television, and going to the movies are constructive forms of relaxation, engaging in excessive fantasy interferes with one's productivity.

A person protects herself from her undesirable feelings and traits by attributing them to others. This defense mechanism is called projection. For example, a student who is unable to answer a test question may claim that the question is unclear. An unsuccessful person who wants to block another's success claims that the colleague is hostile and uncooperative. Projection is a destructive way to meet needs.

Displacement redirects emotions toward ideas, people, or objects other than the source of the emotions. For example, after the supervisor corrects the head nurse, the head nurse may displace her aggression by snapping at the team leaders and staff. Some individuals reacting to conflict may resort to negativism, picking apart every idea and action and putting everything in the worst light.

Fixation is the maintenance of a certain maladaptive behavior even though it is obvious that it is not effective in this situation. One who depends on this escape mechanism will make the same mistake repeatedly.

Withdrawal removes one from the area of frustration. For example, a staff nurse who is frustrated with hospital working conditions may go into teaching. This mechanism can be constructive if the person removes herself from a dangerous situation.

Repression pushes painful information and memories into the subconscious, but the material is not truly forgotten. An individual may revert to earlier, even childish behavior. When regressing, staff members may transfer their attitudes toward their parents to their supervisor and expect the supervisor to act like a parent. Some people may even have temper tantrums. Regression moves one away from the present and is rarely constructive.

An individual may unconsciously convert an emotional conflict into physical symptoms, for example, the common tension headache. Paralysis of an arm to avoid writing a report or losing one's voice to avoid discussing an unpleasant topic are extreme forms of the coping mechanism called conversion.

Everyone uses psychological mechanisms. They are our unconscious defenses against impaired self-esteem, anxiety and guilt, and other threatening or uncomfortable feelings. Defense mechanisms serve a purpose. They become harmful only when excessive.

Stages of conflict. Latent conflict is a phase of anticipation in which antecedent conditions, such as scarcity of resources, predict conflict behavior. When change is required, the manager anticipates differences of opinion about the desirability of the change, how it should be implemented, and how the consequences should be handled.

Perceived conflict, which may or may not be discussed, indicates a cognitive awareness of a stressful situation. One's personal perceptions can contribute to either an accurate or inaccurate assessment of the situation and affect the amount of threat and potential loss the individual anticipates. Conflicts can be perceived when antecedent conditions do not exist, as when individuals have a limited knowledge of the facts or do not know others' opinions and values. For instance, a supervisor may think there are limited resources or that someone else wants to use the same materials when, in fact, there is plenty for everyone or no one else is interested anyway. Personal perceptions also can help to avoid conflict. A suppression mechanism may be used to ignore conflict that involves low potential loss or is only minimally threatening. An attention-focus mechanism helps the individual select which conditions to change and which to ignore.

Affective states such as stress, tension, anxiety, anger, and hostility are present during the felt conflict. Feelings and attitudes may create or avoid conflict. Trust, for example, is a significant factor in the development of a manifest conflict. If the individuals involved possess trusting attitudes, they share information and control and recognize their mutual vulnerability. In the absence of trust, an individual may withhold information so it cannot be used against her or distort communications to her advantage. She may scheme to increase her control over the other and strive to decrease the other person's control over her. Clearly, trusting attitudes may prevent potential conflict, and the lack of them may actually create conflict. Two self-serving individuals are more likely to have manifest conflict than a dominant and submissive pair.

The personalization or depersonalization of the situation affects the evolution of conflict. When the situation is personalized, the individual is threatened or judged negatively. With a depersonalized approach, the behavior rather than the individual is identified as creating the problem. "You are wrong" is personalized, whereas "your views are very different from mine" is depersonalized. Personalized comments increase anxiety; a depersonalized approach is conducive to problem solving.

Manifest conflict is overt behavior resulting from the antecedent, perceived, and felt conflict. It can be either constructive or destructive to problem solving. Unfortunately, aggression, competition, and other defenses are learned unconsciously, whereas problem solving requires a more deliberate, conscious effort.

Conflict resolution

Approaches to conflict resolution. Some common approaches to handling conflict are avoiding, accommodating, compromising, collaborating, and competing. Avoiding creates lose-lose situations through unassertive and uncooperative means. The conflict is simply not addressed. This approach may be appropriate when the other party is more powerful, the issue is unimportant, one has no chance of meeting her goals, or the cost of dealing with the conflict is higher than the benefit of the resolution. It may also be used when it is more appropriate for others to solve a problem, when more information is needed, or when one wishes to reduce tension and gain composure. Withdrawing from a conflict does not resolve it, and the individual who retreats frequently harbors a gnawing anger over a situation that drains energy needed for more constructive purposes.

Accommodating is cooperative but unassertive. It is self-sacrificing—the opposite of competing. The person neglects her own needs to meet the goals of the other party. It is appropriate when the person is wrong, the opponent is more powerful, or the issue is more important to someone else. It can be used when preserving harmony is important or when collecting social credits is necessary for later, more important issues. By complimenting one's opponent and accentuating points of agreement, one may smooth out an agreement on minor issues, but the real problems still have to be dealt with.

Compromising moderates both assertiveness and cooperation. It addresses a problem more effectively than avoidance but less than collaboration. Compromisers are willing to yield less than accommodaters but more than competitors as they seek expedient, mutually acceptable answers. Because both parties feel that they sacrifice something, they are only partially satisfied, and a lose-lose atmosphere results. Compromising is useful for reaching expedient answers for limited periods when the goals are only moderately important and the parties have equivalent power.

Collaborating is assertive and cooperative. It is a win-win strategy. It contributes to effective problem solving because both parties try to find mutually satisfying solutions. This method integrates insights from different perspectives with the commitment developed through participation and the resolution of hard feelings. Problems are identified, alternatives explored, and ramifications considered until difficulties are resolved. Unfortunately, it may take more time than the results are worth. Generally this is a most effective method of conflict resolution.

Competing is a power-oriented mode that is assertive but uncooperative. In competition one is aggressive and pursues her own goals at another's expense. This creates a win-lose situation. Nevertheless, it is appropriate when a quick or unpopular decision is needed, when the person is very knowledgeable about the situation and able to make a sound decision, or when one must protect oneself from other aggressive people. If this strategy is used too often, colleagues may become afraid to admit mistakes and may simply say what they think the aggressor wants to hear. A superior can always fall back on her authority and give orders to a subordinate, but because the resolution is forced, it almost certainly will be unsatisfactory.

A foundation of mutual trust must underlie any attempt to understand alternative views and to actively seek solutions that will allow each party to achieve its goals. This trust creates an atmosphere conducive to successful conflict resolution.

Strategies for conflict resolution. There are three ways of dealing with conflict: the win-lose, lose-lose, or win-win strategy. *Win-lose* methods include the use of position power, mental or physical power, failure to respond, majority rule, and railroading a minority position over the majority. *Lose-lose* strategies include compromise, bribes for accomplishing disagreeable tasks, arbitration by a neutral third party, and resortion to the use of general rules instead of considering the merits of individual cases. In win-lose and lose-lose strategies, the parties often personalize the issues by focusing on each other instead of on the problem. Intent on their personal differences, they avoid the more important matter of how to mutually solve their problem. Solutions are emphasized instead of goals and values. Rather than identifying mutual needs, planning activities for resolution, and solving the problem, each party looks at the issue from her own point of view and strives for total victory.

By contrast, *win-win* strategies focus on goals. They emphasize consensus and integrative approaches to decision making. The consensus process demands a focus on the problem (instead of on each other), on the collection of facts, on the acceptance of the useful aspects of conflict, and on the avoidance of averaging and self-oriented behavior. The group decision is thus often better than the best individual decision.

Problem-solving strategies include identifying both the problem and each party's needs, exploring alternatives, choosing the most acceptable alternative, planning, defining roles, implementing, and evaluating the decision.

Interpersonal conflict. Interpersonal conflict is inevitable, but the supervisor can lessen its impact by coaching subordinates in assertive communication and fair fighting. Engaging in a fair fight demands that the individual with a complaint first ask her opponent for a meeting. Once a time and place are agreed on, both parties should determine whether or not their supervisor should be present. Moreover, a fair fight demands that both parties know the purpose of the meeting so neither will be caught off guard—each can be prepared. The encounter should begin with a statement of the problem. If the supervisor is present, she should act as a mediator, asking the complainer to explain the perceived problem to the opponent. The opponent then should relate her understanding of how the complainer perceives the problem. After each has spoken, each can clarify any differences over the statement of the problem. Next the opponent describes her own perception of the problem; this description then should be followed by the complainer's repeating her understanding of how the opponent perceives the problem. Again, there is a pause for clarification.

A clear statement of the problem helps to shed light on the negative effects of each person's behavior. This feedback process, which requires each party to repeat what the other has just said, forces each to listen carefully. Were it not for such interaction, one might be so busy thinking of what she is going to say next that she fails to hear what is being said. Feedback does not imply parroting, because an understanding of meaning is more important than sheer memorization of words. Differences often begin to disappear when both parties really hear each other for the first time.

By exploring the alternatives to the problem and the ramifications of their options, the parties can identify and request changes in each other's behavior and respond to the other's requests. The discussion should close with an agreement on whether to change and the establishment of the accompanying conditions. A follow-up engagement should be set to discuss the success or failure of the agreement.*

Group conflict. Team development can help prevent and resolve conflict. Planning, goal setting, and rating goals represent the first step in team development. The statement of the core mission of the team is developed by brainstorming and sharing individual mission statements.

The nominal group technique† is very effective for developing team-performance goals and priorities. First, individual group members list on separate pieces of paper what they think team-performance goals should be. The group leader helps keep the group problem centered by presenting the question and avoids interruptions of thoughts by asking participants to work silently and independently. This step allows time for thinking, avoids status and conformity pressures, prevents focusing on a particular idea because of a vocal person, and helps avoid choosing among ideas prematurely.

Next, during a round-robin session, each person in turn states one of her team-performance goals, which is then written on a chalkboard or paper for all to see. It is probable that equalization of participation and sharing of all ideas fosters group creativity. By citing one goal, each member is encouraged to participate equally. By the second round, each member has participated and the precedent is set, and thus competition from aggressive or high-status members is minimized.

---

*Nine steps in a fair fight are presented in Bach, G.R., and Goldberg, H.: Creative aggression: the art of assertive living, New York, 1974, Avon Books, pp. 307-311.
†The nominal group technique is described in detail in Delbecq, A.L., Van de Ven, A.H., and Gustafson, D.H.: Group techniques for program planning: a guide to nominal group and Delphi processes, Glenview, Ill., 1975, Scott, Foresman & Co.

If all an individual's listed goals have been cited, she passes, and other members continue to offer listed goals in turn until all are exhausted. Ideas are not repeated. However, hitchhiking may occur. An idea listed by one member may stimulate another member to have an idea not previously listed. That idea can be added to the member's list and cited during the round-robin session.

It is common for many of an individual's ideas about a problem to remain unspoken because of fear of self-disclosure and embarrassment. When one person states several ideas at once, those ideas tend to be associated with her. However, with the round-robin method, it is difficult to remember who presented what ideas, and full disclosure is encouraged.

The written list can be the basis of recorded minutes and serve as a source of information from which the group continues to work. During this step, the group leader should see that ideas are recorded as rapidly as possible and in the words used by the contributor. The entire list should be made visible to all group members. Tearing completed sheets from a flip chart and taping them on the walls works well, and it is an early reward in that the group can see the array of ideas generated. The written ideas are more objective and less personal than oral comments because the personality and position of the contributors are separated from the written statement. The group leader should encourage the simple listing of ideas by explaining that a discussion period will follow. Discussion of the ideas, arguments about them, and side conversations while the list is being made should not be allowed.

The third step is a serial discussion for clarification. During this step, each listed idea is discussed in order. This provides an opportunity to clarify ideas, state differences of opinion, provide the logic behind ideas, and prevent undue focusing on any one idea. The group leader's responsibility is to clarify the purpose of this step and to pace the group. Arguments can be curtailed by stating that both points of view have been noted and then moving on to the next point. It is better not to ask the contributors to clarify their own items, because such a request can put them on the spot. Instead, the group members can be asked what the items mean to them. The contributor can clarify when appropriate. This method helps reduce identification of items with specific individuals.

The preliminary vote on item importance is the fourth step. In the nominal group process, individuals make independent judgments, express their judgments mathematically by ranking items, use the mean value of the independent judgments for the group's decision, talk over the results, and revote.

Alternative ways to determine a group decision are consensus, majority rule, and independent listing. When using consensus, group members may distort their judgments to maintain group cohesion, and consequently a regression toward the mean may occur. A showing of hands for majority rule

is subject to social pressure, and minority positions do not count. Consequently, it may not truly reflect group preference. Independent listing, however,
overcomes status, personality, and conformity pressures but does not indicate degree of importance. For example, an item listing might look like the
following:

Item	Votes
1	5
2	1
3	2
4	5
5	5
6	5
7	1
8	2

An analysis of the votes suggests that items 1, 4, 5, and 6 are considered the
most important by frequency. Information about degree of importance can be
obtained by having the items ranked. Ranking of the list might look like the
following:

Item	Votes	Totals
1	1-2-5-5-1	14
2	2	2
3	3-2	5
4	4-3-2-4-2	15
5	1-2-1-3-1	8
6	5-5-4-5-4	23
7	1	1
8	3-3	6

Using a scale of 5 as most important and 1 as least important, an analysis of the
votes reveals that items 6, 4, 1, 5, and 8 are considered most important in
descending order from 6 to 8. This method is more likely to reflect the true group
preference.

The group leader asks each individual to select a specific number of most
important items from the list. Individuals seem most able to accurately list five
to nine items. Each member is asked to take that specific number of 3 × 5 index
cards, identify that number of items from the list, place the item number in the
upper left-hand corner, and write some identifying words in the middle of the
card. Then the participants are asked to spread out the cards, choose the item
they consider most important, and put the high number in the lower right-hand
corner of the card and underline it. If five items are being selected, 5 would be
the high number. For nine items, 9 would be the high number. That card
is turned over, the remaining cards are assessed, and a 1 is put in the lower
right-hand corner and underlined for the least important card. That card is
turned over and the next most important item is selected and rated as one

less than the highest number—for instance, 8 for nine items or 4 for five items. Then the next to the lowest item is chosen and marked as 2 and so on until the middle item is left and numbered. This process encourages careful decisions.

An index card illustrating the rank order might appear as follows:

```
┌─────────────────────────────────────────────────────┐
│                                                     │
│  6 (item number from original list)                 │
│                                                     │
│                                                     │
│              setting goals for the unit             │
│                 (identifying words)                 │
│                                                     │
│                                                     │
│                                        2            │
│                                (rank order number)  │
│                                                     │
└─────────────────────────────────────────────────────┘
```

When the card ranking is complete, the group leader collects and shuffles the cards and records the votes on the written list of items.

The fifth step is a discussion of the preliminary vote. Inconsistent voting patterns can be examined, and items receiving many or few votes can be discussed. A discussion will probably allow for correction of misinformation, misunderstandings, and unequal information, thereby offering a more accurate indication of preferences than voting only.

The final step is the revote, which determines the outcome of the process, documents the group judgment, and closes the nominal group process.

Role negotiations—the process of preventing role conflicts, role ambiguities, and role overload—become important once priorities have been set. During this process group members clarify each individual's role on the team and help to resolve any disagreements over the team members' roles. Each member initially sends one written message to each team member indicating that for her to act, she needs the other team member to do more, less, or to continue her previous performance. *To whom* and *from whom* are essential parts of the message. The number of role messages sent to any one individual should be limited to prevent an information overload. The message must clearly state how the sender wants the receiver to behave and how a change will help the sender. Each role message must indicate the need for more, less, or the same of some activity. More than one message in the "same" category indicates support for the other person.

ROLE MESSAGE FORM

To:_____

From:_____

In order for me to _____, I need you to do

Less of:

Same of:

More of:

The receiver responds by indicating what she can or cannot do, explaining why, and offering alternative solutions, for example, "I can't do x, but I can do y, which should help solve your problem," or "If I do x, I would like you to do y." The receiver analyzes the role messages she receives in the "do more, do less, and do the same" categories and according to who sent the message and her response to that message. Does she know what is expected of her? Do different people want her to do more *and* less of the same activity at the same time? Does the receiver have time to meet all the demands made of her? Role definition helps identify role ambiguity, role conflict, and role overload. After roles are negotiated, a contract (p. 226) is written that defines the problem, identifies what each involved person will do, and sets a date for a follow-up check.

Negotiating involves good communication skills. One can identify needs, ideas, and information by using open-ended probes to clarify. Closed probes can be used to pinpoint specifications and to confirm understanding. One should indicate her intent ("I support your idea") when she offers ideas of information. It is preferable to present reasons before conclusions, as they seem to be heard better that way, and the speaker is more likely to be considered reasonable. To build on ideas, one should acknowledge the connection ("Bill's comment made me think of . . . ") and then add value. To criticize constructively, merits should be stated before concerns. One should then ask for ways to retain merits and eliminate concerns. Confront counterproductive tactics by confirming the behavior and expressing its impact. ("That seemed like a personal attact. Is that

---

ROLE CONTRACT

1. Problem:

2. Person x agrees to:

3. Person y agrees to:

4. Others agree to:

We agree that a follow-up check will be done by _____.
(date)

Signatures

_____
x

_____
y

_____
others

---

what you intended? I feel angry when I am treated that way.") To break an impasse, one can indicate her desire to continue and then initiate a change of pace: "Let's go get a cup of coffee and then try to solve this problem."

To come to the terms of an agreement, the purpose of the meeting and review the situation should be discussed. The needs and restrictions to develop, examine ideas from both points of view, and to determine the best alternative, should be explored. The discussion can be closed by summarizing the agreement and confirming the next steps.*

Decision charting is the next major phase of team development and is concerned with who should be involved in decision making and with the nature of that involvement. To determine who should be involved in decision making, one should assess who has the information necessary to make a sound decision

---

*Negotiating skills can be practiced in Negotiating self-taught, Stamford, Conn., 1984, Learning International.

and who is responsible for implementing that decision. The latter needs to understand the decision and be committed to it.

People can be involved in decision making in a variety of ways. Some are directly involved because they have the necessary information and are responsible for implementing the decision. The involvement of some may be limited to input or consultation. Others need to be informed about the decision, and someone must be responsible for managing the overall decision-making process.

A decision chart helps one to visualize the decision-making process. Decisions to be made are listed down the side of the page and the involved people across the top in a grid pattern: placing an *M* in a square indicates who manages the process; *D* indicates who is directly involved; *C* indicates who should be consulted; and *I* indicates who should be informed. Anyone who is expected to implement the decision obviously must be informed.*

DECISION CHART

Names

Tasks

M, Manages the process; C, consulted before the decision; D, makes the decision; I, informed of the decision.

Group process is critical for team development. How the group functions, communicates, and sets and achieves objectives are all related to group dynamics. Both task-oriented behavior and maintenance-oriented behavior are necessary for adequate team development.

People who assume group-task roles coordinate and facilitate the group's efforts to identify the problem, explore alternative options, identify the ramifications of the options, choose the most viable option, and implement and evalu-

*Team development is described in detail in Rubin, I.M., Plovnick, M.S., and Fry, R.E.: Improving the coordination of care: a program for health team development, Cambridge, Mass., 1975, Ballinger Publishing Co., and Managing human resources in health care organizations: an applied approach, Reston, Va., 1978, Reston Publishing Co.

ate the plan. There are numerous group-task roles, and any member of the group may fulfill a number of these roles in successive participation.

The *initiator-contributor* proposes new ideas or different ways of approaching a problem. Her task is to identify the problem, clarify the objectives, offer solutions, suggest agenda items, and set time limits. The *information seeker* searches for factual information about the problem, whereas the *opinion seeker* clarifies values pertinent to the problem and its solutions. Unlike the information seeker, the *information giver* identifies facts, shares her experiences, and makes generalizations. The *opinion giver* states her beliefs and what she thinks the group should value. Her focus is on values rather than on facts. The *elaborator* develops suggestions, illustrates points, and predicts outcomes. Relationships are clarified by the *coordinator*. The *orienter* summarizes the discussion, activities, and points of departure to provide perspective on the group's progress toward its goal. Evaluation of the problem, content, and process is done by the *critic*, who may measure the group's achievement against a set of standards. The *energizer* stimulates the group to increase the quantity and quality of their work. The *procedural technician* facilitates group action by arranging the room for the meeting, distributing the materials, working the audiovisual equipment, and generally functioning as the "go-for"—the person who goes for what is needed. An account of the discussion, suggestions, and decisions is kept by the *recorder*.

The roles of group building and group maintenance focus on how people treat each other while accomplishing a task. The *gatekeeper* regulates communication and takes actions to assure everyone an opportunity to be heard. The *encourager* radiates warmth and approval. She offers commendation and praise and indicates acceptance and understanding of others' ideas and values. The *harmonizer* creates and maintains group cohesion, relieving tension through her sense of humor and helping others reconcile their disagreements. The *compromiser* promotes group process by yielding status, admitting mistakes, modifying her ideas for the sake of group cohesiveness, maintaining self-control for group harmony, or by generally making compromises to keep the group action oriented. The *follower*, acting as a passive audience, goes along with the group. The *group observer* keeps records of the group process and gives interpretations for evaluation of the proceedings. The quality of the group process is compared with standards by the *standard setter*.

Some members of the group may try to satisfy their individual needs irrespective of the group tasks or maintenance roles. For example, the *aggressor* meets her needs at the expense of others by disapproving of others and deflating their status. The *dominator* asserts authority or superiority through flattery, interrupting others, and by giving directions authoritatively. The *recognition-seeker* calls attention to herself by boasting and acting in unusual ways. The *special interest pleader* speaks for an interest group and addresses issues that best meet that need. The *blocker* is negative, resistant, and disagreeable without apparent reason and brings issues back to the floor after the group has rejected them. The *self-confessor* uses the group to express personal feelings, while the *help-seeker* expresses depreciation, insecurity, and personal confusion that elicit sympathy responses. The *playboy* has a lack of involvement in the group process and appears nonchalant. A high incidence of individual roles in a group requires self-diagnosis to suggest what group-training efforts are needed. Having a trained observer record who is fulfilling what roles during a meeting can be revealing. On a form similar to the following, an observer records each time a participant plays a certain role.

Names

Roles								
Initiator-contributor								
Information seeker								
Opinion seeker								
Information giver								
Opinion giver								
Elaborator								
Coordinator								
Orienter								
Critic								
Energizer								
Procedural technician								
Recorder								
Gatekeeper								
Encourager								
Harmonizer								
Compromiser								
Follower								
Group observer								
Standard setter								
Aggressor								
Dominator								
Recognition seeker								
Special interest pleader								
Blocker								
Self-confessor								
Help-seeker								
Playboy								

Intergroup conflict. Intergroup conflict is common and can be dysfunctional. As with interpersonal conflict, intergroup resistance may result from low trust, poor communications, and false assumptions. People resist what they perceive as threatening. Intergroup actions may threaten territorial rights and contribute to role overload and conflict. By avoiding win-lose situations, emphasizing the organization's goals and effectiveness, rotating personnel among groups to facilitate understanding, and increasing interaction and communication between groups, one can help reduce intergroup conflict.

When a group recognizes its need to solve some intergroup conflict, it must first decide how to begin. A study of the organizational chart will determine who should be involved. Who should represent the group—a person or a committee? Someone who is already friendly with members of the other group? Someone with strong or moderate feelings about the position? What is the group's position and how much negotiation is acceptable? It helps to emphasize common goals and discuss constraints. The same process used in interpersonal conflict should be used in group conflict situations: setting and rating goals, negotiating roles, and making decisions.

Organizational conflict. Organizations in conflict display the collective symptoms of their members, and the symptoms can be numerous. Personnel feel frustration at work. If they do not think their skills are being used, they experience a loss of self-esteem and a sense of impotence, both of which lead to withdrawal from the situation instead of an attempt to solve the problems. Group members also engage in backbiting and blame others for the problems. Subgroup formations are common. Members of the organization identify the same task and group maintenance problems but act contrary to the information, thereby increasing their frustrations. However, personnel do not have the same frustrations or exhibit the same dysfunctional behavior outside the organization.

Consultation may be sought to deal with organizational conflict. The consultant must analyze the organization's structure, the leadership and authority of the institution, the communication patterns, the amount of intergroup cooperation and competition, the group's norms and goals, the group's problem-solving and decision-making processes, and various individual roles and functions within the group. Organizational research can help to provide the information necessary to solve the problem.

After data have been collected and analyzed, the consultant offers feedback. Members of the organization can publicly note whether or not they agree with the consultant's views. A public vote facilitates ownership of ideas. If there is disagreement, the consultant helps the group clarify the reasons for the differences and modifies the statement until it reflects the group's thinking.

The consultant then asks each member to write a few sentences about how she contributes to the situation so that each can recognize her own part in the problem. Individuals are likely to maintain the status quo for fear of serious consequences if they confront the issues. The consultant shares her theory with the group, helps develop an awareness of dysfunctional behavior, helps individuals cope with their feelings, encourages fantasy and reality testing, and coaches group members toward new behaviors.

Prevention of conflict. Careful development of an organization's structure, strategic and comprehensive planning, management and organizational development, and careful selection and placement of personnel help prevent organizational conflict. The same strategies also prevent intergroup, group, and interpersonal conflict. Although conflict can be reduced, it cannot be totally avoided. Conflict can be constructive or destructive. By capitalizing on the positive aspects, the negative features can seem more bearable.

MOTIVATION OF PERSONNEL

Why do people work? Why do some employees achieve high productivity while others are content with mediocrity or less? What can a manager do to stimulate intrinsic and extrinsic motivation? These questions are important to the manager. They elicit complex and uncertain answers. Unfortunately, there are no simple rules that a supervisor can follow to stimulate her staff.

Taylor's monistic theory

Monistic theory is derived from the principles of scientific management. Frederick Taylor, a pioneer in this field, believed that if an energetic person with high productivity learned that she earned no more than a lazy worker who did as little as possible, she would lose interest in yielding her optimum. Taylor argued that an incentive was needed to prevent this loss. It should be possible to earn more by producing more, so that pay would be dependent on productivity. Incentives such as merit increases, bonus systems, profit sharing, savings sharing, and piece rates are examples of monistic methods. With implementation of payment by piece rate, the employer must be certain that wage costs do not increase more rapidly than production. This system can place considerable pressure on the worker and create tensions that lead to undesirable behavior. Payment by piece rate almost certainly guarantees that some workers will be paid more than others. A larger paycheck may increase one's self-esteem and even serve as a status symbol, but the amount of motivation provided by money is questionable.

Maslow's hierarchy-of-needs theory

In contrast to Taylor's belief that money is a primary motivator, A.H. Maslow maintained that people are motivated by a desire to satisfy a hierarchy of needs. Maslow hypothesized that satisfaction of the basic physiological needs triggers the emergence of more abstract needs and that a satisfied need is no longer a motivator. The five basic needs he identified are physiological, safety, love, esteem, and self-actualization.

Physiological needs. The body needs water, food, oxygen, elimination, rest, exercise, sex, shelter, and protection from the elements. People have a strong drive for self-preservation, and whenever their basic physiological needs are threatened, the needs become prepotent. These needs are relatively independent and must be met repeatedly to remain fulfilled. In an affluent society, the physiological needs are probably not the most common motivators. The nurse manager should determine whether physiological needs are being met. Personnel should not be overworked. Meal breaks and rest breaks should be provided. Pay should be adequate for food, shelter, health care, and recreation.

Safety needs. People need physical, emotional, and financial safety. They need a stable environment in which they are protected against the threats of danger and deprivation. People do not want to worry about inadequate income because of loss of job, accident, or old age. Therefore, arbitrary management actions, favoritism toward or discrimination against employees, and unpredictable administration of policy are dangerous to safety needs and should be avoided.

Love needs. Love needs include a feeling of belonging, acceptance by one's peers, recognition as an accepted member of a group, being an integral part of the operation, giving and receiving friendship, and affectionate relations with others. A cohesive work group is likely to be more effective than an equal number of people working separately. Yet management, fearing hostility toward its objectives, may control situations to prevent esprit de corps. Thwarting of the social needs, however, may stimulate resistance and antagonism that further defeat management's objectives.

Esteem needs. Achievement, competence, knowledge, independence, status, recognition, prestige, appreciation, reputation, and respect contribute to one's self-confidence and self-esteem. Management can help meet these needs by giving praise when it is deserved and through the use of constructive evaluations, pay raises, and titles. Unlike the lower physiological and safety needs, the esteem needs are not so easily satisfied.

Self-actualization. It is doubtful that one ever achieves all that of which she is capable. Feelings of accomplishment, responsibility, importance, challenge, advancement, and new experiences and opportunities for growth contribute to self-fulfillment.

Alderfer's modified need hierarchy

Clayton Alderfer proposes a modified need hierarchy theory that collapses Maslow's five hierarchical levels into three. His ERG theory (existence-relatedness-growth) suggests that in addition to a satisfaction-progression process, in which an individual is constantly frustrated in her attempts to satisfy one level of needs, she can redirect her energy toward a lower level need. Alderfer's model is less rigid than Maslow's and suggests that more than one need may be operative.

Maslow	Alderfer
Self-actualization Esteem needs	Growth needs
Love needs	Relatedness needs
Safety needs Physiological needs	Existence needs

McClelland's basic needs theory

David McClelland has identified three basic needs that all people have in varying degrees: the need for achievement, power, and affiliation. The need for achievement involves a desire to make a contribution, to excel, and to succeed. People with high achievement needs are eager for responsibility, take calculated risks, and desire feedback about their performance. People who have a high need for power want to be in control and desire influence over others. They are more interested in personal prestige and power than effective performance. For contrast, people with high affiliation needs desire working in humane environments and seek out meaningful friendships. They want to be respected and avoid decisions or actions that oppose group norms. They are more interested in high morale than productivity. Managers should match personnel needs with assignments. If a project has well-defined objectives and specific tasks, a person with a high achievement need may be appropriate. If a project involves unpleasant tasks with personnel (such as retrenchment), a person with high power needs may do the job best. A person with high affiliation needs would not want to make decisions that would alienate peers but would be good for fostering morale.

Herzberg's motivation-hygiene theory or two-factor theory

Frederick Herzberg found that work motivators include achievement, growth, responsibility, advancement, recognition, and the job itself. According to Herzberg, if someone is satisfied with her job, she is receiving positive feedback, developing skills, and improving her performance. Herzberg maintains that an employee can be motivated by giving her challenging work in which she can assume responsibility.

Dissatisfaction results when one perceives that she is being treated unfairly in pay, benefits, status, job security, supervision, and interpersonal relationships. Herzberg classifies all of the above as hygiene factors and argues that they are not motivators because they do not cause any improvement in attitudes or performance. They can only prevent dissatisfaction and poor morale. Hygiene factors do not make a job more interesting. If a person is highly motivated and finds her job interesting and challenging, she can tolerate dissatisfaction with hygiene factors.

Argyris's psychological energy theory

Chris Argyris believes that people will exert more energy to meet their own needs than those of the organization. The greater the disparity between the individual's and the organization's goals, the more likely it is that the employee will feel dissatisfaction, tension, conflict, apathy, or subversion. Argyris suggests that management match personnel and jobs by taking advantage of people's talents and interests, make jobs interesting and challenging, help personnel satisfy their needs for self-actualization, improve interpersonal relationships, and use a management style consistent with Theory Y (discussed later).

Vroom's expectancy theory

Victor Vroom popularized the expectancy theory during the 1960s. It is based on Kurt Lewin's field theory and has been expanded by Lyman Porter and others. Expectancy theory states that motivation is dependent on how much someone wants something and her estimate of the probability of getting it.

$$\text{Motivation} = \text{Valence} \times \text{Expectancy}$$

Valence is the strength of one's preference for something. It may be negative as well as positive. If one does not want something, there is a negative valence. If the person is indifferent, the valence is 0. A positive valence indicates a desire for something.

Valence

$$- 1 \underline{\hspace{3cm} 0 \hspace{3cm}} + 1$$

Expectancy is the probability of getting something through specific actions. If a person believes that an action will result in an outcome, expectancy has a value of 1. If no probability is perceived, the expectancy is 0. Expectancy varies from one situation to another.

Expectancy

$$0 \underline{\hspace{4cm}} + 1$$

If someone has a high valence and a high expectancy, the motivation will be high. If there is a low valence and a low expectancy, the motivation will be low. If one is high and the other low, moderate motivation will result.

$$M = EP \times PO \times V$$

M = Motivation
EP = Belief that effort will lead to desired performance
PO = Anticipation that performance will lead to particular outcome
V = Value of reward

The expectancy theory has been further developed to include the value of the outcome factor. To be highly motivated, a person needs to find an outcome attractive, believe that certain actions will lead to the desired outcome, and assess that the result is worth the effort. Consequently, to motivate personnel, managers should clarify connections between work and outcome and should reward desirable behavior.

Skinner's positive reinforcement theory

Operant conditioning or behavior modification are other names for Skinner's positive reinforcement theory. Behavior may be strengthened or weakened depending on what follows it. Positive reinforcement strengthens behavior. Withholding positive reinforcers weakens behavior, whereas intermittent reinforcement increases resistance to extinction. Punishment will help reduce behavior, but it cannot teach new behaviors, and it may condition avoidance.

Accentuating the positive with plenty of praise and positive feedback may increase the frequency of desired behavior. If, however, a subordinate admits to less than desirable behavior, the supervisor may respond, "I appreciate your honesty," while reminding the worker of the goal. When desired results are not obtained, the supervisor should analyze the situation. First she should assess the working environment for interference. Does the employee have adequate time to complete the task? Does the system allow the nurse to maximize her efficiency, or must she spend most of her time running to central supply to gather materials that should have been readily available? If the supervisor does not locate the cause of the problem in the environment, then she must ask herself if the employee has been properly utilized. Does she have the knowledge and skills necessary to do the job? If not, can she be taught? If she cannot be taught, can she be replaced and assigned other duties?

Equity theory

During the 1960s, Jo Stacy Adams and others studied perceptions of equity and inequity. They found that employees assess fairness by considering their input and the psychological, social, and financial rewards in comparison with those of others. Perceived inequity causes tension. The amount of the tension was found to be proportional to the magnitude of the perceived inequity. Tension motivates people to reduce its cause. Consequently, the strength of the motivation to reduce the perceived inequity is proportional to the cognitive dissonance. To reduce the inequity, a person may alter input or outcome, cognitively distort input or output, change the basis for comparison, or leave. If a person feels overworked and underpaid, she is likely to decrease her productivity. Less often, employees feel overrewarded and strive to improve their performance. People resist changing their bases of comparison or distorting their perceptions. People do not usually leave an organization unless there is extreme inequity. If the comparison is equal, the person feels that she is treated fairly. If not, the person is motivated to take corrective action. The manager should be attentive to the perceived equity of the reward system.

Intrinsic motivation

Edward L. Deci has studied intrinsic motivation. He found that some activities are ends in themselves, not just means to ends. There is no apparent reward except the activity itself. Intrinsically motivated behavior seems to be stimulated by people's needs for feeling competent and self-determining. When there is no stimulation, people will seek it. When they are overstimulated, they back away, regroup, and reaffirm competence. People engage in a process of seeking and conquering to feel competent and self-determined. When a person's feelings of competence and self-determination are enhanced, her intrinsic motivation will increase. If her perception of competence and self-determination are diminished, her intrinsic motivation will decrease. Extrinsic rewards have a controlling aspect that may decrease intrinsic rewards. Insufficient extrinsic rewards tend to increase intrinsic motivation because people try to reduce cognitive dissonance. Consequently, managers should foster stimulation through means such as continuing education and special projects.

McGregor's Theory X and Theory Y

Douglas McGregor has classified traditional management theories as Theory X. They are based on the assumption that people will avoid work if possible because they dislike it; consequently, most people must be directed, controlled, coerced, and threatened. Theory X assumes that people want direction, have little ambition, avoid responsibility, but want security. A manager with a Theory X philosophy would probably use fear and threats to motivate personnel, supervise closely, delegate little responsibility, and not consider personnel participation in planning.

McGregor maintains that if people behave as described in Theory X it is because of what the system has done to them—not because of their inherent nature. He believes that as long as managerial strategies are based on Theory

X, managers will fail to discover, let alone utilize, the potentials of their personnel.

McGregor classifies the newer developments in management as Theory Y. In this theory McGregor makes the assumption that people like and enjoy work, are self-directed, and seek responsibility. It maintains that most people have imagination, ingenuity, creativity, and other intellectual capacities that are only partially utilized. A manager with a Theory Y philosophy will use positive incentives such as praise and recognition, give general supervision, provide opportunities for individual growth, delegate responsibilities, and encourage participation in problem solving. Job enlargement and decentralization are additional motivational techniques that may stimulate personnel's performance to the extent that it exceeds the requirements stated in the job description.

Likert's participative management theory

Rensis Likert believes that an effective manager is highly sensitive to her subordinates, uses communication to keep the group working as a unit, and fosters supportive relationships among all group members. Participative management is a human relations theory that may use management by objectives and job-enrichment approaches.

Theory Z

The Japanese form of participative management is known as Theory Z. The major firms of Japan are organized into *Zaibatsu*, small groups of twenty to thirty firms representing each important industrial sector. Each firm hosts satellite companies that provide a service or manufacture a subassembly for the host firm. Employees are hired to work for the host firm until retirement. After slow evaluation and promotion in nonspecialized careers, employees are retired at age 55. They then work on a part-time basis for a satellite company. Women work temporarily and serve as a buffer to the job security of the male work force. Their schedules are flexible so they can care for their families, and they are laid off in slack periods.

Concern for the worker is apparent. Japanese companies form inclusive personal and professional relationships and provide social support. Because personnel anticipate lifetime relationships, they are cautious about interpersonal conflicts. Cooperation is stressed. Collective decision making is practiced. Through the ritual of *ringi*, ideas pass from manager to manager for approval. This helps establish trust and cooperation. Objectives and the procedures to achieve them are implicitly described. Quality circles are formed when two to ten employees meet to identify problems, explore options, and make decisions. Quality circles have increased worker productivity, enhanced job satisfaction, and reduced turnover in addition to solving identified problems. Decisions are made by consensus. Because it takes so much time to come to a consensus, only policy and behavior changes are dealt with. Responsibility is also collective. An emphasis is placed on developing all aspects of the employees, and they are rewarded with regular pay bonuses based on the company's performance.

The Japanese Theory Z managers focus on the four soft S's of management: staff, skills, style, and superordinate goals. Staff is the workers. Skills are the capabilities of the organization or key personnel. Style refers to the cultural style of the organization or how managers achieve goals. The superordinate goals are the guideposts as determined by the personnel.

Less attention is given to the hard S's: system, structure, and strategy. The system is the mechanism whereby information circulates through the organization. Structure is the organization, and strategy is the plan of action.

Historical development of motivation theory

Traditional management theory is based on McGregor's Theory X. Traditional theory addresses itself to Maslow's primary physiological and safety needs and employs the monistic theory for reinforcement. The latter, according to Herzberg, helps meet some of the hygiene needs but does not provide motivation.

Newer developments in management are based on McGregor's Theory Y. Maslow's secondary needs of love, esteem, and self-actualization are more prepotent than the primary needs for most personnel. Because a satisfied need is no longer a motivator, hygiene factors such as money and working conditions do not serve as motivators. People are more interested in autonomy, responsibility, achievement, recognition, variety in work, and efforts for self-actualization. Argyris has suggested that personnel may become more self-actualized if their personal goals are consistent with the goals of the organization. Talents and interests should be considered when assigning jobs. And then, according to Skinner, positive reinforcement will further increase desired behaviors.

Participation is a major factor in newer management techniques. Personnel are encouraged to contribute to decisions, goals, and plans. Decentralization is supported to the point of management by objectives, allowing personnel to define their own objectives and to determine how they plan to achieve them. The supervisor approves the goals, makes sure they are consistent with the organization's goals, and evaluates personnel using their own objectives as the standard. The modern manager delegates duties and assists others to work more effectively. She helps each person develop her own talents and tries to maintain a close relationship between the interests and skills of the individual and the requirements of the job. Job enrichment and job rotation may be used to help develop personnel fully. When personnel are actively striving toward esteem and self-actualization and when their goals are consistent with those of the organization, there is likely to be a noticeable effect on the accomplishment of the organization's goals and productivity.

Job satisfaction*

Job dissatisfaction contributes to higher turnover rates and decreased productivity. Considerable time and money are required to recruit and select a replacement for someone who leaves a position. It takes time to socialize the new employee to the organization's norms. This orientation period is expensive because of educational expenses and decreased productivity. Other employees must carry more than their share of the load until the new individual can work to capacity, and group redevelopment is necessary after each change in membership. For all these reasons job satisfaction is a concern for nursing administrators.

Job dissatisfaction has been shown to be correlated with absenteeism and turnover. Herzberg maintains that satisfiers and dissatisfiers are mutually exclusive; he classifies the sense of achievement, recognition for achievement, the work itself, responsibility, advancement potential, and possibility of growth as motivators or satisfiers and matters such as working conditions, policies, supervision, interpersonal relations, salary, status, and job security as hygiene factors or dissatisfiers. He concludes that hygiene factors cannot motivate employees but can only prevent dissatisfaction. Herzberg's work remains controversial.

Through a systems approach, Wernimont has shown how extrinsic factors (dissatisfiers) cause intrinsic factors (satisfiers). Maslow's theory shows further insight into Herzberg's findings. It suggests that hygiene factors can be motivators and that only when hygiene factors are satisfied do satisfiers such as responsibility become motivators. Several research studies have indicated that people at lower educational, socioeconomic, and occupational levels and minority members tend to place more emphasis on hygiene or extrinsic job factors, whereas people at higher educational, socioeconomic, and occupational levels and whites are more concerned with motivators or intrinsic factors. In accordance with Maslow's theory, physiological and safety needs are apparently prepotent for lower socioeconomic groups, whereas these needs have probably been satisfied for people at higher educational and occupational levels, such as nurses, for whom esteem and self-actualization needs have become prepotent.

---

*From Marriner, A.: Contemporary nursing management, St. Louis, 1982, The C. V. Mosby Co., pp. 242-258.

Researchers disagree about the effects of supervision on job satisfaction. Employees' attitudes toward supervision are influenced by their perception of the supervisor's role, their self-perception, and their level of development. These individual differences necessitate that supervision be an adaptive leadership process.

The desire for influence in decision making is also affected by individual differences. Even though people presumably desire some control over their environment, this desire is not equally strong for all people. Vroom found that authoritarians are relatively unaffected by participating in decision making but that participation in decision making generally has favorable effect on job satisfaction. Role ambiguity, the result of a failure to inform an individual of what is needed to do the job, is relatively common. Even if the role is clear, an employee in that role may resign if role conflict is present and persists. Role conflicts may result from a number of factors and are affected by individual differences. Likewise, job satisfaction is multidimensional and subject to individual differences.

Women seem to show more variation than men in their job attitudes. Women emphasize working conditions, hours and ease of work, supervision, and social aspects of the job, whereas men emphasize wages, opportunity for advancement, company management and policies, and task interest. College-educated women rank the importance of motivators such as achievement, recognition, and responsibility significantly higher than female clerical workers without college degrees. People tend to have more job satisfaction before the age of 20 years and after the age of 35 years than during the period between. Younger people tend to be more interested in income, whereas older people are interested in security.

Nurses surveyed about their sources of satisfaction identify a sense of achievement, recognition, challenging work, responsibility, advancement potential, autonomy, authority, pleasant work environment, agreeable working hours, and adequate staffing all as satisfiers. Nurses stress the importance of respected hospital administrators, supportive nursing administrators, trustful supervisors, fair evaluations, and adequate feedback. Poor planning, poor communication, inadequate explanations of decisions affecting jobs, unclear rules and regulations, unreasonable pressure, too much work, work load negatively affecting work quality, understaffing, uncooperative physicians, nonnursing duties, and unqualified supervisors are all sources of dissatisfaction. Reduced productivity, increased absenteeism, and rapid turnover are expensive consequences of job dissatisfaction but can be reduced if the nursing administrator fosters job satisfaction through organization and management.

COMMUNICATION

Communication process

All of the manager's functions involve communication. The communication process involves six steps.

Ideation → Encoding → Transmission → Receiving → Decoding → Response ⌐
Response ← Decoding ← Receiving ← Transmission ← Encoding ←⌐

The first step, ideation, begins when the sender decides to share the content of her message with someone, senses a need to communicate, develops an idea, or selects information to share. The purpose of communication may be to inform, persuade, command, inquire, or entertain. Whatever the reason, the sender needs to know her goal and think clearly, or the message may be garbled and meaningless.

Encoding, the second step, involves putting meaning into symbolic forms— speaking, writing, or nonverbal behavior. One's personal, cultural, and professional biases affect the goals and encoding process. Use of clearly understood symbols and communication of all the receiver needs to know are important.

The third step, transmission of the message, must overcome interference, such as garbled speech, unintelligible use of words, long complex sentences, distortion from recording devices, noise, and illegible handwriting.

Receiving is next. The receiver's senses of seeing and hearing are activated as the transmitted message is received. People tend to have selective attention (hear the messages of interest to them but not others) and selective perception (hear the parts of the message that conform with what they want to hear) that cause incomplete and distorted interpretation of the communication. Sometimes people tune out the message because they anticipate the content and think they know what is going to be said or are so busy formulating their response that they do not hear the message. The receiver may be preoccupied with other activities and consequently not be ready to listen. Poor listening is one of the biggest barriers in the communication process.

Decoding of the message by the receiver is the critical fifth step. The receiver defines words and interprets gestures during the transmission of speech. Written messages allow more time for decoding, as the receiver assesses the explicit meaning and implications of the message based on what the symbols mean to her. The symbols are subject to interpretation based on one's personal, cultural, and professional biases and may not have the same meaning to the receiver as to the sender. The communication process is dependent on the receiver's understanding of the information.

Fig. 4-6. Communication systems—chain, Y, wheel, circle, all-channel.

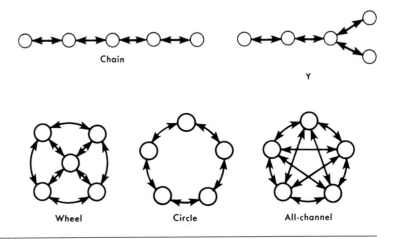

Response, or feedback, is the final step. It is important for the supervisor or sender to know that the message has been received and accurately interpreted.

Communication systems

Study of small-group process has revealed various communication networks (Fig. 4-6). The chain system is fast and accurate for simple problems. The middle person in the chain emerges as the leader, and the leadership position is stable. Unfortunately, morale is low and so is the flexibility for problem solving.

The leader emerges at the location of highest centrality, which is the fork of the Y and the hub of the wheel. Both provide fast, accurate problem solving. The coordinator, who is centrally located, is generally satisfied, but the peripheral members are less satisfied than members in less efficient systems. The wheel is an efficient, effective communication structure for simple problems.

The circular structure is slow and inaccurate. The structure does not influence the emergence of a leader. Because no one can communicate with everyone, there is no coordinator. However, morale is high, and there is considerable flexibility for problem solving.

When free to do so, groups tend to evolve to the all-channel network as problems become complex and shift back to a wheel structure as problems become simple. Greater amounts of information must be processed as task uncertainty and complexity increase. Consequently, an adaptive structure like the all-channel system is best for completing complicated and unpredictable tasks.

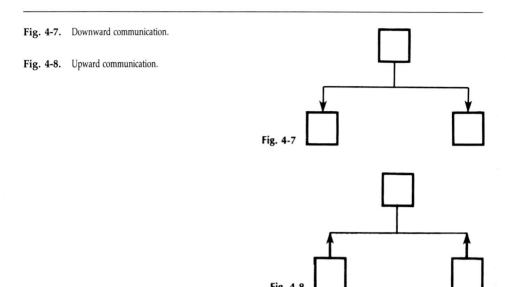

Fig. 4-7. Downward communication.

Fig. 4-8. Upward communication.

Fig. 4-7

Fig. 4-8

Essentially, the right network is the structure that facilitates the communication necessary to accomplish the task.

Downward communication

The traditional line of communication is from the superior to the subordinate down through the levels of management (Fig. 4-7). This downward communication is primarily directive and helps coordinate the activities of different levels of the hierarchy by telling the subordinate what to do and by providing the information needed by the subordinate to relate her efforts to the organization's goals. It includes oral and written indoctrination, education, and other information to influence the attitudes and behaviors of subordinates. Common forms of downward communications are employee handbooks, operating manuals, job description sheets, performance appraisal interviews, employee counseling, a loudspeaker system, letters, memos, messages circulated with paychecks, posters, bulletin boards, information racks, company newspapers, annual reports, the chain of command, the grapevine, and unions. Downward communication contributes to greater subordinate dissatisfaction than upward communication, regardless of the quality of the message.

Upward communication

Newer management techniques encourage delegation of authority and more personal involvement in decision making, thus creating a need for accurate upward communication (Fig. 4-8). Upward communication provides a means

Fig. 4-9. Lateral communication.

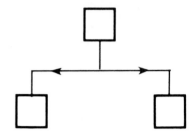

for motivating and satisfying personnel by allowing employee input. The supervisor summarizes information and passes it upward to the next level for use in decision making. That level then summarizes its action and transmits information to the next level. Because each level tends to bias the report by embellishing it with information that puts that level in the best light, there is a natural filtering process as information moves upward. By the time it reaches top management, it is highly refined.

In spite of this bias, the subordinate is often in a position to assess the situation more accurately than are her superiors. An employee may have a better solution to a problem than the first-line supervisor; the first-line supervisor may know more about a situation than a middle manager, and so on. Consequently, accurate upward communication is important for effective problem solving. Subordinates must feel free to upwardly communicate both solicited and unsolicited information and must have opportunity to do so, or management will lack needed information, and both managers and subordinates will become frustrated. Common means for upward communication include face-to-face discussions; open-door policies; staff meetings; task forces; written reports; performance appraisals; grievance procedures; exit interviews; attitude surveys; suggestion boxes; counseling; the chain of command; ombudsmen; informers; the grapevine; unions; and participative, consultative, and democratic management in general.

Lateral communication

Lateral or horizontal communication is between departments or personnel on the same level of the hierarchy and is most frequently used to coordinate activities (Fig. 4-9). The need for lateral communication increases as interdependence increases. For instance, it becomes more important when one worker starts a job and someone else finishes it. It is also used by staff to transmit technical information to line authorities, and it may contain subjective and emotional aspects. Committees, conferences, and meetings are often used to facilitate horizontal communication.

Fig. 4-10.   Diagonal communication.

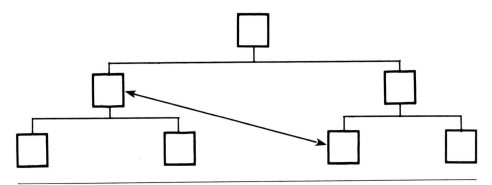

Diagonal communication

Diagonal communication occurs between individuals or departments that are not on the same level of the hierarchy (Fig. 4-10). Informal in nature and frequently used between staff groups and line functions and in project-type organizations, it is another facet of multidirectional communication, which is common when communications often flow in all directions at the same time.

The grapevine

Informal methods of communication coexist with formal channels and are referred to as the grapevine. Informal communication is often rapid and subject to considerable distortion. The grapevine transmits information much faster than the formal channels because it uses cluster chain pathways involving three or four individuals at a time instead of going from one person to another as in superior-subordinate relationships. Communication passes at an increasing rate as individuals from clusters inform other small groups of people who work near each other or have contact with each other. Information spreads most quickly through the grapevine when it is recent, affects personnel's work (for example, pay increases or changes in policies), and involves people they know. People who work near each other or come in contact with each other are likely to be on the same grapevine.

Information gets distorted for a number of reasons. Grapevine information is often fragmentary and incomplete. Consequently, there is a tendency to supply the missing pieces. Some people seize this opportunity to express feelings of self-importance, thus compensating for feelings of insecurity but also distorting the message. Because the grapevine is informal with no formal lines of accountability, the individual does not have to answer to her superior for misinforming others.

Managers can learn much by listening to the grapevine and can remedy distortions by using the informal channels to pass on correct information.

Barriers to communication

Faulty reasoning and poorly expressed messages are major barriers to communication. Lack of clarity and precision resulting from inadequate vocabulary, poorly chosen words, platitudes, jargon, awkward sentence structures, poor organization of ideas, and lack of coherence are common. Talking too fast or too slow, slurring words, and not emphasizing important points lead to the faulty transmission of ideas. Memos that are poorly organized, ramble, and lack summaries also complicate the communication process. Words mean different things to different people. Communication is complicated when the sender uses words with which the receiver is not familiar, does not communicate on the receiver's level, or makes the message long and complicated.

If the sender lacks information or omits facts she does know, she will pass on a distorted or filtered message. Filtering, whether intentional or unintentional, involves a biased choice of what is communicated. For instance, distortion is more likely when a subordinate desires promotion, for she may pass on information about her merits and suppress less successful aspects of her work. Fear of the consequences of full disclosure contributes to such omissions. At other times individuals may not communicate some information because they do not believe it is important enough to do so. The receiver becomes confused when nonverbal cues, such as facial expressions and posture, conflict with the verbal communication or when the sender does not admit to the intent of, or to the emotions underlying, the message.

People use selective perception to hear what they want to hear based on their biases. Values, attitudes, and assumptions affect one's perception of the message. Making a value judgment about the worth of a message based on one's opinion of the sender or the expected meaning of the message allows the receiver to hear what she wants to hear. An attitude is a feeling toward someone or something that is based on experience or the lack thereof and it is a common barrier to communication because of its screening effect. Uncommunicated assumptions are common and can make a considerable difference between the message sent and the one received. For instance, when program evaluation is mandated, personnel may fear that the results will be used to terminate workers, whereas management's actual intention is to use the results for recruiting purposes. Trust or distrust of the sender also influences how the message is received.

The sender is judged along with the message because the receiver has difficulty separating what she hears from how she feels about the sender. If fact, nonexistent motives can be attributed to the sender. Messages from higher echelons are often considered authoritative, even when they are not intended to be.

The higher up in the hierarchy a message originates, the greater are its chances of being accepted because of the status of the sender. If the sender has status with the listener, her message is usually considered credible. If she does not, the message may be discounted.

Subordinates tend to pay attention to communications from superiors, thus facilitating downward communication. Unfortunately, superiors may give verbal and nonverbal cues about how busy and unapproachable they are. They probably value communications from superiors more than from subordinates and may not reward subordinates for communications. In fact, subordinates are sometimes punished for communicating. Subordinates will be reluctant to report problems or potential problems when they believe these will be viewed as a weakness in their performance appraisal. Similarly, the middle manager may not report problems that would reflect unfavorably on her managerial skills.

Status symbols magnify role and status barriers by increasing the psychological distance and the perceived organizational distance. Time pressures also become barriers that prevent communication. Managers do not have time to see all of their subordinates as much as desired, and the subordinates may not take the time to report to the supervisor. Time pressures are also used as an excuse for not listening. Premature evaluation of what is going to be said, preoccupation with oneself, lack of readiness to hear, lack of receptivity to new ideas, and resistance to change interfere with listening. Physical distance, organizational complexity, temperature, noise, physical facilities (such as offices, meeting rooms, and an informal coffee shop), and technical facilities (such as telephones, loudspeakers, and duplicating equipment) also affect communications.

Improving communications

Ideas should be clear before one speaks. What is the purpose of the message? Is it to seek information, inform, persuade, or initiate action? To formulate a message, one must gather the information needed and seek consultation from others as appropriate. Considering the goals and attitudes of the receivers helps the sender convey something of help or value to the receivers. One must also determine the mode of communication—by written or oral messages or through gestures. Face-to-face contact involves nonverbal behavior that further clarifies intent and allows for feedback to validate understanding of the message. Feedback through mutual exchange decreases the chance for misunderstanding. A climate that allows people to say what they think facilitates feedback.

One must also consider the setting in which she communicates and time her messages for maximal impact. Should the communication be made in public or private? What is the social climate and what effect will that have on the tone of the communication? What are the customs and practices of the audience and how does one's message conform to its expectations? It is helpful for the message to refer to something the person has experienced and for it to be timed for immediate use by the receiver. For example, a building evacuation plan will be better received during fire prevention week when personnel are expecting a fire drill than at most other times.

Communications should be well organized and expressed in simple words, a clear style, and the shortest sentences possible. Redundancy—the repetition of the message verbatim or its presentation in several different ways—ensures that the message is understood. The amount of redundancy is dependent on the content of the message and the experience and background of the receiver. Repetition is especially important when the information is important and the directions are complicated. However, redundancy can become a barrier to communication if the message is simple and personnel are familiar with it. Employees are likely to stop listening because they know what is going to be said.

Because actions speak louder than words, the message is more forceful if the sender acts congruously. Communications should be followed up to make sure they were understood, and one should seek to understand as well as to be understood.

Listening—an active process that requires conscious attention—is critical to good communication. Trust is a prerequisite, because nurses will not share feelings with people they do not trust. The speaker must be convinced that disclosures will be kept confidential, feelings will be respected and not judged, and that the information will be used appropriately and not used against the speaker.

Once trust is established, empathetic listening is needed. We think faster than we talk. Consequently, when listening to another talk, we have time left over for thinking, time that is frequently misused. There is less time for irrelevant thoughts when one concentrates on what is being said. One can think ahead of the speaker, try to guess the points that will be made next, consider what the conclusion will be, listen between the lines, try to understand the speaker's point of reference, review, and summarize the points made.

Active listening involves refraining from talking while trying to understand the speaker's attitude and feelings. One should listen to the whole story, talking as little as possible and avoiding leading questions, arguing, or giving advice. Silent pauses encourage the speaker to continue. Attentiveness is indicated by comments such as "yes," "uh huh," "go on," restatement (repeating what was said), paraphrasing (saying what was said in different words), clarifying (asking the speaker what was meant), reflecting (responding to the feelings communicated), and summarizing (reviewing the major points made). By saying little, the receiver can concentrate on listening instead of on what she is going to say in return.

Written communications usually have the advantage of being more carefully formulated than oral communications. They also may save time and money and can be retained as legal records and reference sources. Written communications are sent downward, upward, or horizontally. Policies, procedures, handbooks, annual reports, bulletin boards, and house newspapers are usually directed downward. Attitude and morale surveys, suggestion systems, and written grievances are directed upward. Letters, memos, and reports may be upward, downward, or horizontal communication. Between department heads they are horizontal.

Before writing, one must first consider the purpose of the communication. For a planned and organized message, the writer develops thoughts logically, gives evidence to back up statements, and carefully selects her words. The writer must ask herself if the communication answers who, what, when, where, and why questions and should appraise the tone of the document. Because writing is not easy, one should expect to edit original drafts.

Dictation is a valuable communication skill. Dictating probably requires more effort at first, but it can soon become easier than writing in longhand. In dictation one must again consider the purpose of the communication and plan and organize her remarks. One starts dictation by indicating who is dictating what (letter or memo), the subject, type of paper needed (letterhead stationery, memo pad), and the number of copies needed. One should state the format (headings, double space, tabular outline, new paragraph), punctuation (capitalization, hyphen, period, commas, question mark, italics), and spell out unusual or unfamiliar words. Conversational instructions are given as one dictates. For example, "Mary, list the following statements and precede each with a dash." One should not smoke, eat, or chew gum while dictating. Background noises should be reduced as much as possible. Closing the office door during dictation can eliminate interference. Dictation should be given at a normal talking speed, with the words pronounced clearly and correctly. The sender can conclude dictation by saying "end of memo." If one cannot complete the dictation, instructions for the incomplete correspondence should be dictated. The dictator may want to keep a list of what is dictated and mark the items off as they are processed.

Communications are critical for the functioning of an organization. Nurses need to be familiar with the communication process, communication systems, and directions communications can take. There are numerous barriers to communication. Managers need to know them and ways to overcome them.

COMMUNICATING WITH DIFFICULT PEOPLE

One requires special communication skills in order to deal with some personalities, including hostile-aggressive, complaining, negative, unresponsive, and overly nice. Some hostile-aggressive types seem to attack in an abrupt, abusive, intimidating manner that pushes others to acquiesce against their better judgment. These people tend to know what others should do, need to prove themselves right, and lack trust and caring. One must stand up to a hostile-aggressive person or feel overrun and frustrated. It is important to do this without fighting, or the conflict will escalate. It is advantageous to give the hostile-aggressive person time to run down for a while and then interrupt to stand up for oneself. There may be no opportunity to speak between sentences, thus making it necessary to interrupt before the other person has finished speaking. It is also likely that she may interrupt. Then one must state firmly, "you interrupted me," and start again, preferably with a smile. One needs to get her attention to do problem solving. Calling the person by her name (not a name) helps get her attention. Deliberately dropping a book is a more dramatic way to get attention. By standing up, one may also get attention and will likely find the other person less aggressive if she will sit down. Then one needs to state ideas forcefully in a friendly manner that does not belittle the other person. It is important to avoid fighting with the hostile-aggressive person because such a battle will likely be lost. Even if the battle is won, her righteous anger will likely increase, and the war may be lost. When one stands up to the bully, she is likely to become a friend. When dealing with hostile-aggressive people, it is important to stand up for oneself without fighting.

Exploders are another type of hostile-aggressive personality. Adult tantrums are the grown-up version of childhood tantrums that are a defense mechanism to cope with fear, helplessness, and frustration. Adult tantrums are sudden, almost automatic, responses to feeling threatened. The exploder typically feels angry first and then blaming or suspicious. People act on their perceptions, but people are likely to perceive the same situation differently. Consequently, the object of the tantrum may be unaware that the exploder has been threatened and be surprised by the outburst. The exploder should be given time to run down and regain self-control. If she does not run down, a neutral statement like "Stop" may interrupt the tantrum. Then show that she is taken seriously by a comment like, "I can see this is important to you. I want to discuss this with you but not like this." Possibly change the pace by getting a cup of coffee and seeking a private place for a problem-solving session.

Sniping is an aggressive response to an unresolved problem. It causes distress rather than any positive actions. Unfortunately, the unsolved problems become worse, and the resulting stress causes more difficult behavior such as innuendoes, not-too-subtle remarks, and nonplayful teasing.

First of all, it is important to expose the attack by such comments as, "That sounded like a put-down, did you mean it that way?" Usually snipers will deny any attack. Sniping is not possible without a camouflage that works. Standing up to the attack without escalating it will help one proceed with problem solving.

It gives the sniper an alternative to a direct contest. It is appropriate to get other points of view that confirm or deny the sniper's criticism, then try to solve any problems that have surfaced. Sniping can be prevented by establishing regular problem-solving meetings.

Complainers may dump directly on you or may complain about other awful people. Complaining helps the person appear blameless and innocent, at least to herself. One should listen attentively to the complaints, paraphrase as acknowledgment of what you heard, and confirm one's perception of how the complainer feels. One should not agree with or apologize for the allegations and avoid the accusation-defense-reaccusation pattern. It is preferable to simply state and acknowledge the facts without comment, then proceed with problem solving.

Negatively thinking people believe that any task that is out of their hands will fail and that others do not care and are self-serving. One should beware of being dragged down by their despair. One can make optimistic but realistic comments about past successes in similar situations but should not try to argue the negativist out of her pessimism. It is better not to offer solution-alternatives until the problem has been thoroughly discussed or to ask people to act before they feel ready. During the problem-solving session, the negative events that could occur if the option were implemented should be explored. Be ready to take independent action if the group refuses to do so, and announce these plans without equivocation.

Unresponsive people can not or will not speak when input is needed from them. It is difficult to know what their silence means. The most important strategy is to get the silent person to speak by asking open-ended questions, waiting calmly for a response, and not talking to fill the silence. If an open-ended question gets no response, one should comment on what is happening, for example, "I'm not getting any feedback from you," and end the observation with another open-ended question like "What are you thinking?" Attention should be given when the person does speak. If the person never speaks, one should terminate the meeting by stating what will be done because no discussion occurred.

Superagreeable people are equally difficult people because they lead one to believe that they are in agreement but let one down when it comes to taking action. They have strong needs to be liked and accepted and help others feel approved in order to get approval themselves. They run into trouble when their need for approval conflicts with negative aspects of reality. They commit themselves to actions that they do not complete. Once again, problem solving is important. One must try to learn what prevents the person from taking action and letting her know that she is valued by telling her so and by asking questions about her interests, hobbies, and family to get to know her better. One should ask her what is not as good as she would like it to be and what could interfere with good relationships. Listening to her humor for hidden messages in teasing remarks and being prepared to do problem solving is also important.*

ASSERTIVENESS
Barriers to assertiveness

Communication styles are either passive, aggressive, or assertive. Assertiveness is the best style for the nurse manager and the one she should foster in her personnel. However, there are barriers that nurses must overcome to become assertive. The most pervasive barrier is female sex role socialization. Whereas men are characterized as aggressive, competitive, independent, objective, analytical, task oriented, confident, self-disciplined, and emotionally controlled, women are expected to be passive, dependent, subjective, intuitive, empathetic, sensitive, interpersonally oriented, weak, inconsistent, and emotionally unstable.

The nursing socialization process and the nature of nursing are additional barriers. Both nursing schools and health agencies have organizational hierarchies with authority and power concentrated at the top. This arrangement usually promotes compliance and conformity. Nurses are taught to value sacrifice, humility, and service to others. They have been taught not to state their thoughts or feelings. Although they give intimate physical nurturing, they are not to become emotionally involved with clients. Nurses have been socialized into a subservient role. They are expected to follow physicians' orders and to be professional but not to anticipate equal financial reimbursement for their education and responsibilities. They are expected to be a part of the health team but not to make decisions or policies. They tend to keep so busy that they ignore their own rights.

In addition to these male-female role competition problems, nurses face female-female relationship problems. Men are more competitive with women than with other men, and women are more competitive with women than with men. Consequently, attempts to develop support systems for nurses are not usually successful. Instead, the queen bee and the trashing syndrome emerge.

The queen bee identifies with men, enjoys being told that she is different from most women, and feels superior to other women. The queen bee usually has to work very hard to become a success in a male-dominated society. She is likely to need to be cooperative and nonthreatening to achieve and maintain her successful position. She probably feels little animosity toward the system and the men who allowed her to become successful. Consequently, she is likely to

---

*For a more extensive discussion, see Branson, R.M.: Coping with difficult people, Garden City, N.Y., 1981 Anchor Press.

identify with her male colleagues instead of with other women. However, protective of her own position and aware of the high price she paid for it, she makes it no easier for other women to succeed.

Trashing is a form of character assassination that divides women against one another. It is self-destructive and leads to impotent rage. Rather than exposing disagreements to resolve differences, trashing is done to destroy. It can be done to one's face or behind one's back, in public or in private. It questions one's motives, stresses one's worthlessness, and breaches one's integrity. The victim may be ignored, or anything she says or does may be interpreted in the most negative manner. Others' unrealistic expectations about her assure failure. The trasher may give misinformation to others about what the victim does and thinks or tell her lies about what others think of her. Whatever method is used, it is manipulative, dishonest, and destructive. Women in general and nurses specifically need to become aware of what they are doing to each other, commit themselves to supportive instead of destructive behavior, learn to analyze interpersonal communication, and learn assertive behavior.

Transactional analysis

Transactional analysis is a technique that can be used by nurses for analyzing and understanding behavior. It was developed by Eric Berne and popularized by Thomas Harris, Muriel James, and Dorothy Jongeward. Transactional analysis is an outgrowth of the Freudian concepts of id, ego, and superego—elements of the psyche that stimulate, monitor, and control behavior. Berne calls these ego states parent, child, and adult.

The parent ego state controls and is the source of values, opinions, rules, regulations, and social conscience. The two major types of parent ego states are nurturing parent and critical parent. The nurturing parent guides, teaches, advises, and supplies "how to" information. The critical parent prohibits and supplies "should" and "should not" information. The parent ego state is a result of cultural traditions, social programming, and responsibilities. Parental judgments are drawn heavily from natural parents, older siblings, teachers, and other parent figures.

The child ego state is dominated by emotions and is the feeling state. It is the id ego state where strong feelings are triggered by immediate experiences. A person is in the child state when she is experiencing childlike natural impulses, such as joy, delight, gaiety, or anger, hostility, and rage. The child ego state may be happy or destructive. The natural child is spontaneous, trusting, joyful, living, creative, and adventurous. The adapted child is suppressed and may express anger, rebellion, fear, or conformity.

The adult is the ego state that monitors one's behavior. It is the unemotional, thinking, problem-solving state. The adult ego state collects information, sets

Fig. 4-11. Transactions. **A**, Complementary, **B**, Crossed.

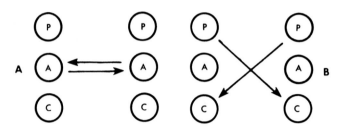

goals, compares alternatives, makes decisions and plans, and tests reality. The adult ego state is an unemotional state in which rational decision making takes place.

Every individual exhibits behavior from the three ego states at different times. A healthy individual maintains a balance between them. Unfortunately, some people are dominated by one or two of the ego states and are likely to create problems for managers. Parent-dominated individuals may not participate in problem solving because they think they already have the answer and know what is right and wrong. The child-dominated individual does not engage in rational problem solving either. Screaming and being emotional have helped the child get what she wanted before. It is likely to be very difficult to reason with someone dominated by the child ego state. Working with adult-dominated individuals may be boring because they work so hard. A balance among the three ego states produces the healthiest worker.

When people interact, they participate as parent, child, or adult (Fig. 4-11). A transaction or an observation unit is an exchange between people that consists of at least one stimulus and one response. Transactional analysis is done to identify the participant's ego state and consists of complementary or crossed types. The basic principle of the complementary type is that the response to the stimulus is predictable and expected.

Adult-to-adult transactions are the manner in which much business is conducted (Fig. 4-12). For instance, a supervisor says, "Would you please give Mr. Jones his PRN medication before you give Mrs. Smith her 8 AM medications?" A staff nurse replies, "Yes, I understand that Mr. Jones is complaining of surgical pain."

Parent-to-parent interaction is often a short-term sharing of opinions (Fig. 4-13). One staff nurse says to another, "Those new graduate nurses sure don't know how to function." The other nurse replies, "That's for sure."

Child-to-child interactions usually involve an emotional exchange (Fig. 4-14). As long as both parties are in a child ego state, they are unable to think rationally

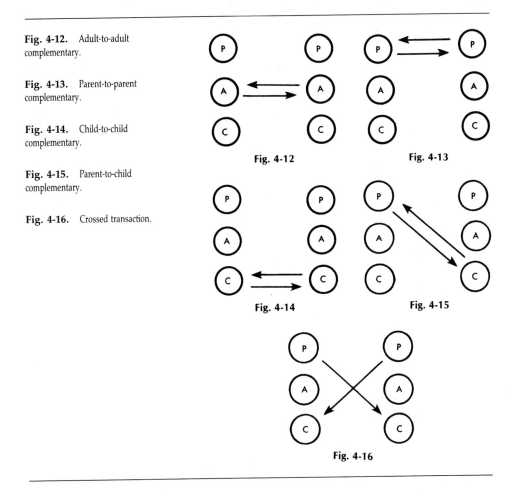

Fig. 4-12. Adult-to-adult complementary.

Fig. 4-13. Parent-to-parent complementary.

Fig. 4-14. Child-to-child complementary.

Fig. 4-15. Parent-to-child complementary.

Fig. 4-16. Crossed transaction.

Fig. 4-12

Fig. 4-13

Fig. 4-14

Fig. 4-15

Fig. 4-16

and solve problems. The first staff nurse says, "I just gave Mrs. Smith her 8 AM medications, and when I went to chart them, you had signed for giving them. Why don't you sign right after you give medications so they won't be repeated!" The second nurse answers, "Why don't you give me a chance to sign before you go and give them again!"

In parent-to-child interactions, one person takes a psychologically superior position over the other (Fig. 4-15). Supervisor says, "I want to see you in my office." Staff nurse answers, "Yes, ma'am."

Crossed transactions result in closing communications at least temporarily (Fig. 4-16). The response may be inappropriate or unexpected and may confuse or threaten the sender of the stimulus. Supervisor says, "Miss Jones, could I see you about this in my office right away?" Miss Jones replies, "No! Can't you see I'm busy? You'll have to wait."

Transactions usually proceed in a programmed series with rituals and procedures being the simplest kinds. Rituals are a series of simple complementary transactions that provide mutual stroking with no real commitment. Most rituals have been used so often that the form has become more important than the content, but they provide structure for greeting people and expressing religious beliefs. Greeting rituals, such as "Hi," "How are you?" "I am fine," are not intended to supply information. The person who goes from office to office participating in rituals may get promoted because she is "a good guy." Rituals work for the person who can still get her job done. People who work hard to develop themselves may become apathetic when they realize socializing is more effective for obtaining promotions than hard work. Rituals may have started as a series of complementary adult transactions intended to manipulate reality, but they have lost their procedural validity over time.

Pastimes are pleasant ways to pass time with others to learn if you have enough in common to warrant further interaction. Common small talk includes topics such as cooking, fashions, costs, sports, recreation, and mutual acquaintances. There is no goal or emotional closeness involved. People who spend too much time participating in pastimes may sense that their lives are happy but empty, while the person who spends too little time making small talk may not have much fun and may feel harassed. Pastimes become a problem for the organization when they are an alternative to work.

In *Games People Play*, Eric Berne writes: "A game is an ongoing series of complementary ulterior transactions progressing to a well-defined, predictable outcome."* Games have a high stroke or recognition potential, but the payoff is usually negative. Games have hidden agendas that prevent both people and organizations from becoming winners. While playing games, people dwell on their own sorrows and inadequacies, make mistakes, catch others making mistakes, pass the buck, and fail to meet their obligations. People receive negative strokes and get hurt while real problems go unsolved. Productivity is limited because people use their energies to play games instead of to get the job done. Attention is given to past events rather than to the present. While realities of the current situation go unperceived, problems go unsolved.

People need strokes, and negative strokes are better than no strokes. Consequently, in work environments that do not provide positive strokes, people have a need to play games. People who are bored with their jobs are also likely to play games. Games discourage openness, honesty, and intimacy. They take many forms. Games that blame others include "If it weren't for you" and "See what you made me do." Games that attack others include "Blemish," "Now I've got you, you SOB," "Bear Trapper," "Corner," "Rapo," "Uproar," and

---

*Berne, E.: Games people play, New York, 1964, Grove Press, p. 48.

"Let's You and Him Fight." Self-pity is reinforced by games such as "Poor me," "Kick me," "Stupid," "Wooden leg," "Harried," and "Lunch bag."

"If it weren't for you" is a blaming game in which people who feel inadequate blame others for their inability to achieve. People who blame their inability to be innovative on rigid policies may fear their own creative abilities. "If it weren't for . . ." is a clue that the game is being played. When a manager hears an employee saying this, she should suspect that the complainer would not function better under different circumstances but would likely become frustrated and request a transfer or quit. Changes may be made on a trial basis to test suspicions.

"See what you made me do" and "You got me into this" are closely related blaming games. The player avoids responsibility by being vindictive. It is common for workers to blame managers for problems, and for democratic managers to blame workers for mistakes or poor decisions. The manager decides whether or not to use the input from the workers and needs to accept that responsibility.

Many games attack others. The "Blemish" player looks for inconsequential, unimportant flaws. Instead of looking at purposes, the player concentrates on minutiae and zeroes in on trivial mistakes. Any positive stroke is discounted with a blemish. "Blemish" players also play "I was only trying to help you." The victims become resentful and may become the persecutor by playing "Now I've got you, you SOB." In this game the persecutor waits for the victim to make a mistake or sets the victim up for failure. The manager may be indulging in this game by setting standards too high to achieve, assigning people to work they are not qualified for, creating impossible working conditions, or giving incomplete or unclear instructions. The worker may use grievance procedures or law suits against managers playing this game.

The "Bear trapper" often baits someone with false promises and then lets the trap fall. Organizations play this game in hiring practices when glamorous job descriptions are presented. This tends to result in high turnover. Workers learn the shortcomings of the job and become disillusioned. Presenting both the advantages and disadvantages of jobs is a more realistic approach.

The "Corner" player's victim is in a lose-lose situation. No matter what the victim does, it is wrong. A woman manager is damned if she is aggressive because that is not considered feminine and damned if she is not because aggressiveness is a desired managerial quality. A manager can corner someone into not completing work on time by not accepting the work that is done.

"Corner" can lead to "Uproar." Uproar often starts with a critical remark and results in an attack-defense dialogue that is often loud.

"Rapo" is a sexual game. A woman may wear revealing clothing and move in provocative ways. When a man responds, she rejects him. This game is problematic when men and women work together. Organizations need to concentrate on equality and utilization of human resources regardless of sex.

In "Let's you and him fight," one person gets a second and third person into a fight. When one person tells a second person the "bad" things a third person said about the second, the first person is fostering a fight.

There are several versions of self-pity games. "Kick me" players provoke put-downs and make comments such as, "I could kick myself for that." "Stupid" players collect put-downs about their intelligence. Managers need to give immediate feedback and take corrective actions to prevent the "Stupid" game. The "Wooden leg" player uses a physical or social handicap to avoid work. A deprived background may be used as an excuse to underachieve. The manager needs to set and maintain standards to minimize this game.

Managers play "Poor me" games also. "Harried" executives work hard to maintain the sense of being OK. They are likely to work nights and weekends to appear competent and confident. "I'm not OK" feelings are hidden by appearing super OK.

The "Harried" executive may also participate in the "Lunch bag game." The manager carries leftovers in a used paper bag and eats at his desk instead of going out to lunch with peers. This technique can be used to make other people feel guilty.

Games always involve putting someone down. To decrease games in organizations, one must stop putting herself and others down. One should not play the complementary role, but should give and receive positive strokes and invest time in activities and intimacy. Managers should integrate the goals of the workers and the organization and decrease boredom through job enrichment and personnel development. With good organization and management, positive strokes can become an intrinsic part of the job. Managers should foster an "I'm OK, you're OK" atmosphere.

Activities such as working and learning are goal directed and have a high stroke potential. They are a highly rewarding way to spend time. Workers must be careful not to take on so many activities that they neglect rituals and pastimes, and managers should not overload themselves with activities and leave the workers with idle time.

Intimacy is an open sharing of experience with others, usually by people with close relationships but sometimes by strangers. It is the most rewarding way to spend time. It is also the most risky. Although intimacy is without ulterior motives or exploitation, one needs high self-esteem to risk the openness of intimacy. It requires and fosters the "I'm OK, you're OK" atmosphere.

Life positions

Life positions are more permanent than ego states. As individuals mature, they make assumptions about themselves and others. They consider themselves as OK or not OK and see others as OK or not OK. Four positions result: "I'm

OK, you're OK," "I'm OK, you're not OK," "I'm not OK, you're OK," and "I'm not OK, you're not OK." OK feelings are associated with a sense of power, personal worth, well-being, capability, and lovableness. Not-OK feelings result from a sense of inability, weakness, helplessness, worthlessness, anxiety, and a feeling of being insignificant and unlovable. Most people develop a basic life position early in childhood that tends to be reinforced by the person's selective perceptions and reactions to experiences.

In the I'm OK, you're OK position, individuals feel interdependent with others and the environment. They are happy, active people with a positive outlook on life who like reinforcement for being OK but are not dependent on it. They use the happy child and nurturing parent ego states. Because they feel OK about themselves, they have little difficulty feeling others are OK.

People in the I'm OK, you're not OK position do not believe they can rely on anyone but themselves. They think people are worthless and are likely to be enemies and consequently tend to blame others. The critical parent ego state is dominant. A manager in this position possesses a Theory X philosophy, implements a Likert type I system, and supervises people closely because they cannot be trusted.

People in the I'm not OK, you're OK position are burdened with self-defeating attitudes and a lack of confidence. They take a psychologically inferior stand to others and assume that they are less competent and less influential than others.

Individuals in the I'm not OK, you're not OK position are maladjusted. They think they are worthless and so are others. Lacking confidence in themselves and trust in others, they are suspicious and anxious, disconnected from others, alienated from the environment, miserable, and tend to give up.

During infancy individuals have a mixture of OK and not-OK feelings, with the not-OK feelings predominating. The infant feels OK when physical needs are met and positive strokes are received. Most of an infant's experiences provide negative strokes and not-OK feelings. Because adults can satisfy the infant's needs, they are viewed as OK. Consequently, for most people the I'm not OK, you're OK position is established early and continues into adulthood. Socialization of women and nurses particularly reinforces the position that they are not OK. Therefore they need a lot of positive reinforcement to move to an I'm OK, you're OK position. Assertiveness can help one achieve and maintain that position. Once it is learned, there will be less passive-aggressive behavior.

Assertive techniques

Communication styles are commonly passive, aggressive, or assertive. A passive person is often self-denying, inhibited, and allows others to choose for her. Consequently, her goals are not achieved and she feels hurt, anxious, and frustrated. The aggressive person is self-enhancing at others' expense. She is expressive, chooses for others, depreciates others, and achieves her goals by using others. Aggressive behavior generates hatred and sometimes revenge. The assertive person is self-enhancing. She is expressive, chooses for herself, and can achieve her goals. Consequently, she is likely to feel good about herself.

The passive person tends to be at a loss for words, does not say what she really means, uses many apologetic words, and hopes people will understand what she wants without telling them. She tends to have a weak, hesitant voice, downcast eyes, fidgety hands, and she nods frequently.

The aggressive person is loud, uses loaded subjective words, makes accusations, and sends "you" messages that blame others. A flippant, sarcastic style with an air of superiority and rudeness is common. The person is likely to stand with hands on hips, feet apart, narrowed eyes, pointing a finger and talking in a superior, demanding, authoritarian manner.

The assertive person says what she wants in direct statements that say what she means. She uses objective words, sends "I" messages, and makes honest statements about her feelings. She is an attentive listener who gives the impression of caring. She uses eye contact and spontaneous verbal expressions with appropriate gestures and facial expressions while speaking in a well-modulated voice.

The style used governs how situations will be handled. Suppose, for instance, that a manager has noticed that one of her staff nurses has been coming to work late for the past 3 days. The passive manager may not mention the problem at all. The aggressive manager might say, "How about getting here on time or looking for a new job? What do you think we pay you for anyway?" The assertive manager would be likely to speak to the staff nurse in private. She may say, "I've noticed you have been late the past 3 days. Why haven't you been getting to work on time?" The last approach gives an impression of caring and facilitates problem solving.

Assertiveness is the most desirable style for a nurse manager. To achieve assertiveness, one must substitute verbal persistence for silent passivity or verbal abuse. Broken record is a technique the manager can use to reach a compromise by indicating what she wants and by keeping other people from talking her into what they want to do. With the broken-record technique the manager keeps repeating what she wants.

Manager: *I expect you to get to work on time.*

Staff nurse: *But I'm a night person. I stay up late, and it's difficult to get up so early to come to work. I'm so tired that I shut off my alarm and go back to sleep. Then when I do get up, I stumble around in the dark to find my clothes so I won't wake my husband.*

Manager: *You are scheduled to work the day shift this rotation, and I expect you to be at work on time. If you are a night person, would you like to be assigned to the night shift permanently?*

Staff nurse: *No. I wouldn't be able to see my husband then. He works 9 AM to 9 PM and gets home about 9:30 PM. I would have to come to work at 10:30 and I could only see him for about an hour. I would get home just in time for him to go to work.*
Manager: *You are scheduled to work the day shift this rotation, and I expect you to be to work on time. However, we could assign you to the evening shift permanently. Would you want that?*
Staff nurse: *Working the evening shift would allow me to see my husband after work and to sleep in. Yes, I would prefer the evening shift.*
Manager: *I will see how quickly we can get your schedule changed to permanent evenings. I do expect you to be here by 7 AM until we get your schedule changed.*

Fogging, negative assertion, and negative inquiry are techniques for dealing with criticism whether it is self-directed or from another source, real or imagined. They help minimize the negative emotional response of anxiety to criticism that manipulates us into defending what we want to do instead of doing it. Consequently, the person feels less at conflict with herself and more comfortable with both the negative and positive aspects of her personality.

Fogging is agreeing with the truth, agreeing in principle, or agreeing with the odds rather than denying the criticism, getting defensive, or counterattacking with criticism. It helps desensitize one to criticism and leads to a reduction in the frequency of criticism from others. It sets up psychological distance, is a passive skill, and does not encourage the other person to assert herself. It also encourages a person to listen to what the critic says, to respond only to what the critic says rather than to what is implied, and to consider probabilities. For example:

Staff nurse: *You scheduled me to double back from evenings to days twice in a 2-week time schedule.*
Supervisor: *I see that I scheduled you to double back the first Wednesday and the second Friday (agreeing with the truth).*
Staff nurse: *When I double back, I have less than 7 hours for sleep. I get tired, have trouble functioning, and fear making mistakes.*
Supervisor: *I understand that you get tired when you double back and fear making mistakes. It seems logical that one would make more mistakes when tired than when alert (agreeing with the odds).*
Staff nurse: *We need a policy to prevent having just one shift off between shifts.*
Supervisor: *I agree. We do need staffing policies that would provide for adequate rest periods between shifts (agreeing in principle).*

With negative assertion a person assertively accepts negative aspects about herself. This reduces the need to seek forgiveness for one's mistakes or the need to counterattack with criticism.

Staff nurse: *Your new uniform really reveals how fat you are.*
Supervisor: *I'm overweight because I eat too much. I eat just about everything in sight except the kitchen sink. I've even seen the cat get worried (negative assertion).*
Staff nurse: *Well, that new uniform sure makes you look like a blimp.*
Supervisor: *These new styles don't compliment my figure (negative assertion).*

Negative assertion is not appropriate for physical or legal conflicts or for relating to people on a close interpersonal basis. The persistence of the critic will determine if one needs to use other assertive techniques.

Negative inquiry fosters assertiveness in the critic. The criticized person in an unemotional manner asks for more information about herself that may be negative. This provides a basis for problem solving and consequently reduces repetitive criticism.

Staff nurse: *You don't look good today.*
Supervisor: *Is it me or what I'm wearing?*
Staff nurse: *It's your face. You look so tired.*
Supervisor: *I don't feel tired. What about my face makes me look tired?*
Staff nurse: *Your eyes look so tired. They're so dark. There are black bags under them.*
Supervisor: *What can I do to make them look less tired?*
Staff nurse: *If the problem isn't fatigue, I guess you could use a white creme cosmetic over the bags so they won't look so dark and use light instead of dark-colored eye shadow.*

Assertive behavior is more than demanding one's rights from others and keeping others from manipulating. In a social sense, assertiveness is the ability to communicate with others about who you are, how you live, what you do, and what you want and the ability to make them feel comfortable talking about themselves. Free information—information offered without being asked for—gives you something to talk about and reduces awkward silences. Self-disclosure reveals how you think, feel, and react to others' free information. This social conversation allows one to discover mutually rewarding relationships or to identify people with whom one has few common interests.

Nurse leaders should behave assertively to achieve positive self-images and maintain an I'm OK position. Assertiveness techniques facilitate professional productivity and social satisfaction.

LEARNING ACTIVITIES

1

Write your philosophy of management and discuss it with a class-mate.

2

Practice team development with a group of classmates. Set goals and priorities by using nominal group process. Negotiate roles. One or more students may analyze the communication process. One or more other students may do transactional analysis of class-mates' interactions. Other students may analyze conflict escala-tion and de-escalation techniques used during the process.

3

List five major desires. In which categories of Maslow's hierarchy of needs do they belong? Do your needs fluctuate from time to time?

4

Make a list of what was happening when you felt job satisfaction and another list of what was happening when you felt job dis-satisfaction. Compare and contrast the lists. Do they support Herzberg's motivation-hygiene theory?

5

Keep a diary of some of your interactions with others. Do trans-actional analysis on them and analyze if you were passive, ag-gressive, or assertive. If you were passive or aggressive, decide how you could have behaved assertively.

BIBLIOGRAPHY

Books

Albers, H.H.: Principles of management: a modern approach, New York, 1974, John Wiley & Sons, Inc.

Alberti, R.E., and Emmons, M.L.: Your perfect right: a guide to assertive living, ed. 5, San Luis Obispo, Calif., 1986, Impact Publishers, Inc.

Alberti, R.E., and Emmons, M.L.: Stand up, speak out, talk back! New York, 1984, Pocket Books.

Alexander, E.L.: Nursing administration in the hospital health care system, ed. 2, St. Louis, 1978, The C. V. Mosby Co.

Alinsky, S.D.: Rules for radicals, New York, 1972, Random House, Inc.

Arndt, C., and Daderian Huckabay, L.M.: Nursing administration: theory for practice with a systems approach, ed. 2, St. Louis, 1980, The C. V. Mosby Co.

Ashley, J.: Hospitals, paternalism, and the role of the nurse, New York, 1976, Teachers College Press.

Bach, G.R., and Goldberg, H.: Creative aggression: the art of assertive living, New York, 1983, Doubleday Publishing Co.

Baer, J.: How to be an assertive (not aggressive) woman in life, in love, and on the job, New York, 1976, New American Library.

Bagwell, M., and Clements, S.: A political handbook for health professionals, Boston, 1985, Little, Brown & Co.

Berger M.S., et al., editors: Management for nurses, ed. 2, St. Louis, 1980, The C. V. Mosby Co.

Berne, E.: Games people play, New York, 1978, Ballantine Books.

Berne, E.: What do you say after you say hello? New York, 1975, Bantam Books, Inc.

Beyers, M., and Phillips, C.: Nursing management for patient care, ed. 2, Boston, 1979, Little, Brown & Co.

Billings, V.: The womansbook, Greenwich, Conn., 1974, Fawcett World Library.

Bittel, L.R.: What every supervisor should know, ed. 5, New York, 1984, McGraw-Hill Book Co.

Blake, R.R., and Mouton, J.S.: The managerial grid, ed. 3, Houston, 1984, Gulf Publishing Co.

Blake, R.R., Shepard, H.A., and Mouton, J.S.: Managing intergroup conflict in industry, Houston, Tex., 1964, Gulf Publishing Co.

Blau, P.M.: Exchange and power in social life, New Brunswick, N.J., 1986, Transaction Books.

Bloom, L.Z., Coburn, K., and Pearlman, J.: The new assertive woman, New York, 1976, Dell Publishing Co., Inc.

Blum, M.L., and Naylor, J.C.: Industrial psychology: its theoretical and social foundations, New York, 1968, Harper & Row, Publishers.

Bonner, H.: Group dynamics: principles and applications, New York, 1959, Ronald Press Co.

Boshear, W.C., and Albrecht, K.G.: Understanding people: models and concepts, La Jolla, Calif., 1977, University Associates, Inc.

Bower, S.A., and Bower G.H.: Asserting yourself: a practical guide for positive change, Reading, Mass., 1976, Addison-Wesley Publishing Co.

Bradford, L.P.: Group development, ed. 2, La Jolla, Calif., 1978, University Associates, Inc.

Bramson, R.M.: Coping with difficult people, Garden City, N.Y., 1981, Anchor Press.

Brooten, D.A.: Managerial leadership in nursing, Philadelphia, 1984, J.B. Lippincott Co.

Buchholz, R.A.: Essentials of public policy for management, Englewood Cliffs, N.J., 1985, Prentice-Hall, Inc.

Burke, W.W., editor: New technologies in organizational development, La Jolla, Calif., 1972, University Associates, Inc.

Burke, W.W., and Hornstein, H.A.: The social technology of organization development, La Jolla, Calif., 1972, University Associates, Inc.

Charns, M.P., and Schaefer, M.J.: Health care organizations: a model for management, Englewood Cliffs, N.J., 1983, Prentice-Hall, Inc.

Chenevert, M.: Special techniques in assertiveness training for women in the health professions, ed. 2, St. Louis, 1983, The C. V. Mosby Co.

Christian, W.P., and Hannah, G.T.: Effective management in human services, Englewood Cliffs, N.J., 1983, Prentice-Hall, Inc.

Clark, C.C., and Shea, C.A.: Management in nursing: a vital link in the health care system, New York, 1979, McGraw-Hill Book Co.

Claus, K.E., and Bailey, J.T.: Power and influence in health care: a new approach to leadership, St. Louis, 1977, The C. V. Mosby Co.

Cohen, H.: You can negotiate anything, New York, 1983, Citadel Press.

Connor, P.E.: Dimensions in modern management, ed. 3, Boston, 1982, Houghton Mifflin Co.

Cowart, M., and Allen, R.F.: Changing conceptions of health care, Grove Road, 1981, Charles B. Black, Inc.

Dale, E.: Management: theory and practice, ed. 4, New York, 1978, McGraw-Hill Book Co.

Davis, K., and Newstrom, J.: Human behavior at work, ed. 7, New York, 1985, McGraw-Hill Book Co.

De Vito, J.A.: Communication: concepts and processes, ed. 3, Englewood Cliffs, N.J., 1981, Prentice-Hall, Inc.

Deci, E.L.: Intrinsic motivation, New York, 1975, Plenum Press.

Deep, S.: Human relations in management, Encino, Calif., 1978, Glencoe Publishing Co., Inc.

Delbecq, A.L., Van de Ven, A.H., and Gustafson, D.H.: Group techniques for program planning: a guide to nominal group and Delphi processes, Glenview, Ill., 1975, Scott, Foresman & Co.

Deloughery, G., and Gebbie, K.M.: Political dynamics: impact on nurses and nursing, St. Louis, 1975, The C. V. Mosby Co.

Di Vincenti, M.: Administering nursing service, ed. 2, Boston, 1977, Little, Brown & Co.

Donnelly, J.H., Jr., Gibson, J.L., and Ivancevich, J.M.: Fundamentals of management: functions, behavior, models, Austin, Tex., 1971, Business Publications, Inc.

Donovan, H.M.: Nursing service administration: managing the enterprise, St. Louis, 1975, The C. V. Mosby Co.

Durbin, R.L., and Springall, W.H.: Organization and administration of health care: theory, practice, environment, St. Louis, 1974, The C. V. Mosby Co.

Dyer, W.: Your erroneous zones, New York, 1977, Avon Books.

Eckles, R.W., Carmichael, R.L., and Sarchet, B.R.: Essentials of management for first-line supervision, New York, 1974, John Wiley & Sons, Inc.

Eddy, W.B., et al., editors: Behavioral science and the manager's role, ed. 2, La Jolla, Calif., 1980, University Associates, Inc.

Epstein, C.: The nurse leader: philosophy and practice, Norwalk, Conn., 1982, Appleton & Lange.

Feldman, D.C., and Arnold, H.J.: Managing individual and group behavior in organizations, New York, 1983, McGraw-Hill Book Co.

Fensterheim, H.: Don't say yes when you want to say no, New York, 1975, Dell Publishing Co., Inc.

Fiedler, F.E.: A theory of leadership effectiveness, New York, 1967, McGraw-Hill Book Co.

Fiedler, F.E., and Chemers, M.M.: Leadership and effective management, Glenview, Ill., 1974, Scott, Foresman & Co.

Fiedler, F.E., Chemers, M.M., and Mahar, L.: Improving leadership effectiveness: the leader match concept, ed. 2, New York, 1984, John Wiley & Sons, Inc.

Filley, A.C.: Interpersonal conflict resolution, Glenview, Ill., 1975, Scott, Foresman & Co.

Filley, A.C., and House, R.J.: Managerial process and organizational behavior, Glenview, Ill., 1969, Scott, Foresman & Co.

Flippo, E.B.: Management: a behavioral approach, Boston, 1970, Allyn & Bacon, Inc.

Fisher, R., and Ury, W.: Getting to yes: negotiating agreement without giving in, Boston, 1983, Penguin Books.

Franklin, J.L., Wissler, A.L., and Spencer, G.J.: Survey-guided development. III. A manual for concepts training, La Jolla, Calif., 1977, University Associates, Inc.

French, W.L.: The personnel management process, Boston, 1982, Houghton Mifflin Co.

Friday, N.: My mother myself, ed. 5, New York, 1988, Dell Publishing Co., Inc.

Frieze, I.H., et al.: Woman and sex roles: a social psychological perspective, New York, 1978, W.W. Norton & Co.

Frost, J.H., and Wilmot, W.W.: Interpersonal conflict, Dubuque, Iowa, 1978, William C. Brown Co., Publishers.

Ganong, J.M., and Ganong, W.L.: Nursing management, ed. 2, Rockville, Md., 1980, Aspen Systems Corp.

George, C.S., Jr.: The history of management thought, ed. 2, Englewood Cliffs, N.J., 1972, Prentice-Hall, Inc.

Gibson, J.L., Ivancevich, J.M., and Donnelly, J.H.: Organizations: behavior, structure, processes, Plano, Tex., 1985, Business Publications, Inc.

Gillies, D.A.: Nursing management: a systems approach, Philadelphia, 1982, W.B. Saunders Co.

Goodstein, L.D., Lubin, B., and Lubin, W.: Organizational change sourcebook. II. Cases in conflict management, La Jolla, Calif., 1979, University Associates, Inc.

Grissum, M., and Spengler, C.: Woman power and health care, Boston, 1976, Little, Brown & Co.

Hagen, E., and Wolff, L.: Nursing leadership behavior in general hospitals, New York, 1961, Institute of Research and Service in Nursing Education, Teachers College, Columbia University.

Haimann, T., and Scott, W.G.: Management in the modern organization, Boston, 1974, Houghton Mifflin Co.

Hall, R.H.: Organizations: structure, process, and outcomes, ed. 4, Englewood Cliffs, N.J., 1987, Prentice-Hall, Inc.

Hampton, D.R.: Contemporary management, New York, 1977, McGraw-Hill Book Co.

Hampton, D.R., Summer, C.E., and Webber, R.A.: Organizational behavior and the practice of management, ed. 5, Glenview, Ill., 1986, Scott, Foresman & Co.

Hand, L.: Nursing supervision, Norwalk, Conn., 1980, Appleton & Lange.

Harragan, B.L.: Games mother never taught you: corporate gamesmanship for women, New York, 1977, Warner Books, Inc.

Harris, T.: I'm OK—you're OK, New York, 1967, Harper & Row, Publishers.

Haynes, W.W., and Massie, J.L.: Management: analysis, concepts, and cases, Englewood Cliffs, N.J., 1969, Prentice-Hall, Inc.

Hein, E.C.: Communication in nursing practice, Boston, 1986, Little, Brown & Co.

Hennig, M., and Jardim, A.: The managerial woman, Garden City, N.Y., 1981, Doubleday Publishing Co.

Hepner, J.O., and Hepner, D.M.: The health strategy game: a challenge for reorganization and management, St. Louis, 1973, The C. V. Mosby Co.

Herman, S.L.: Becoming assertive: a guide for nurses, New York, 1978, D. Van Nostrand Co.

Hersey, P., and Blanchard, K.: Management of organizational behavior: utilizing human resources, ed. 4, Englewood Cliffs, N.J., 1982, Prentice-Hall, Inc.

Herzberg, F., Mausner, B., and Snyderman, B.B.: The motivation to work, New York, 1959, John Wiley & Sons, Inc.

Hicks, H.G.: The management of organizations, ed. 4, New York, 1981, McGraw-Hill Book Co.

Hodgetts, R.M.: Management: theory, process,

and practice, Orlando, Fla, 1985, Academic Press.

Holle, M.L., and Blatchley, M.E.: Introduction to leadership and management in nursing, ed. 3, Monterey, Calif., 1987, Jones & Bartlett Publishers, Inc.

Huseman, R.C., Logue, C.M., and Freshley, D.L., editors: Readings in interpersonal and organizational communication, Boston, 1969, Holbrook Press, Inc.

James, M., and Jongeward, D.: Born to win, Reading, Mass., 1978, New American Library.

Jandt, F.E.: Conflict resolution through communication, New York, 1973, Harper & Row, Publishers.

Jongeward, D.: Everybody wins: transactional analysis applied to organizations, Reading, Mass., 1973, Addison-Wesley Publishing Co.

Jongeward, D.: Women as winners: transactional analysis for personal growth, Reading, Mass., 1976, Addison-Wesley Publishing Co.

Joos, I.M., Nelson, R., and Lyness, A.: Man, health, and nursing: basic concepts and theories, Norwalk, Conn., 1985, Appleton & Lange.

Josefowitz, N.: Paths to power, Reading, Mass., 1980, Addison-Wesley Publishing Co.

Kaluzny, A.D., et al.: Management of health services, Englewood Cliffs, N.J., 1982, Prentice-Hall, Inc.

Karrass, C.L.: Give & Take, New York, 1974, Thomas Y. Crowell Co.

Kast, F.E., and Rosenzweig, J.E.: Organization and management: a systems and contingency approach, ed. 4, New York, 1984, McGraw-Hill Book Co.

Katz, D., and Kahn, R.L.: The social psychology of organizations, ed. 2, New York, 1978, John Wiley & Sons, Inc.

Kazmier, L.J.: Management: a programmed approach, New York, 1980, McGraw-Hill Book Co.

Keane, C.B.: Management essentials in nursing, Norwalk, Conn., 1980, Appleton & Lange.

Kelley, C.: Assertion training: a facilitator's guide, La Jolla, Calif., 1979, University Associates, Inc.

Kelly, J.: Organizational behaviour, ed. 3, Homewood, Ill., 1980, Richard D. Irwin, Inc.

Koontz, H., and O'Donnell, C.: Principles of management: an analysis of managerial functions, New York, 1972, McGraw-Hill Book Co.

Korda, M.: Power! How to get it, how to use it, New York, 1976, Ballantine Books.

Kurtz, R., and Prestera, H.: The body reveals: an illustrated guide to the psychology of the body, New York, 1984, Harper & Row, Publishers.

Lange, A., and Jakubowski, P.: Responsible assertive behavior, Champaign, Ill., 1976, Research Press.

Langford, T.L.: Managing and being managed, Norwalk, Conn., 1981, Appleton & Lange.

Levey, S., and Loomba, N.P.: Health care administration: a managerial perspective, ed. 2, Philadelphia, 1984, J.B. Lippincott Co.

Likert, R., and Likert, J.G.: New ways of managing conflict, New York, 1976, McGraw-Hill Book Co.

Litterer, J.A.: The analysis of organizations, New York, 1973, John Wiley & Sons, Inc.

Longest, B.B.: Management practices for the health professional, ed. 3, Norwalk, Conn., 1984, Appleton & Lange.

Margulies, N., and Wallace, J.: Organizational change: techniques and applications, Glenview, Ill., 1973, Scott, Foresman & Co.

Marriner, A.: Contemporary nursing management: issues and practice, St. Louis, 1982, The C. V. Mosby Co.

Mason, D.J., and Talbott, S.W.: Political action handbook for nurses, Menlo Park, Calif., 1985, Addison-Wesley Publishing Co.

May, R.: Power and innocence, New York, 1972, W.W. Norton & Co., Inc.

McBride, A.B.: Living with contradiction: a married feminist, New York, 1976, Harper & Row, Publishers.

McCelland, D.C.: Power: the inner experience, New York, 1979, Irvington Publishers, Inc.

McConnell, C.R.: The effective health care supervisor, Rockville, Md., 1982, Aspen Systems Corp.

McFarland, D.: Management principles and practice, New York, 1974, Macmillan, Inc.

McGregor, D.: The human side of enterprise, New York, 1960, McGraw-Hill Book Co.

Meininger, J.: Success through transactional analysis, New York, 1974, New American Library.

Miller, J.B.: Toward a new psychology of women, Boston, 1976, Beacon Press.

Molloy, J.T.: The woman's dress for success book, New York, 1977, Warner Books.

Newman, W.H., Warren, E.K., and Kirby, E.: The process of management, ed. 5, Englewood Cliffs, N.J., 1981, Prentice-Hall, Inc.

Newport, M.G.: The tools of managing: functions, techniques, and skills, Reading, Mass., 1972, Addison-Wesley Publishing Co.

O'Brien, M.J.: Communications and relationships in nursing, ed. 2, St. Louis, 1978, The C. V. Mosby Co.

Osborn, R.N., Hunt, J.G., and Jauch, L.R.: Organization theory: an integrated approach, New York, 1980, R.E. Krieger Publishing Co.

Osborn, S.M., and Harris, G.G.: Assertive training for women, Springfield, Ill., 1978, Charles C Thomas, Publisher.

Ouchi, W.G.: Theory Z, New York, 1982, Avon Books.

Pascale, R.T., and Athos, A.G.: The art of Japanese management, New York, 1982, Warner Books.

Peters, T.J., and Waterman, R.H.: In search of excellence, New York, 1984, Warner Books.

Phelps, S. and Austin, N.: The assertive woman, ed. 2, San Luis Obispo, Calif., 1985, Impact Publishers, Inc.

Porter, L.W., and Lawler, E.E.: Managerial attitudes and performance, Homewood, Ill., 1968, The Dorsey Press.

Randolph, W.A.: Understanding and managing organizational behavior, Homewood, Ill., 1985, Richard D. Irwin, Inc.

Ringer, R.J.: Winning through intimidation, New York, 1977, Fawcett Books.

Robbins, S.P.: Managing organizational conflict: a nontraditional approach, Englewood Cliffs, N.J., 1974, Prentice-Hall, Inc.

Robbins, S.P.: Organizational behavior: concepts, controversies, and applications, Englewood Cliffs, N.J., 1983, Prentice-Hall, Inc.

Robbins, S.P.: Organizational theory: the structure and design of organizations, ed. 3, Englewood Cliffs, N.J., 1986, Prentice-Hall, Inc.

Rogers, C.: On personal power, New York, 1977, Delacorte Press.

oRowland, H.S., and Rowland, B.L.: Nursing administration handbook, ed. 2, Germantown, Md., 1985, Aspen Systems Corp.

Rubin, I.M., Plovnick, M.S., and Fry, R.E.: Improving the coordination of care: a program for health team development, Cambridge, Mass., 1975, Ballinger Publishing Co.

Rubin, I.M., Plovnick, M.S., and Fry, R.E.: Managing human resources in health care organizations: an applied approach, Reston, Va., 1978, Reston Publishing Co., Inc.

Scanlan, B.K.: Principles of management and organizational behavior, New York, 1973, John Wiley & Sons, Inc.

Schaef, A.W.: Women's reality: an emerging female system in the white male society, New York, 1986, Harper & Row, Publishers.

Schein, E.H.: Process consultation: its role in organization development, Reading, Mass., 1969, Addison-Wesley Publishing Co.

Schweiger, J.L.: The nurse as manager, New York, 1980, John Wiley & Sons, Inc.

Sheehy, G.: Passages: predictable crises of adult life, New York, 1976, E.P. Dutton & Co., Inc.

Sheridan, R.S., Bronstein, J.E., and Walker, D.D.: The new nurse manager: a guide to management development, Rockville, Md., 1984, Aspen Systems Corp.

Simms, L.M., Price, S.A., and Ervin, N.E.: The professional practice of nursing administration, New York, 1985, John Wiley & Sons, Inc.

Sisk, H.L.: Management and organization, Cincinnati, 1973, South-Western Publishing Co.

Smith, M.J.: When I say no, I feel guilty, New York, 1985, Bantam Books.

Steers, R.M., and Porter, L.W.: Motivation and work behavior, New York, 1979, McGraw-Hill Book Co.

Stevens, B.J.: The nurse as executive, ed. 2, Germantown, Md., 1980, Aspen Systems Corp.

Stevens, B.J.: First-line patient care management, ed. 2, Germantown, Md., 1983, Aspen Systems Corp.

Stone, S., et al., editors: Management for nurses: a multidisciplinary approach, St. Louis, 1986, The C. V. Mosby Co.

Sullivan, E.J., and Decker, P.J.: Effective management in nursing, Reading, Mass., 1985, Addison-Wesley Publishing Co.

Swingle, P., editor: The structure of conflict, New York, 1970, Academic Press.

Taubman, B.: How to become an assertive woman, New York, 1976, Pocket Books.

Terry, G.R.: Principles of management, ed. 8, Homewood, Ill., 1982, Richard D. Irwin, Inc.

Veninga, R.L.: The human side of health administration, Englewood Cliffs, N.J., 1982, Prentice-Hall, Inc.

Voich, D., and Wren, D.A.: Principles of management: resources and systems, New York, 1968, Ronald Press Co.

Walton, R.E.: Interpersonal peacemaking: confrontations and third-party consultation, Reading, Mass., 1969, Addison-Wesley Publishing Co.

Watson, D.L., and Tharp, R.G.: Self-directed behavior: self-modification for personal adjustment, ed. 4, Monterey, Calif., 1985, Brooks/Cole Publishing Co.

Wieczorek, R.R., editor: Power, politics, and policy in nursing, New York, 1984, Springer Publishing Co.

Wren, D.A.: The evolution of management thought, New York, 1979, John Wiley & Sons, Inc.

Yura, H., Ozimek, D., and Walsh, M.B.: Nursing leadership: theory and process, ed. 2, Norwalk, Conn., 1981, Appleton & Lange.

Zurlage, C., editor: The nurse as personnel manager, Chicago, 1982, S-N Publications.

Journals

Leadership

Anderson, A.M.: Concepts of leadership, N.Z. Nurs. J. 60:7-10, March 1967.

Blake, R.R., and Mouton, J.S.: Should you teach there's only one best way to manage? Training HRD 15:24-29, April 1978.

Blake, R.R., and Mouton, J.S.: What's new with the grid? Training Dev. J. 32:3-8, May 1978.

Borgatta, E.F., Bales, R.F., and Couch, A.S.: Some findings relevant to the great-man theory of leadership, Am. Sociol. Rev. 19:755-759, 1954.

Calkin, J.D.: Using management literature to enhance new leadership roles, J. Nurs. Adm. 10:24-30, April 1980.

Colton, M.R.: Nursing's leadership vacuum, Supervisor Nurse 7:29-37, October 1976.

Corona, D.F.: Followship: the indispensable corollary to leadership, Nurs. Leadership 2:5-8, June 1979.

Cutler, M.J.: Nursing leadership and management: an historical perspective, Nurs. Adm. Q. 1:7-19, Fall 1976.

Diers, D.: Leadership problems and possibilities in nursing, Am. J. Nurs. 72:1447-1448, August 1972.

Diers, D.: Lessons on leadership, Image 11:67-71, October 1979.

Donovan, H.M.: Toward an understanding of leadership and supervision, Supervisor Nurse **3**:22-24, October 1972.

Eggers, E.T.: The essence of leadership, Supervisor Nurse **3**:23-27, December 1972.

Erickson, E.H.: The nursing service director, 1880-1980, J. Nurs. Adm. **10**:6-13, April 1980.

Evans, M.G.: The effects of supervisory behavior on the path-goal relationship, Organizational Behav. Hum. Perform. **5**:277-298, May 1970.

Fagin, C.M.: Refocus on leadership, Nurs. Leadership **2**:6-13, December 1979.

Fielder, F.E.: Engineer the job to fit the manager, Harvard Business Rev. **43**:115-122, September-October 1965.

Fiedler, F.E.: The effects of leadership training and experience: a contingency model interpretation, Adm. Sci. Q. **17**:453-470, December 1972.

Fine, R.B.: Application of leadership theory, Nurs. Clin. North Am. **13**:139-153, March 1978.

Freund, C.M.: The tenure of directors of nursing, J. Nurs. Adm. **15**:11-15, February 1985.

Fuller, S.: Humanistic leadership in a pragmatic age, Nurs. Outlook **27**:770-773, December 1979.

Heller, F.A.: Leadership, decision making, and contingency theory, Industrial Relations pp. 183-199, May 1973.

Hendricks, D.E.: Avoiding cultural myopia: what the Japanese can teach nurses about management, Nurs. Leadership **5**:11-15, June 1982.

Henry, B.M., and Moody, L.E.: Nursing administration in small rural hospitals, J. Nurs. Adm. **16**:37-44, July-August 1986.

Hersey, P., Blanchard, K.H., and LaMonica, E.L.: A situational approach to supervision: leadership theory and supervising nurse. I. Supervisor Nurse **7**:17-22, May 1976.

Hoogendijk, L.: Vision quest: qualities for nurse leaders, Nurs. Success Today **3**:4-7, August 1986.

House, R.J.: A path goal of leader effectiveness, Adm. Sci. Q. **16**:321-338, September 1971.

House, R.J., and Mitchell, T.R.: Path-goal theory of leadership, J. Contemporary Business **3**:81-97, Fall 1974.

Katz, R.L.: Skills of an effective administrator, Harvard Business Rev. **52**:90-102, September-October 1974.

Keaveny, M.E.: Leadership: what is it? Can the supervisor evaluate it? Supervisor Nurse **4**:28-39, January 1973.

Kooker, B.M.: The corporate image of a nurse executive, Nurs. Management **17**:52-55, February 1986.

Kron, T.: How to become a better leader, Nurs. 76 **6**:67-78, October 1976.

Leininger, M.: The leadership crisis in nursing: a critical problem and challenge, J. Nurs. Adm. **4**:28-34, March-April 1974.

Lundborg, L.B.: What is leadership? J. Nurs. Adm. **12**:32-33, May 1982.

Marriner, A.: Theories of leadership, Nurs. Leadership **1**:13-17, December 1978.

McConnel, E.A.: How to choose a leadership style, career guide, Nursing 80 **10**:105-112, March 1980.

McGee, R.: Leadership styles, Nurs. Success Today **1**:25-32, March-April 1984.

McNally, J.M.: Gentleness: an attribute for administrators, Supervisor Nurse **7**:70-71, October 1976.

Mealy, S., et al.: Shared leadership: no head nurse! Nurs. Adm. Q. **1**:81-93, Fall 1976.

Merton, R.K.: The nature of leadership, Int. Nurs. Rev. **16**:310-319, 1969.

Munn, H.E.: Measure your nursing supervisor leadership behaviors, Hosp. Top. **54**:14-18, November-December 1976.

Murray, M.: The nursing service administrator, Nurs. Management **12**:59-62, November 1981.

O'Donovan, T.R.: Leadership dynamics, J. Nurs. Adm. **5**:32-35, September 1975.

Poulin, M.A.: The nurse executive role: a structural and functional analysis, J. Nurs. Adm. **14**:9-14, February 1984.

Rosswurm, M.A.: A human resource framework for administrative practice, Supervisor Nurse **9**:52-55, August 1978.

Sargent, A.G.: The androgynous manager, Supervisor Nurse **10**:23-30, March 1979.

Schurr, M.: A comparative study of leadership in industry and the nursing profession. I. Int. Nurs. Rev. **16**:16-30, 1969.

Schurr, M.: A comparative study of leadership in industry and the nursing profession. II. Int. Nurs. Rev. **16**:115-132, 1969.

Schweiger, J.L.: The see-saw administrator, Nurs. Management **14**:26-27, April 1983.

Silber, M.B.: Right stuff: clinical services leaders, Nurs. Management **17**:46-47, July 1986.

Simms, L.M., Pfoutz, S.K., and Price, S.C.: Caring for older people: a challenge for nurse administrators, Nurs. Outlook **34**:145-148, May-June 1986.

Singleton, E.K., and Nail, F.C.: Developing relationships with the board of directors, J. Nurs. Adm. **16**:37-42, January 1986.

Tannenbaum, P., and Schmidt, W.H.: How to choose a leadership pattern, Harvard Business Rev. **51**:162-180, May-June 1973.

Thomas, L.A.: How to become a witch, Nurs. Outlook **22**:40-42, January 1974.

Thorton, N.F.: Change—over to head nurse, Nurs. Management **13**:52-53, March 1982.

Thorpe, R.: Supervision: is a master's degree really necessary? Supervisor Nurse **10**:33-35, January 1979.

Trainor, M.A.: A helping model for clinical supervision, Supervisor Nurse **9**:30-36, January 1978.

Tyndall, A.: Situational leadership theory, Nurs. Leadership **2**:25-29, June 1979.

Walsh, M., and Yura, H.: Super-vision, Supervisor Nurse **2**:18-26, March 1971.

White, H.C.: Some perceived behavior and attitudes of hospital employees under effective and ineffective supervisors, J. Nurs. Adm. **1**:49-54, January-February 1971.

White, H.C.: Perceptions of leadership styles by nurses in supervisory positions, J. Nurs. Adm. **1**:44-51, March-April 1971.

Wiley, L.: The spaghetti theory of leadership and other saucy ideas, Nursing 76 **6**:89-94, February 1976.

Wilsea, M.M.: Nursing leadership crisis: proposal for solution, Supervisor Nurse **11**:47-48, April 1980.

Zorn, J.M.: Nursing leadership for the '70s & '80s, J. Nurs. Adm. **7**:33-35, October 1977.

Theory Z

Adair, M.N., and Nygard, N.K.: Theory Z management: can it work for nursing? Nurs. Health Care **3**:489-491, November 1982.

Alexander, C.P.: A hidden benefit of quality circles, Personnel J. pp. 54-58, February 1984.

Brand, J.: Quality circles may substantially improve hospital employees' morale, Modern Healthcare, 70-74, September 1981.

Brody, E.W.: Japan's quality-control circles fall flat for American hospital industry, Modern Healthcare, p. 96, January 1982.

Cline, N., and Palau, D.: Quality circle in the

recovery room, Nurs. Health Care **3**:494-496, November 1982.

Haggard, A.: Quality circles, Nurs. Management **14**:32-34, February 1983.

Johnson, D.E.L.: Quality circles put workers in charge of their productivity, Modern Healthcare, pp. 68-69, September 1981.

Metz, E.J.: Caution: quality circles ahead, Training Dev. J. pp. 71-76, August 1981.

NLN Division of Continuing Education Services and National Forum for Administrators of Nursing Service: The quality circle process, Nurs. Health Care **3**:492-493, November 1982.

Smith, H.L., Reinow, F.D., and Reid, R.A.: Japanese management: implications for nursing administration, J. Nurs. Adm. **14**: 33-39, September 1984.

Waszak, J.J.: Adapting QCs to health care: some special challenges, Hosp. Prog. pp. 47-51, August 1982.

Younger, J.B.: Theory Z management and health care organizations, Nurs. Econ. **1**:40-45, 69, July-August 1983.

Management

Bargagliotti, L.A.: Misconceptions of a cc manager, Nurs. Management **13**:14-16, June 1982.

Behrens, A.D.: The pleasures and problems of the director of nursing in a small hospital, J. Nurs. Adm. **5**:31-34, February 1975.

Bopp, W.J., and Rosenthal, W.P.: Participatory management, Am. J. Nurs. **79**:671-672, April 1979.

Brown, B.J.: The role of nursing administrator in patient care delivery systems, Nurs. Adm. Q. **1**:1-6, Fall 1976.

Colton, M.R.: What is the manager's function in a health care facility? Supervisor Nurse **10**:54-61, September 1979.

Davidhizar, R., and Farabaugh, N.: The new manager: finding *your* place—and *theirs*, Nurs. Management **77**:43-49, April 1986.

Deines, E.: Participative management, Nurs. Management **12**:50-53, November 1981.

Dooley, S.L., and Hauben, J.: From staff nurse to head nurse: a trying transition J. Nurs. Adm. **9**:4-7, April 1979.

Elliott, K.: Am I still a nurse? Supervisor Nurse **10**:60-63, July 1979.

Foster, C.: You've joined the management team? Nurs. Management **12**:16-18, October 1981.

Freeman, R., Sr.: The responsibility of supervisors in personnel management, Dimen. Health Serv. **52**:41-43, April 1975.

Ganong, W., and Ganong, J.: The head nurse as hospital integrator, Supervisor Nurse **8**:27-39, March 1977.

Genovich-Richards, J., and Carissimi, D.C.: Developing nurses' managerial competence, Nurs. Management **17**:36-38, March 1986.

Hanson, R.L.: Managing human resources, J. Nurs. Adm. **12**:17-23, December 1982.

Hayes, P.M.: Redefining the role of the clinical supervisor, Nurs. Leadership **2**:29-33, December 1979.

Hill, B.S.: Participative management: a valid alternative to traditional organizational behavior, Supervisor Nurse **7**:19-21, March 1976.

Holland, M.G.: Can managerial performance be predicted? J. Nurs. Adm. **11**:17-20, June 1981.

Holle, M.L.: Staff nurse yesterday, nurse manager today, Supervisor Nurse **11**:52-56, April 1980.

Hopper, S.A.: Becoming an administrator—overnight! Nurs. Outlook **23**:752-754, December 1975.

Jenkins, J.W.: Good nurse or good manager—what's the difference? Supervisor Nurse **9**:48-50, November 1978.

Kepler, T.L.: Mastering the people skills, J. Nurs. Adm. **10**:15-20, November 1980.

Kinzer, J.: Does nursing administration affect patient care? Supervisor Nurse **9**:84-90, September 1978.

Koontz, H.: The management theory jungle, J. Acad. Management **4**:174-188, December 1961.

Kucha, D.H.: The human relations approach to nursing administration, Nurs. Forum **9**:162-168, Spring 1970.

Lapping, E.A.: Human relations management on a burn unit, Supervisor Nurse **12**:48-51, August 1981.

Levenstein, A.: Art and science of management: developing their independence, Nurs. Management **13**:50-53, July 1982.

Mackenzie, R.A.: The management process in 3D, J. Nurs. Adm. **9**:30-31, November 1979.

Marriner, A.: Development of management thought, J. Nurs. Adm. **9**:21-31, September 1979.

Marriner, A.: Management moves, Nurs. Success Today **3**:8-13, August 1986.

McClure, M.L.: Managing the professional nurse. I. The organizational theories, J. Nurs. Adm. **14**:15-21, February 1984.

McClure, M.L.: Managing the professional nurse. II. Applying management theory to the challenges, J. Nurs. Adm. **14**:11-17, March 1984.

McMillin, B.A.: On being a manager in rural Montana, Nurs. Management **14**:34-36, August 1983.

Miller: How to succeed in nursing management, Supervisor Nurse **8**:18-19, October 1977.

Mohney, S.J.: Why participative management in the modern hospital? Supervisor Nurse **11**:36-38, May 1980.

Monte, R.: Parenting aspects of nursing supervision, Nurs. Management **12**:39-41, October 1981.

Monti, J.E.: Management by individualization, Supervisor Nurse **11**:45-46, June 1980.

Murphy, E.C.: Practical management course: module 17: whole-brain management. I. Nurs. Management **16**:66-70, March 1985.

Murphy, E.C.: Practical management course: module 13: Murphy's law: lessons from folklore for nurse managers, Nurs. Management **15**:47-49, August 1984.

Niederbaumer, L.: The director of nursing service: a participant in top management, Supervisor Nurse **10**:22-27, December 1979.

Niessner, P.: Participative management in the ICU, Supervisor Nurse **9**:41-44, March 1978.

O'Neal, E.: How supervisors become real, Supervisor Nurse **9**:29-31, October 1978.

Peterson, G.G.: The director of nursing should be a nurse, Am. J. Nurs. **73**:1902-1904, November 1973.

Poulin, M.A.: The nurse administrator: survival in the executive jungle, Nurs. Digest **5**:56-58, Spring 1977.

Robbins, S.E.: Nursing service administration in the small hospital, Supervisor Nurse **9**:48-51, August 1978.

Seday, A.J.: Developing nurses' ability to manage: the roles of trust, participation and commitment, J. Continuing Education Nurs. **5**:7-12, January-February 1974.

Sherman, V.C.: Nursing's management crisis, Supervisor Nurse **11**:31-33, October 1980.

Sherman, V.C.: Taking over: notes to the new executive, J. Nurs. Adm. **12**:21-23, May 1982.

Smith, S.N., and Bohnet, N.: Organization and administration of hospice care, J. Nurs. Adm. **13**:10-16, November 1983.

Stagnitto, M.R.E.B.: Nursing supervision: leadership or police work? Supervisor Nurse **10**: 17-19, January 1979.

Stahl, L.D.: Demystifying critical care management. I. J. Nurs. Adm. **15**:27-32, October 1985.

Stahl, L.D.: Demystifying critical care management. II. J. Nurs. Adm. **15**:14-20, November 1985.

Stevens, B.J.: The problem in nursing's middle management, J. Nurs. Adm. **2**:35-38, September-October 1972.

Stevens, B.J.: The head nurse as manager, J. Nurs. Adm. **4**:36-40, January-February 1974.

Stevens, B.J.: Management tools needed, Am. Nurse **7**:9, April 1975.

Stevens, B.J.: Improving nurses' managerial skills, Nurs. Outlook **27**:774-777, December 1979.

Westphal, B.C., Jenkins, R., and Miller, M.C., III: Charge nurse: where staff and management meet, Nurs. Management **17**:56-58, April 1986.

White, H.C., and Wolfe, M.N.: Nursing administration and personnel administration, J. Nurs. Adm. **13**:15-19, July-August 1983.

Whitsett, D.A.: Making sense of management theories, Personnel **52**:44-52, May-June 1975.

Wilkinson W.R.: Effective management, Supervisor Nurse **12**:44-45, January 1981.

Wine, J.A., and Baird, J.E., Jr.: Improving nursing management and practice through quality circles, J. Nurs. Adm. **13**:5-10, May 1983.

Zaleznik, A.: Managers and leaders: are they different? J. Nurs. Adm. **11**:25-31, July 1981.

Power and authority

Ashley, J.: This I believe about power in nursing, Nurs. Outlook **21**:637-641, October 1973.

Beck, C.T.: The conceptualization of power, Adv. Nurs. Sci. pp. 1-17, January 1982.

Bernal, H.: Power and interorganizational health care projects, Nurs. Outlook **24**:418, July 1976.

Bowman, R.A., and Culpepper, B.L.: Power Rx for change, Am. J. Nurs. **74**:1054-1056, June 1974.

Boyle, K.: Power in nursing: a collaborative approach, Nurs. Outlook **32**:164-167, May-June 1984.

Brown, B.J., Gebbie, K., and Moore, J.F.: Affecting nursing goals in health care, Nurs. Adm. Q. **2**:17-31, Spring 1978.

Clary, T.C., and Luke, R.A., Jr.: Organizational and individual power, Training Dev. J. **29**:41-50, April 1975.

Conway, M.E.: The acquisition and use of power in academia: a dean's perspective, Nurs. Adm. Q. **2**:83-90, Spring 1978.

Courtade, Sister S.: The role of the head nurse: power and practice, Supervisor Nurse **9**:16-23, December 1978.

Courtemanche, J.B.: Powernomics: a concept every nurse should know! Nurs. Management **17**:39-41, July 1986.

Curtin, L.L.: Nurse power . . . maybe! (editorial) Supervisor Nurse **11**:7, April 1980.

Dahl, R.A.: The concept of power, Behav. Sci. **2**:201-215, 1957.

Del Bueno, D.J.: Power and politics in organizations, Nurs. Outlook **34**:124-128, May-June 1986.

DeSantis, G.: Power, tactics, and the professionalization process, Nurs. Health Care **3**:14-24, January 1982.

Dickoff, J., and James, P.: Power, Am. J. Nurs. **68**:2128-2132, October 1968.

Diers, D.: A different kind of energy: nurse-power, Nurs. Outlook **26**:51-55, January 1978.

Doona, M.E.: A nursing unit as a political system, J. Nurs. Adm. **7**:28-32, January 1977.

Elsberry, N.L.: Power relations in hospital nursing, J. Nurs. Adm. **2**:75-77, September-October 1972.

Gorman, S., and Clark, N.: Power and effective nursing practice, Nurs. Outlook **34**:129-134, May-June 1986.

Graham, D., and Reeve, D.: There's power in numbers: statistical analysis can pinpoint problems and help solve them, Nurs. Management **15**:48-51, September 1984.

Hendricks, D.E.: The power problem, Nurs. Management **13**:23-24, October 1982.

Hott, J.R.: The struggles inside nursing's body politic, Nurs. Forum **15**:325-340, Fall 1976.

Johnson, R.L.: Characteristics of a power broker, J. Nurs. Adm. **11**:50, November 1980.

Kalisch, B.J.: The promise of power, Nurs. Outlook **26**:42-46, January 1976.

Kotter, J.P.: Power, dependence, and effective management, Harvard Business Rev. **55**:125-136, July-August 1977.

Lamar, E.K.: Communicating personal power through nonverbal behavior, J. Nurs. Adm. **15**:41-44, January 1985.

Langford, T.: Impotence may be curable: an essay, Nurs. Leadership 1:29-33, June 1978.

Leininger, M.: Political nursing: essential for health service and educational systems of tomorrow, Nurs. Adm. Q. 2:1-16, Spring 1978.

Levenstein, A.: Art and science of management: the uses of power, Nurs. Management 12:24-25, October 1981.

Levenstein, A.: Art and science of management: tactics of persuasion, Nurs. Management 13:40-41, November 1982.

Lieb, R.: Power, powerlessness, and potential: nurse's role within the health care delivery system, Image 10:75-83, October 1978.

Masson, V.: On power and vision in nursing, Nurs. Outlook 27:782-784, December 1979.

McClelland, D.C.: Two forces of power, J. Int. Affairs 24:29, 1970.

McFarland D.E.: Power and the nursing administrator, J. Nurs. Adm. 8:19-23, March 1978.

Mechanic, D.: Sources of power of lower participants in complex organizations, Adm. Sci. Q. 7:349-364, December 1962.

Munn, Y.: Power: how to get it and use it in nursing today, Nurs. Adm. Q. 1:95-103, Fall 1976.

Peterson, G.G.: Power: a perspective for the nurse administrator, J. Nurs. Adm. 9:7-10, July 1979.

Salancik, G.R., and Pfeffer, J.: Who gets power and how they hold onto it: a strategic contingency model of power, Organizational Dynamics 5:3-21, Winter 1977.

Shiflett, N., and McFarland, D.E.: Power and the nursing administrator, J. Nurs. Adm. 8:19-23, March 1978.

Silber, M.B.: Nurse power: projecting self and ideas, Supervisor Nurse 12:65-68, July 1981.

Stevens, B.J.: Power and politics for the nurse executive, Nurs. Health Care 1:208-212, November 1980.

Storlie, F.J.: Power: getting a piece of the action, Nurs. Management 13:15-18, October 1982.

Conflict

Bickford, J.: The crisis, Supervisor Nurse 10:28-29, January 1979.

Booth, R.Z.: Conflict resolution, Nurs. Outlook 30:447-453, September-October 1982.

Burke, R.J.: Methods of resolving superior-subordinate conflict: the constructive use of subordinate differences and disagreements, Organizational Behav. Hum. Perform. 5:393-411, 1970.

Carey, M.C.: Staff disunity: a destructive force, Am. J. Nurs. 69:2375-2377, November 1969.

Cochran, R.B.: Don't let tactics trip you up, Am. J. Nurs. 83:844, May 1983.

de Lodzia, G., and Greenhalgh, L.: Creative conflict management in a nursing environment, Supervisor Nurse 4:33-41, July 1973.

Deutsch, M.: Trust and suspicion, J. Conflict Resolution 2:265-279, 1958.

Deutsch, M.: Trust, worthiness, and the F-scale, J. Abnorm. Social Psychol. 61:138-140, 1960.

Ellis, D.E., and Fisher, A.: Phases of conflict in small group development: a Markov analysis, Hum. Commun. Res. 1:195-212, 1975.

Evan, W.M., and MacDougall, J.A.: Interorganizational conflict: a labor-management bargaining experiment, J. Conflict Resolution 11:398-413, 1967.

Fay, M.S., and Morrill, A.K.: The grievance-arbitration process: the experience of one nursing administration, J. Nurs. Adm. 15:11-16, June 1985.

Ganong, W.L., and Ganong, J.M.: Reducing organizational conflict through working committees, J. Nurs. Adm. 40:50-57, November-December 1974.

Glaser, I., and Horvath, K.: A tool for dealing with nursing problems, Supervisor Nurse 10:46-52, April 1979.

Glennon, T.K.: Practitioner vs. bureaucrat: professions in conflict, Nurs. Management 16:60-65, March 1985.

Haw, M.A.: Conflict resolution and the communication myth, Nurs. Outlook, 28:566-570, September 1980.

House, R.J.: Role conflict and multiple authority in complex organizations, Calif. Management Rev. 12:53-60, Summer 1970.

Isaac, S.: Professional growth: 5 ways to resolve conflict, Nurs. 86, 16:89-91, March 1986.

Kay, M.J.: Handling complaints and grievances, Supervisor Nurse 3:72-76, April 1972.

Kramer, M., and Schmalenberg, C.E.: Conflict: the cutting edge of growth, J. Nurs. Adm. 6:19-25, October 1976.

Laser, R.J.: I win-you win negotiating, J. Nurs. Adm. 11:24-29, November-December 1981.

Levenstein, A.: The art and science of supervision: resolving conflict, Supervisor Nurse 7:44-46, February 1976.

Levenstein, A.: Negotiation vs. confrontation, Nurs. Management **15**:52-53, January 1984.

Lewis, J.H.: Conflict management, J. Nurs. Adm. **6**:18-22, December 1976.

Lutjens, L.R.: The name of this game is conflict, Nurs. Management **14**:23-24, June 1983.

Marriner, A.: Conflict theory, Supervisor Nurse **10**:12-16, April 1979.

Marriner A.: Conflict resolution, Supervisor Nurse **10**:46-54, May 1979.

Marriner, A.: Managing conflict, Nurs. Management **13**:29-31, June 1982.

Miles, R.H.: Role requirements as sources of organizational stress, J. Appl. Psychol. **61**:172-179, April 1976.

Nash, A.: Conflict relations between nursing supervisors, practical nurses and attendants, J. Nurs. Adm. **7**:9-12, July-August 1977.

Notz, W.W., and Starke, F.A.: Final-offer versus conventional arbitration as means of conflict management, Adm. Sci. Q. **23**:189-203, June 1978.

O'Toole, A.W., and O'Toole, R.: Negotiating cooperative agreements between health organizations, J. Nurs. Adm. **13**:33-38, December 1983.

Rizzo, J.R., House, R.J., and Lirtzman, S.I.: Role conflict and ambiguity in complex organizations, Adm. Sci. Q. **15**:150-163, June 1970.

Schulz, R., and Johnson, A.C.: Conflict in hospitals, Hosp. Adm. **16**:36-50, 1971.

Stein, A.A.: Conflict and cohesion, J. Conflict. Resolution **20**:143-165, March 1976.

Thurkettle, M.A., and Jones, S.L.: Conflict as a systems process: theory and management, J. Nurs. Adm. **13**:39-43, January 1978.

Tosi, H.: Organization stress as a moderator of the relationship between influence and role response, Acad. Management, J. **14**:7-20, March 1971.

Veglahn, P.A.: Making the grievance procedure work, Personnel J. **56**:122-150, March 1977.

Veninga, R.: The management of conflict, J. Nurs. Adm. **3**:12-16, July-August, 1973.

Walton, R.E., and Dutton, J.M.: The management of interdepartmental conflict: a model and review, Adm. Sci. Q. **14**:73-83, March 1969.

Whetten, D.A.: Coping with incompatible expectations: an integrated view of role conflict, Adm. Sci. Q. **23**:254-270, June 1978.

Zand, D.E.: Trust and managerial problem solving, Adm. Sci. Q. **17**:229-239, 1972.

Politics

Archer, S.E., and Goehner, P.A.: Acquiring political clout: guidelines for nurse administrators, J. Nurs. Adm. **11**:49-55, November-December 1981.

Cavanaugh, D.E.: Gamesmanship: the art of strategizing, J. Nurs. Adm. **15**:38-4l, April 1985.

Curtin, L.: Political savvy (editorial), Nurs. Management **13**:7-8, March 1982.

Davis, C.K., Oakley, D., and Sochalski, J.A.: Leadership for expanding nursing influence on health policy, J. Nurs. Adm. **12**:15-21, January 1982.

Donley, Sister R.: An inside view of the Washington health scene, Am. J. Nurs. **79**:1946-1949, November 1979.

Doona, M.E.: A nursing unit as a political system, J. Nurs. Adm. **7**:28-32, January 1977.

Ehrat, K.S.: A model for politically astute planning and decision making, J. Nurs. Adm. **13**:29-35, September 1983.

Kalisch, B.J., and Kalisch, P.A.: A discourse on the politics of nursing, J. Nurs. Adm. **6**:29-34, March-April 1976.

Lake, R.S.: Legislators' opinions about nursing: results of a pilot study, Nurs. Health Care **5**:204-207, April 1984.

Leininger, M.: Political nursing: essential for health service and educational systems of tomorrow, Nurs. Adm. Q. **2**:1-16, Spring 1978.

Longest, B.B.: Institutional politics, J. Nurs. Adm. **5**:38-41, March-April 1975.

Maraldo, P.: Politics: a very human matter, Am. J. Nurs. **82**:1104-1105, July 1982.

Moore, E., and Oakley, D.: Nurses, political participation, and attitudes toward reforms in the health care system, Nurs. Health Care **4**:504-507, November 1983.

The name of the game is politics, Hospitals **48**:67-71, August 16, 1974.

Nursing representation on hospital governing boards, Regan Rep. Nurs. Law **13**:1, June 1972.

Rowell, P.A., and Knauss, P.J.: The legislative task force: a method to increase nurses' political involvement, Nurs. Outlook **29**:715-716, December 1981.

Underly, N., Doxsey, K., and Reeves, D.M.:

Establishing a nursing legislation subcommittee, Nurs. Outlook **29**:717-719, December 1981.

Team and organizational development

Beer, M., and Huse, E. F.: A systems approach to organization development, J. Appl. Behavioral Sci. **8**:79-101, January-February 1972.

Callaway, J.: Developing a cohesive team in a critical care unit, Nurs. Management **17**:34B-34F, February 1986.

Cohen, M.H., and Ross, M.E.: Team building: a strategy for unit cohesiveness, J. Nurs. Adm. **12**:29-34, January 1982.

Fisher, D.W.: A review of organizational development, J. Nurs. Adm. **10**:31-36, October 1980.

Greiner, L.E.: Red flags in organization development, Business Horizons **15**:17-24, June 1972.

Hendricks, D.E.: Opportunity for managerial growth, Nurs. Management **13**:40-42, April 1982.

Jacobsen-Webb, M.: Team building: key to executive success, J. Nurs. Adm. **15**:16-20, February 1985.

Nelson, G.M., and Schaefer, M.J.: An integrated approach to developing administrators and organizations, J. Nurs. Adm. **10**:37-42, February 1980.

Parrish, D.M., and Cleland, V.S.: Characteristics of a professional nursing practice climate: a survey, J. Nurs. Adm. **11**:40-45, April 1981.

Pointer, D.D., Strum, D.W., and Scalzi, C.C.: Strengthening the top-level management team, J. Nurs. Adm. **11**:45-48, February 1981.

Rubin, I., et al: Improving the coordination of care: an educational program, Hosp. Health Services Adm. **7**:57-70, Spring 1977.

Thomas, R.M.: Management team assessment: a learning style inventory, Nurs. Management **17**:39-48, March 1986.

Wallace, M.J., Ivancevich, J.M., and Lyon, H.L.: Measurement modifications for assessing organizational climate in hospitals, Acad. Management J. **18**:82-97, March 1975.

Weisbord, M.R.: Why organization development hasn't worked (so far) in medical centers, Health Care Management Rev. **1**:17-28, Spring 1976.

Willis, M.M.: Uniting the management team, Supervisor Nurse **12**:40-41, September 1981.

Motivation

Adams, J.S.: Toward an understanding of inequity, J. Abnorm. Social Psychol. **67**:422-436, November 1963.

Axne, S., Boniger, G., and Dodson, D.: Staff motivation through a self-help design, Supervisor Nurse **7**:65-68, October 1978.

Batey, M.V., and Lewis, F.M.: Clarifying autonomy and accountability in nursing service. I. J. Nurs. Adm. **12**:13-18, September 1982.

Bracken, R.L., and Christman, L.: An incentive program designed to develop and reward clinical competence, J. Nurs. Adm. **8**:8-18, October 1978.

Bragg, T.L.: Motivation and dissatisfaction, Nurs. Management **13**:20-22, August 1982.

Buchanan, B.: To walk an extra mile, Organizational Dynamics **4**:67-80, Summer 1975.

Burton, G.E.: What motivates hospital supervisors? Hosp. Top. **54**:30-34, November-December 1976.

Cady, L.: The "don't give a damn" syndrome, Occupational Health Nurs. **21**:12-13, August 1973.

Case, B.B.: Moving your staff toward excellent performance, Nurs. Management **14**:45-48, December 1983.

Chopra, A.: Motivation in task-oriented groups, J. Nurs. Adm. **3**:55-60, January-February 1973.

Edwards, F.G.: The growing needs for motivated nurses, Hosp. Adm. **16**:44-53, Winter 1971.

Fitzgerald, T.H.: Why motivation theory doesn't work, Harvard Business Rev. **49**:37-44, July-August 1971.

Fleishman, R.: Human resource motivation, Supervisor Nurse **9**:57-60, November 1978.

Fleming, A.S.: Motivating others: what works, what doesn't. I. Nurs. 75 **5**:85-88, March 1975.

Ganong, J., Ganong, W., and Huenefeld, J.: Motive force: a key to evaluating nurse managers, Nurs. Digest. **5**:26-28, Fall 1977.

Giblin, E.J.: Motivating employees: a closer look, Personnel J. **55**:68-84, February 1976.

Gordon, G.K.: Motivating staff: a look at assumptions, J. Nurs. Adm. **12**:27-28, November 1982.

Gordon, G.K.: Developing a motivating environment, J. Nurs. Adm. **12**:11-16, December 1982.

Herzberg, F.: One more time: how do you motivate employees? Harvard Business Rev. **46**: 53-62, January-February 1968.

Howell, D.L., and Boxx, W.R.: Motivating workers on routine jobs, Supervisor Nurse **4**:44-52, May 1973.

Hunt, J.G., and Hill, H.W.: The new look in motivational theory for organizational research, Hum. Organization **28**:100-109, Summer 1969.

Jehring, J.J.: Motivational problems in the modern hospital, J. Nurs. Adm. **2**:34-41, November-December 1972.

Jenkins, R.L., and Henderson, R.L.: Motivating the staff: what nurses expect from their supervisors, Nurs. Management **15**:13-14, February 1984.

Joiner, C., et al.: The motivating potential in nursing specialties, J. Nurs. Adm. **12**:26-30, February 1982.

Kenwood, N.J., and Martens, L.C.: Morale problems, Nurs. Management **13**:37-39, July 1982.

Kistler, J.F., and Kistler, R.C.: Motivation and morale in the hospital, Supervisor Nurse **11**:26-29, February 1980.

Lasca, Sister L.: Motivation, evaluation, and leadership, J. Nurs. Adm. **2**:12-21, September-October 1972.

Lawrence, A.C.: Individual differences in work motivation, Hum. Relations **25**:327-335, 1972.

Leidecker, J.K., and Hall, J.: Motivation: good theory—poor application, Training Dev. J. **28**:3-7, June 1974.

Levenstein, A.: Feedback improves performance, Nurs. Management **15**:64-66, February 1984.

Levinson, H.: Asinine attitudes toward motivation, Harvard Business Rev. **51**:70-76, January-February 1973.

Livingston, J.S.: Pygmalion in management, Harvard Business Rev. **47**:81-89, July-August 1969.

Lupascu, D.: Changing TGIF to TGIM, Nurs. Management **12**:25-27, September 1981.

Lysaught, J.P.: No carrots, no sticks: motivation in nursing, J. Nurs. Adm. **2**:13-20, September-October 1972.

Marcus, J., and Marcus, R.: "Nursing" the organization, Supervisor Nurse **8**:8-12, October 1977.

Marriner, A.: Motivation of personnel, Supervisor Nurse **7**:60-63, October 1976.

Murphy, E.C.: Module 9: what motivates people

to work? Nurs. Management **15**:58-63, February 1984.

New tool: "reinforcement" for good work, Business Week, December 18, 1971, pp. 76-77.

Nusinoff, J.R.: How to motivate your employees toward more effective patient care, Hosp. Top. **54**:50-52, March-April 1976.

O'Donovan, T.R.: Dealing with impact needs, Supervisor Nurse **2**:30-41, February 1973.

Pinkelton N.: Commitment to nursing and to self, Nurs. Management **13**:39-41, February 1982.

Roach, K.L.: Production builds on mutual respect, Nurs. Management **15**:54-56, February 1984.

Rosenthal, R.: The pygmalion effect lives, Psychol. Today **7**:56-63, September 1973.

Schmitz, H.H.: Participative management: a technique for employee motivation, Hosp. Prog. **52**:50-54, November 1971.

Schwab, D.P., and Cummings, L.L.: Theories of performance: a review, Industrial Relations **9**:408-430, October 1970.

Schweiger, J.F.: Dealing with apathy in nursing, Supervisor Nurse **7**:42-44, July 1976.

Sherwin, D.S.: Strategy for winning employee commitment, Harvard Business Rev. **50**:37-47, May-June 1972.

Silber, M.B.: The motivation pyramid in nurse retention, Supervisor Nurse **12**:45-46, April 1981.

Skinner, W.: Big hat, no cattle: managing human resources. I. J. Nurs. Adm. **12**:27-29, July-August 1982.

Skinner, W.: Big hat, no cattle, managing human resources. II. J. Nurs. Adm. **12**:32-35, September 1982.

Sossong, A.: Motivating others, Nurs. Management **13**:26-28, June 1982.

Taylor, M.: Motivation at all levels, Aust. Nurses' J. **2**:28-31, February 1973.

Timmreck, T.C., and Randall, P.J.: Motivation, management and the supervisory nurse, Supervisor Nurse **12**:28-31, March 1981.

Warren, J.C.: Motivating and rewarding the staff nurse, J. Nurs. Adm. **8**:4-7, October 1978.

Watkin, B.: Management topics: motivation, Nurs. Mirror **138**:75, April 5, 1974.

Job satisfaction

Baldonado, A.A.: Making job satisfaction a reality for nurses, Supervisor Nurse **11**:39-40, May 1980.

Bayley, E.W.: Breaking a turnover cycle: a successful approach, Supervisor Nurse 12:19-21, March 1981.

Behling, O.C., and Kosmo, R.: Reducing nursing turnover, Hospitals 45:124-144, February 1, 1971.

Benton, D.A., and White, H.C.: Satisfaction of job factors for registered nurses, J. Nurs. Adm. 2:55-63, November 1972.

Brief, A.P.: Personnel management: turnover among hospital nurses—a suggested model, J. Nurs. Adm. 6:55-58, October 1976.

Brief, A.P., Aldag, R.J., and Jacox, A.: A study: the impact of task characteristics on employee response in hospital nursing, Nurs. Adm. Q. 2:107-114, Summer 1978.

Cronin-Stubbs, D.: Job satisfaction and dissatisfaction among new graduate staff nurses, J. Nurs. Adm. 7:44-49, December 1977.

Feldman, H.R.: The organization game, Nurs. Management 16:47-49, September 1985.

Flowers, V.S., and Hughes, C.L.: Why employees stay, Harvard Business Rev. 51:49-60, July-August 1973.

Godfrey, M.A.: Working conditions: how do yours compare with other nurses? Nursing 75 5:85-102, May 1975.

Godfrey, M.A.: Job satisfaction—or should that be dissatisfaction? How nurses feel about nursing, I, Nursing 78 8:89-91, April 1978.

Godfrey, M.A.: Job satisfaction—or should that be dissatisfaction? How nurses feel about nursing, II, Nursing 78 8:105-120, May 1978.

Godfrey, M.A.: Job satisfaction—or should that be dissatisfaction? How nurses feel about nursing, III, Nursing 78 8:81-92, June 1978.

Heinen, B.: Job satisfaction for the float staff, Supervisor Nurse 10:48-51, January 1979.

Hertel, M., Keibert, C., and DeJoseph, J.F.: The photographic image process, Supervisor Nurse 11:36-38, November 1980.

Hunter, J.K., et al.: Job satisfaction: is collective bargaining the answer? Nurs. Management 17:56-60, March 1986.

Katz, R.: Job longevity as a situational factor in job satisfaction, Adm. Sci. Q. 23:204-223, June 1978.

Kovner, C.T., and Oliver, R.S.: Directors of nursing: satisfaction and dissatisfaction, Nurs. Adm. Q. 2:57-63, Fall 1977.

Larson, E., et al.: Job satisfaction: assumptions and complexities, J. Nurs. Adm. 14:31-38, January 1984.

Lemler, S.F., and Leach, A.K.: The effect of job satisfaction on retention, Nurs. Management 17:66-68, April 1986.

Lenz, E.R., and Waltz, C.F.: Patterns of job search and mobility among nurse educators, J. Nurs. Educ. 22:267-273, September 1983.

Levenstein, A.: The art and science of supervision: job satisfaction and hospital loyalty, Supervisor Nurse 6:8-12, June 1975.

Levenstein, A.: The art and science of supervision: a source of dissatisfaction, Supervisor Nurse 7:68-69, November 1976.

Levenstein, A.: The art and science of supervision: the tragedy of turnover, Supervisor Nurse 8:74-75, February 1977.

Longest, B.B.: Job satisfaction for registered nurses in the hospital setting, J. Nurs. Adm. 4:46-52, May-June 1974.

MacDonald, M.R.: Matching personalities with position: a study of job satisfaction, Supervisor Nurse 6:43-50, April 1975.

Marriner, A., and Craigie, D.: Job satisfaction and mobility of nursing educators in baccalaureate and higher degree programs in the West, Nurs. Research 26:349-360, September-October 1977.

McCloskey, J.: Influence of rewards and incentives on staff nurse turnover rate, Nurs. Res. 23:239-247, May-June 1974.

Miller, D.S., and Norton, V.M.: Absenteeism: nursing service's albatross, J. Nurs. Adm. 16:38-42, March 1986.

Nichols, G.A.: Important, satisfying, and dissatisfying aspects of nurses' jobs, Supervisor Nurse 5:10-15, January 1974.

Rozell, V.: The head nurse as a staff nurse satisfaction factor, Nurs. Adm. Q. 2:65-69, Fall 1977.

Scanlan, B.K.: Determinants of job satisfaction and productivity, Personnel J. 53:12-14, January 1976.

Seybolt, J.W., Pavett, C., and Walker, D.D.: Turnover among nurses: it can be managed, J. Nurs. Adm. 8:4-9, September 1978.

Slavitt, D.B., et al.: Nurses' satisfaction with their work situation, Nurs. Res. 27:114-120, March-April 1978.

Stember, M.L., et al.: Job satisfaction research: an aid in decision making, Nurs. Adm. Q. 2:95-105, Summer 1978.

Strilaeff, F.: Supervision and turnover of general staff nurses, Dimen. Health Serv. 53:36-39, November 1976.

Stryker-Gordon, R.: Minnesota study suggests means of reducing turnover rates in nursing homes, J. Nurs. Adm. **9**:17-20, April 1979.

Ullrich, R.A.: Herzberg revisited: factors in job dissatisfaction, J. Nurs. Adm. **8**:19-24, October 1978.

Watson, L.A.: Keeping qualified nurses, Supervisor Nurse **10**:29-34, October 1979.

Wernimont, P.F.: A systems view of job satisfaction, J. Appl. Psychol. **56**:173-176, April 1972.

What do you like . . . and dislike . . . about nursing? Nurs. 77 7:48-53, September 1977.

White, C.H., and Maquire, M.C.: Job satisfaction and dissatisfaction among hospital nursing supervisors: the applicability of Herzberg's theory, Nurs. Res. **22**:25-30, January-February 1973.

Wolf, G.A.: Nursing turnover: some causes and solutions, Nurs. Outlook **29**:233-236, April 1981.

Communication

Bloom, M.T.: The great communications dilemma, J. Nurs. Adm. **1**:29-36, November-December 1971.

Brunner, N.A.: Communications in nursing service administration, J. Nurs. Adm. **7**:29-32, October 1977.

Calabrese, R.: Interaction skills for nurse managers, Nurs. Management **13**:29-30, May 1982.

Chartier, M.R.: Clarity of expression in interpersonal communication, J. Nurs. Adm. **11**:42-46, July 1981.

Chiavetta, L.: Group communication: when I speak no one listens, Nurs. Management **13**:36-37, May 1982.

Davis, A.J.: Body talk, Supervisor Nurse **9**:36-37, June 1978.

DeBell, C.M., and Costello, M.K.: Starting a reprint filing system, J. Nurs. Adm. **15**:38-42, December 1985.

Elliott, T.G., Everly, G.S., and Everly, G.S.: Communication: a program design, Supervisor Nurse **9**:12-18, February 1979.

Evans, C.S.: Communication in infection control, Supervisor Nurse **8**:48-49, September 1977.

Evans, R.O.: Upward communications, Supervisor Nurse **2**:23-24 +, December 1971.

Geutzkow, H., and Simon, H.A.: The impact of certain communication nets upon organization and performance in task-oriented groups, Management Sci. **1**:233-250, April-July 1955.

Gibb, J.R.: Defensive communication, J. Nurs. Adm. **12**:14-22, April 1982.

Harris, C.C., Stern, P., and Paris, N.F.: The troubleshooter's guide to media, Nurs. Outlook **34**:28-33, January-February 1986.

Lancaster, J.: Public speaking can be improved, J. Nurs. Adm. **15**:31-35, March 1985.

Levenstein, A.: Art and science of management: one to one, Nurs. Management **12**:45-46, December 1981.

Miltz, R.J.: Nurses improve their personal communication, Supervisor Nurse **8**:13-15, December 1977.

Mlynczak, B.A.: Improving management, Nurs. Management **13**:45-49, July 1982.

Murphy, E.C.: Practical management course: module 14.: communication and wellness: managing patient/staff relationships, Nurs. Management **15**:64-68, October 1984.

Ness, J.W.: Meetings can improve nurse-physician relations, Supervisor Nurse **12**:24-26, January 1981.

Orr, E.P.: Communication crisis, Aust. Nurses' J. **2**:32-34, February 1973.

O'Sullivan, P.S.: Detecting communication problems, Nurs. Management **16**:27-30, November 1985.

Pincus, J.D.: Communication: key contributor to effectiveness—the research, J. Nurs. Adm. **16**:19-25, September 1986.

Rogers, C.R., and Roethlisberger, F.J.: Barriers and gateways to communication, Harvard Business Rev. **30**:46-52, July-August 1952.

Rosenblum, E.H.: Groupthink: one peril of group cohesiveness, J. Nurs. Adm. **12**:27-31, April 1982.

Salome, P.B.: Developing a department newsletter, J. Nurs. Adm. **15**:36-41, March 1985.

Sevel, F.: Are you prepared to meet the media? J. Nurs. Adm. **16**:21-24, March 1986.

Somers, J.B.: Information systems: the process of development, J. Nurs. Adm. **9**:53-58, January 1979.

Veehoff, D.C.: Standing ovation: a holistic approach to successful speaking, J. Nurs. Adm. **15**:34-39, October 1985.

Veninga, R.: Interpersonal feedback: a cost-benefit analysis, J. Nurs. Adm. **5**:40-43, February 1975.

Veninga, R.: Interpersonal feedback: a cost-benefit analysis, Nurs. Digest **5**:54-57, Fall 1977.

Wang, R.Y., and Hawkins, J.W.: Interpersonal feedback for nursing supervisors, Supervisor Nurse **11**:26-28, January 1980.

Watkin, B.: Management topics: effective communication, Nurs. Mirror **139**:54, July 5, 1974.

Wlody, G.S.: Effective communication techniques, Nurs. Management **12**:19-23, October 1981.

Wolf, G.A.: Communication: key contributor to effectiveness—a nurse executive responds, J. Nurs. Adm. **16**:26-28, September 1986.

Worthington, J.: The art of effective communication, Nurs. Management **13**:47-49, November 1982.

Assertiveness

Armstrong, D.: Nurse-doctor games, AORN J. **17**:61-65, June 1973.

Bakdash, D.P.: Becoming an assertive nurse, Am. J. Nurs. **78**:1710-1712, October 1978.

Belanger C.: Do you confront the boss? Supervisor Nurse **9**:36-40, December 1978.

Broveman, I.K., et al.: Sex-role stereotypes and clinical judgments of mental health, J. Consulting Clin. Psychol. **34**:1-7, 1970.

Broveman, I.K., et al.: Sex-role stereotypes: a current appraisal, J. Social Issues **28**:59-78, 1972.

Cady, L.M.: Nurse-nurse games, AORN J. **17**:56-60, June 1973.

Christy, T.: Equal rights for women: voices from the past, Am. J. Nurs. **71**:288-293, February 1971.

Clark, C.C.: Assertiveness issues for nursing administrators and managers, J. Nurs. Adm. **9**:20-24, July 1979.

Cleland, V.: Sex discrimination: nursing's most pervasive problem, Am. J. Nurs. **71**:1542-1547, August 1971.

Curry, J.L.: Assertiveness training for supervisory nurses, Supervisor Nurse **9**:43-50, September 1978.

Edelstein, R.G.: Equal rights for women: perspectives, Am. J. Nurs. **71**:294-298, February 1971.

Etzkowitz, H.: The male sister: sexual separation of labor in society, J. Marriage Family **33**:431-434, August 1971.

Fretz, C.F., and Hayman, J.: Progress for women: men are still more equal, Harvard Business Rev. **51**:133-142, September-October 1973.

Golick, T.: The amendment: do women need it? Am. J. Nurs. **71**:285-287, February 1971.

Grimm, L.J., and Crawford, J.J.: Viewpoint: assertiveness training for nurses, Nurs. Adm. Q. **2**:59-63, Spring 1973.

Heide, W.S.: Nursing and women's liberation: a parallel, Am. J. Nurs. **73**:824-827, May 1973.

Hutchings, H., and Colburn, L.: An assertiveness training program for nurses, Nurs. Outlook **27**:394-397, June 1979.

Joreen: Trashing: the dark side of sisterhood, Ms **4**:49-51, 92-98, April 1976.

Kilkus, S.P.: Adding assertiveness to the nursing profession, Nurs. Success Today **3**:17-19, August 1986.

Komarovsky, M.: Cultural contradictions and sex roles: the masculine case, Am. J. Sociol. **78**:873-884, January 1973.

Kritek, P., and Glass, L.: Nursing: a feminist perspective, Nurs. Outlook **26**:182-186, March 1978.

LeRoux, R.S.: Sex-role stereotyping and leadership, Nurs. Adm. Q. **1**:21-29, Fall 1976.

Marriner, A.: Assertive behavior for nursing leaders, Nurs. Leadership **2**:14-20, December 1979.

McGillick, K., and Fernandes, R.C.: Reaching for the stars, Nurs. Management **14**:24-26, January 1983.

McKee, J.P., and Sherriffs, A.C.: The differential evaluation of males and females, Personnel **25**:356-371, 1957.

Migut, P.J.: Self-care for nurses: assertiveness, Nurs. Management **13**:13-14, February 1982.

Mischel, H.N.: Sex bias in the evaluation of professional achievement, J. Educ. Psychol. **66**:157-166, 1974.

Moniz, D.: Putting assertiveness techniques into practice, Am. J. Nurs. **78**:1713, October 1978.

Numerof, R.E.: Assertiveness training, Am. J. Nurs. **80**:1796-1799, October 1980.

Pardue, S.F.: Assertiveness for nursing, Supervisor Nurse **11**:47-50, February 1980.

Riley, M.W., Johnson, M.E., and Boocock, S.S.: Woman's changing occupational role: a research report, Am. Behav. Sci. **7**:33-37, May 1963.

Rosen, B.: The influence of sex-role stereotypes on evaluations of male and female supervisory behavior, J. Appl. Psychol. **57**:44-48, 1973.

Rosen, B.: Influence of sex role stereotypes on

personnel decisions, J. Appl. Psychol. **59**:9-14, 1974.

Rosen, B., and Jerdee, T.H.: Effects of applicant's sex and difficulty of job on evaluations of candidates for managerial positions, J. Appl. Psychol. **59**:511-512, 1974.

Schein, V.E.: The relationship between sex role stereotypes and requisite management characteristics, J. Appl. Psychol. **57**:95-100, 1973.

Schein, V.E.: Relationships between sex role stereotypes and requisite management characteristics among female managers, J. Appl. Psychol. **60**:340-344, 1975.

Serber, M.: Teaching the nonverbal components of assertive training, J. Behav. Ther. Exp. Psychiat. **3**:179-183, 1972.

Silber, M.: Daring directors of nursing, Nurs. Management **14**:30-32, January 1983.

Spitzer, R.: The nurse in the corporate world, Supervisor Nurse **12**:21-24, April 1981

Staines, G., Tauris, C., and Jayaratne, T.E.: The queen bee syndrome, Psychol. Today **7**:55-60, January 1974.

Thorpe, R.: Sabotage in nursing, Supervisor Nurse **12**:24-25, May 1981.

Touhey, J.C.: Effects of additional women professionals on ratings of occupational prestige and desirability, J. Pers. Soc. Psychol. **29**: 86-89, 1974.

Transactional analysis

Alvandi, O.M., and Klingbeil, G.A.: Concepts of transactional analysis and anxiety with persons in crisis, J. Psychiatr. Nurs. **13**:5-10, November-December 1975.

Babcock, D.E.: Transactional analysis, Am. J. Nurs. **76**:1153-1155, July 1976.

Bennett, D.: Transactional analysis in management, Personnel **52**:34-44, January-February 1975.

Bunning, R.L.: Victims, persecutors and rescuers, Supervisor Nurse **10**:13-17, November 1979.

D'Angelo, H.: TA for management training: a good idea, Nurs. Homes **25**:6-7, 16, July 1976.

Fulton, K.: Acknowledgment supports effective communication, Supervisor Nurse **12**:37-40, March 1981.

Gowell, E.C.: Transactional analysis strategies for dealing with pain, J. Psychiatr. Nurs. **12**:25-30, September-October 1974.

Hurt, R.: TA for managers, Management World **2**:17-22, October 1973.

Lee, D.K., and Ventres, S.: The nurse: the enabler, Am. J. Nurs. **81**:506-508, March 1981.

Silber, M.B.: Nursing management starts and succeeds with self-esteem, Supervisor Nurse **12**:42-46, March 1981.

Wachter-Shikora, N.: Scapegoating among professionals, Am. J. Nurs. **77**:408-409, March 1977.

Wagner, F.: The stroke bank, Nurs. Care **7**:26, October 1974.

PART 5

CONTROL

OBJECTIVES

After completing this part, the reader will be able to:

Identify three strategies for effecting change.

Describe five methods of personnel evaluation.

Identify at least five principles of disciplinary action.

Discuss four components of a disciplinary action program.

Appraise behavior-modification techniques.

Discuss phases of unionization.

Differentiate between research designs.

Discuss quality assurance.

Identify at least three tools for control.

Practice stress management techniques.

STUDY QUESTIONS

1
What are ways to effect change?

2
What tools are available to evaluate personnel?

3
What are principles of disciplinary action?

4
What are the components of a disciplinary action program?

5
How can one person modify another person's behavior?

6
How are unions formed?

7
What are the pros and cons of various research designs?

8
What is quality assurance and how is it maintained?

9
What are tools for control?

10
What can you do to control your stress level?

NATURE AND PURPOSE OF CONTROLLING

Controlling is the last step in the management process. It involves setting standards, measuring performance against those standards, reporting the results, and taking corrective actions. Controls should be designed for specific situations and should report potential or actual deviations promptly enough for corrective action to be effective. The manager concentrates on the deviations at critical points. The size of the deviation from standards can appear misleading. For instance, a 5% deviation in the personnel budget may be a far more serious problem than a 15% deviation in telephone expenses. Thus, the manager must rank the exceptions in order of importance. Controls must be determinable, verifiable, and flexible. Alternative flexible plans help achieve flexible controls. Controls must be understandable, economical, and must lead to corrective action. Adequate control systems disclose deviations, identify who is responsible, and recommend corrections. Controls are justified by correcting deviations.

MANAGEMENT OF CHANGE

Strategies for effecting change

Whether working with individuals, groups, or systems, the nurse manager is sure to be involved with management of change. Several strategies for managing change have been identified.

Empirical-rational strategies. Empirical-rational strategies are based on the assumption that people are rational and behave according to rational self-interest. It follows then that people should be willing to adopt a change if it is justified and if the person is shown how she can benefit from the change.

The nurse manager who uses empirical-rational strategies is likely to want the appropriate persons for specific positions. Desirous of having well-qualified people performing jobs for which they are well qualified, she gives considerable attention to recruitment and selection of personnel. Staff development through independent study, in-service education, continuing education, and formal degree programs is encouraged. Systems analysis, operations research, and implementation of research findings are consistent with the empirical-rational philosophy, as is long-range futuristic planning.

Normative re-educative strategies. Normative re-educative strategies are based on the assumption that people act according to their commitment to sociocultural norms. The intelligence and rationality of people are not denied, but attitudes and values are also considered. The manager pays attention to changes in values, attitudes, skills, and relationships in addition to providing information.

Believing that the basic unit of the social organization is composed of individuals, the manager fosters the development of staff members through means such as personal counseling, training groups, small groups, and experiential learning because the person needs to participate in her own re-education. Organizational development programs are fostered, and it is typical to collect data about the organization, give data feedback and analysis to appropriate people, plan ways to improve the system, and train managers and internal change agents. The relationships of internal change agents with other personnel can be a major tool in re-educating others.

Power-coercive strategies. Power-coercive strategies involve compliance of the less powerful to the leadership, plans, and directions of the more powerful. These strategies do not deny the intelligence and rationality of people or the importance of their values and attitudes, but rather they acknowledge the need to use sources of power to bring about change. Use of strikes, sit-ins, negotiations, conflict confrontation, and administration decisions and rulings are power-coercive strategies.*

Process of change

Unfreezing, moving, and refreezing are the three phases of change. Unfreezing is the development through problem awareness of a need to change. Even if a problem has been identified, a person must believe there can be an improvement before she is willing to change. Coercion and the induction of guilt and anxiety have been used for unfreezing. Removal of a person from the source of her old attitudes to a new environment, punishment and humiliation for undesirable attitudes, and rewards for desirable attitudes effect change.

Stress may cause dissatisfaction with the status quo and become a motivating factor for change. Points of stress and strain should be assessed. Change may begin at a point of stress but ordinarily should not be started at the point of greatest stress. It is most appropriate for it to start with a policy-making body that considers both formal and informal structures. The effectiveness of the change may depend on the amount of involvement in fact finding and problem solving of all personnel.

Moving is working toward change by identifying the problem or the need to change, exploring the alternatives, defining goals and objectives, planning how to accomplish the goals, and implementing the plan for change.

Refreezing is the integration of the change into one's personality and the consequent stabilization of change. Frequently personnel return to old behaviors

---

*Discussed in detail in Chin, R., and Benne, K.D.: General strategies for effecting changes in human systems. In Bennis, W., Benne, K.D., and Chin, R., editors: The planning of change, New York, 1969, Holt, Rinehart & Winston, pp. 32-59.

after change efforts cease. Related changes in neighboring systems, momentum to perpetuate the change, and structural alterations that support the procedural changes are stabilizing factors.

Types of change

The variables of mutual goal setting, the power ratio between the change-agent and the client system, and the deliberativeness of change are differentiating factors in the change process.

Coercive change. Coercive change is characterized by nonmutual goal setting, imbalanced power ratio, and one-sided deliberativeness.

Emulative chance. In this case, change is fostered through identification with and emulation of power figures.

Indoctrination. Indoctrination uses mutual goal setting, has an imbalanced power ratio, and is deliberative. Subordinates are instructed in the beliefs of the power sources.

Interactional change. This is characterized by mutual goal setting, fairly equal power, but no deliberativeness. Parties may be unconsciously committed to changing one another.

Natural change. These changes include accidents and acts of God. They involve no goal setting or deliberativeness.

Socialization change. This has a direct relationship with interactional change. One conforms to the needs of a social group. When there is greater deliberativeness on the power side, change becomes indoctrination.

Technocratic change. Change is brought about by collecting and interpreting data. A technocrat merely reports the findings of the analysis to bring about change.

Planned change. Planned change involves mutual goal setting, an equal power ratio, and deliberativeness.

Seven phases of planned change have been identified. First, the client must feel a need for change. The manager, as the change agent, can stimulate an awareness of the need to change, help the client become aware of the problems, and indicate that a more desirable state of affairs is possible. Thus, unfreezing occurs.

Next, the helping relationship must be established, and the moving process begun. The manager as a change agent must identify herself with the client's problems while remaining neutral so that she can take an objective view. The change agent needs to be viewed as an understandable and approachable expert. The success or failure of most planned action will be largely dependent on the quality and workability of the relationship between the change agent and the client.

Third, the problem must be identified and clarified. Collecting and analyzing data can facilitate this process. Fourth, alternative possibilities for change should be examined. Goals and objectives are planned. The client's emotional and material resources are examined. Strategies for change are determined. The success of planned change is evaluated by the implementation of the plans. The fifth phase is the active work of modification, which completes the moving process.

The refreezing process occurs during the sixth phase—generalization and stabilization. All too often the client slips back to her old ways after change efforts cease. The spread of change to neighboring systems and to subparts of the same system aids the stabilization process. Change momentum, positive evaluation of the change, rewards for the change, and related procedural and structural changes increase the stabilization.

The helping relationship ends, or a different type of continuing relationship is established in the last phase. Dependency is the major factor determining when the relationship will end.*

Role of the manager as change agent

As a change agent, the manager identifies the problem, assesses the client's motivations and capacities for change, determines alternatives, explores ramifications of those alternatives, assesses resources, determines appropriate helping roles, establishes and maintains a helping relationship, recognizes the phases of the change process and guides the client through them, and chooses and implements techniques for planned change.†

Force-field analysis

Kurt Lewin's force-field analysis provides a framework for problem solving and planned change. Status quo is maintained when driving forces equal the restraining forces, and change will occur when the relative strength of opposing forces changes. Consequently, when planning change, the manager should identify the restraining and driving forces and assess their strengths.

Driving forces may include pressure from the manager, desire to please the

---

*Planned change is discussed in more detail in Lippitt, R., Watson, J., and Westley, B.: The dynamics of planned change, New York, 1958, Harcourt, Brace & World.
†Adapted from Lippitt, R., Watson, J., and Westley, B.: The dynamics of planned change, New York, 1958, Harcourt, Brace & World, p. 126.

manager, perception that the change will improve one's self-image, and belief that the change will improve the situation. Restraining forces include conformity to norms, morals, and ethics; desire for security; perception of economic threat or threat to one's prestige and homeostasis; and regulatory mechanisms for keeping the situation fairly constant.

Once the driving and restraining forces have been identified, the manager determines their relative strengths. Which are the major factors toward or resisting change? Which are important or moderately important? Which have little effect for or against change? These might be listed in columns under "driving" and "restraining" and ranked.

Driving forces		Restraining forces	
Rank	**Factor**	**Rank**	**Factor**
1	Pressure from manager	4	Conformity
4	Please manager	4	Security
2	Improve self-image	2	Economic threat
2	Improve situation	3	Threat to prestige

Scale:
1 = Little strength
2 = Moderate strength
3 = Important strength
4 = Major strength

To help visualize these forces, the manager can draw the following diagram, write in key words to identify the forces, and draw arrows toward the status quo line to represent the strength of the forces. The longer the line, the stronger the force.

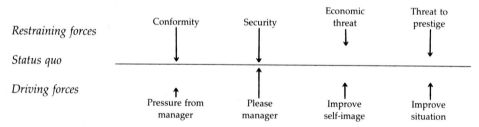

Next the manager plans strategies for reducing the restraining forces and strengthening the driving forces. The manager may do some experiental learning exercises to facilitate the change of group norms, explain each person's role in the change with emphasis on security, and provide some status symbols to reduce the threat to people's prestige. She should also help the workers identify how the change will improve their situation. Steps should be taken to improve self-images. For instance, people may be taught new tasks to prepare themselves for the change, to reduce the threat to their prestige and their fear of making fools of themselves when doing something new, and to improve their self-images. If the manager perceives that the workers want to please her, she may inform them that she desires the change and give positive reinforcement for the desired changes. Keeping the goals in mind, the manager should assess the results of implementing the strategies and revise plans as necessary.

MAPS design technology

MAPS is an acronym for multivariate analysis, participation, and structure. It facilitates the organization's development by applying theories of motivation to create organizational structures. First the organization is designed to determine if the organization's structure is a cause of performance problems. Second, the focus of the change effort must be determined. Will only selected workgroup structures or will the whole organization structure be changed? Third, the objectives of the project must be identified and stated. Fourth, strategies to deal with diagnosed problems and to meet the objectives must be determined. Fifth, a questionnaire that identifies the total range of tasks necessary to achieve the change and a list of the members of the organization or group involved must be composed. Participative collaboration from organizational members and possibly from clients is recommended. Next the questionnaire is administered to all members of the targeted group. They identify their qualifications and preferences for tasks and identify with whom they would prefer to work. Then the questionnaire is analyzed by use of multivariate statistics to identify clusters of tasks and people that reflect sociometric choice. A specific cluster of tasks and people is selected. Resources and support are provided to help the new group develop and do the tasks. The implementation process is monitored so that problems can be detected and resolved easily. Results are evaluated in terms of meeting the objectives. The new structure will then need to be redesigned, because solutions to old problems create new problems.

EVALUATION OF PERSONNEL

Purposes

Performance appraisal is a periodic formal evaluation of how well the nurse has performed her duties during a specific time period. Purposes of the evaluation are (1) to determine job competence, (2) to enhance staff development and motivate personnel toward higher achievement, (3) to discover the employee's aspirations and to recognize her accomplishments, (4) to improve communications between supervisors and staff and to reach an understanding about the objectives of the job and agency, (5) to improve performance by examining and encouraging better relationships among nurses, (6) to aid supervisor's coaching and counseling, (7) to determine training and developmental needs of nurses, (8) to make inventories of talent within the organization and reassess assignments, (9) to select qualified nurses for advancement and salary increases, and (10) to identify unsatisfactory employees.

Common errors in evaluation

Criteria involving judgments are used for performance evaluation. Because human judgment is subject to the influences of prejudice, bias, and other subjective and extraneous factors, the attempt to get objective, accurate evaluations is extremely difficult. There are a number of errors that may affect performance ratings. The supervisor should be aware of the most common errors and try to minimize them.

The halo error is the result of allowing one trait to influence the evaluation of other traits or of rating all traits based on a general impression. A logical error is rating a nurse high on one characteristic because she possesses another characteristic that is logically related. Sometimes a person is given a good rating in the recent past because she did good work in the distant past, or outstanding performance on a recent job may offset a mediocre performance during the rest of the evaluation period. A supervisor is likely to rate personnel who are compatible with her higher than they deserve and may not see certain types of defects that are like her own. The person who does not complain is likely to get higher ratings than the person who does.

The horns error is the opposite of the halo effect. The evaluator is hypercritical. If the supervisor is a perfectionist, she may rate personnel lower than she should. The supervisor may compare how she used to do the job with how it is done now and is more likely to rate people doing jobs with which she is familiar lower than those with whose jobs she is not familiar. A good worker on a weak team is likely to get lower ratings than if she were working on a better team. A person who is not well known may be judged by the company she keeps. A recent mistake may offset a year's good work. If the worker is contrary, the supervisor may vent her irritation by lowering the rating. The nonconformist or person with a personality trait that is not appreciated is likely to be rated lower than her work merits.

The contrast error is produced by the tendency of the supervisor to rate the nurse opposite from how she perceives herself. A small range of scores may be a result of the central tendency error. When the rating on a preceding characteristic influences the rating on the following trait, a proximity error exists. As every rater tends to have her own built-in set of standards or frame of reference on which she makes her evaluation, it becomes a major problem comparing different raters' scores. Some supervisors may be easy and lenient, whereas others may be severe in their judgments.

There are precautions the supervisor can take to minimize judgment errors.

For instance, a forced-distribution technique may be used to overcome the leniency and central tendency errors. A critical incident checklist can reduce the halo effect and logical rating errors. Ranking systems, paired comparisons, and force-choice techniques may be used.

Methods of evaluation

Anecdotal notes. Anecdotal records are objective descriptions of behavior recorded on plain paper or a form. The notations should include who was observed, by whom, when, and where. The notation comprises a description of the setting or background and the incident, and interpretation and recommendations may be included. Value-laden words such as good and bad should be avoided.

Characteristic behavior cannot be determined without several incidents depicting similar behavior. The supervisor, head nurse, or team leader may use time sampling to accumulate observations. The time that is set aside specifically for observations may be divided by the number of staff to be observed. The supervisor then concentrates on the scheduled staff member for a short period of time. It is advisable to make several brief observations over a time span to allow for temporary variables and to identify patterns of behavior.

An advantage of anecdotal recordings is that the description is not coerced into a rigid structure. However, this latitude becomes a problem when the interpreter tries to develop relationships among notations that may have little or no relationship to each other. Although anecdotal records provide a systematic means for recording observations, they do not guarantee that observations will be made systematically or that specific, relevant behaviors will be observed. It also takes considerable time to record the observations.

Checklists. With a checklist the supervisor can categorically assess the presence or absence of desired characteristics or behavior. Checklists are most useful for tangible variables, such as inventory of supplies, but they can be used for evaluation of nursing skills as well. It is advisable to list only the behaviors essential to successful performance, and it is advantageous to determine the behavior to be observed in advance. The same criteria can then be used in each situation. Unfortunately, this does not guarantee that the observed behavior is a persistent one or that a representative situation is being observed. Nor is the checklist practical for evaluating interpersonal relations.

Rating scales. The rating scale does more than just note the absence or presence of desirable behavior. It locates the behavior at a point on a continuum and notes quantitative and qualitative abilities. The numerical rating scale usually includes numbers against which a list of behaviors are evaluated. For example:

Observation of working hours	1 2 3 4 5	
Ability to get along with others	1 2 3 4 5	

This is not a very reliable tool because of the inconsistent value attributed to the number. That fault can be partially overcome by adding a few quantitative terms. For example:

Observation of working hours	**Never**	**Sometimes**	**About half the time**	**Usually**	**Always**
	(1)	(2)	(3)	(4)	(5)

The tool can be made even more reliable by developing a standard scale by using comparative examples to establish a set of standards. The difficulty is finding appropriate comparative standards. To illustrate, a nurse-to-nurse comparison scale might be developed as follows:

Nurse	Observation of working hours				
	Lowest (1)	**Below average** (2)	**Average** (3)	**Above average** (4)	**Highest** (5)
Betty Green	x				
Sara Smith		x			
Pam Peterson			x		
Sue Jones				x	
Anita Anderson					x

As long as the supervisors can agree on the qualifications of a few nurses known to all of them, a comparison scale can be developed that gives a common reference for rating the rest of the staff nurses.

The graphic rating scale is different from the numerical rating scale in that words rather than numbers are used. For example:

	Unsatisfactory	Below average	Average	Above Average	Outstanding

Observation of working hours

Graphic rating scales usually list extremely broad and general personal characteristics that are to be rated from poor to excellent or from low to high. The rater is given little if any guidance about what work behavior qualifies a person for a particular rating and must consequently use her own judgment about how to classify the behaviors.

The following descriptive graphic rating scale is similar to the graphic rating scale except that it presents a more elaborate description of the behavior being rated:

Usually late   Sometimes late   Usually on time

Observation of working hours

BARS is an acronym for behaviorally anchored rating scales, sometimes known as BES, behavioral expectation scales. They are similar to graphic rating scales in that a person is rated on a series of dimensions or qualities. However, BARS differs from graphic rating scales in the ways that the criteria are identified and the alternative responses along the rating scale are anchored or described. BARS evaluates behavior relevant to specific demands of the job and provides examples of specific job behaviors corresponding to good, average, and poor performances. This reduces the amount of personal judgment needed by the rater.

The major disadvantage of BARS is the time and expense required to involve large numbers of employees in determining the dimensions of effective performance and behavioral examples of various levels of performance of each variable. Separate BARS are needed for each job. It is primarily applicable to physically observable behaviors rather than to conceptual skills. However, it should reduce rating errors and provide more reliable, valid, meaningful, and complete data. Employees give more acceptance and commitment to this appraisal system because of their involvement in designing it. Employees have full knowledge of the requirements of the job, and they evidence less defensiveness and conflict because people are evaluated on the basis of specific behaviors rather than personalities. This system thereby identifies performance deficiencies and needs for development.

BOS is an acronym for behavioral observation scales. This system capitalizes on some of the strengths of BARS while avoiding some of the disadvantages. BOS also uses critical incidents of worker behavior. The evaluator lists a number of critical incidents for each performance dimension and rates the extent to which the behavior has been observed on a 5-point scale ranging from almost never to almost always. It too is relatively reliable, well accepted, and understood, provides useful feedback, but is relatively time consuming and expensive to develop.

Punctual
almost never   1   2   3   4   5   **almost always**

Instead of a descriptive choice, a frequency-rating scale provides a quantitative choice. The supervisor may rank the employee's behavior on any given criterion as among the bottom 10% of staff, next 20%, middle 40%, next 20%, or top 10% of staff, as follows:

Observation of working hours

10%	20%	40%	20%	10%
Bottom				Top

To maintain perspective, the supervisor may list staff names down the side of a paper and the behavior to be rated across the top. Rating one behavior at a time, she checks for variation in evaluations because one expects variation in performance. Forced distribution should be used cautiously. It is based on a normal bell-shaped curve with a few people ranked high, a few ranked low, and the majority ranked in the middle. However, this assumes that the group is representative of the total population, which is not true for a group of nurses.

Ranking. Ranking forces the supervisor to rank staff in descending order from highest to lowest even if she does not feel there is a difference. Ranking implicitly requires the supervisor to compare each nurse with others, but that comparison is not systematically built into the method. Paired comparison forces the supervisor to compare each nurse with each other nurse. If the supervisor is ranking four nurses, she must deal with six possible pairs or $N(N - 1)/2 = 4(3)/2 = 12/2 = 6$.

Nurses	Possible pairs	
Anita Anderson	AA with SJ	SJ with PP
Sue Jones	AA with PP	SJ with SS
Pam Peterson	AA with SS	PP with SS
Sara Smith		

Then each pair is presented to the supervisor who must determine which of the two she feels is better. Choices should be marked. For example:

(AA)	vs.	SJ	(SJ)	vs.	PP
(AA)	vs.	PP	(SJ)	vs.	SS
(AA)	vs.	SS	(PP)	vs.	SS

Tally marks can be placed in a matrix to help visualize the ranking.

	More qualified			
Less qualified	AA	SJ	PP	SS
AA				
SJ	1			
PP	1	1		
SS	1	1	1	
TOTAL TIMES PREFERRED	3	2	1	0

The major disadvantages of paired comparisons are that they do not lend themselves to large numbers of staff and take considerable time on the part of the supervisor.

Management by objectives. Management by objectives (MBO) is a tool for effective planning and appraisal. It emphasizes the achievement of objectives instead of personality characteristics. It focuses attention on individual achievement, motivates individuals to accomplishment, and measures performance in terms of results. MBO is a managerial method whereby the supervisor and staff nurse identify major areas in which the nurse will work, set standards for performance, and measure results against those standards. It determines the results that the nurse is to achieve in a given time frame.

To develop management by objectives, the nurse should first review the mission and group objectives. The nurse can determine the mission and objectives by analyzing what she does or what she thinks she should do. She describes her job and clarifies its purpose. This helps identify major job responsibilities.

Next she lists her major job responsibilities. Results expected rather than activities should be listed. This can be accomplished by asking oneself why the activity is being done or why it is important. For example:

What is the task? To help team members organize their work for the day.

Why? To improve utilization of their time.

Why? To be as productive as possible.

Why? To give good, cost-effective nursing care by completing the work identified on nursing care plans efficiently.

Major job responsibilities of a nurse manager are related to productivity, quality of care, morale, turnover, staff development, self-development, and affirmative action.

Once the major job responsibilities are identified, expected levels of accomplishment are determined. Criteria for expected levels of accomplishment should be results oriented, established before the fact, time bound, realistic and attainable, measurable and verifiable, written, and agreed on by both the superior and the subordinate. Common errors to avoid when developing objectives are writing too many objectives, too complex objectives, too high or too low standards, too long or too short a time period, imbalanced emphasis, objectives that are not measurable, or objectives for which the cost of measurement is too high.

After the subordinate has reviewed the mission and group objectives and determined her major job responsibilities and the expected levels of accomplishment, she should meet with her superior to establish priorities and to develop plans for the accomplishment of the objectives. The supervisor will determine whether the objectives are compatible with the overall goals of the organization. The supervisor and subordinate should hold periodic reviews to check the progress and make adjustments. An annual review should be held to compare the actual results with the expected levels of accomplishment and to set the objectives for the next time period.

The underlying philosophy is a belief that people perform best and develop most in an environment of participative management, high performance standards that build on individual strengths, prompt feedback that accentuates the positive, and appropriate rewards. Staff is encouraged to "do their thing" while maintaining individual accountability. The supervisor is a listener and clarifier who readjusts responsibilities based on individual differences.

Higher frequencies of appraisal are associated with a more favorable attitude toward MBO, higher goal success, improvement of superior-subordinate relationships, clarity of goals, an opinion that the supervisor was helpful and supportive, the attitude that the subordinate had influence in matters affecting her, and esteem and satisfaction for the superior. More praise and less criticism of the objectives by the supervisor are associated with higher goal success. It is advisable to use an incentive system that rewards effective planning as well as goal achievement when using MBO.

Advantages of MBO for the staff nurse are that the standard of evaluation is based on the characteristics of a specific person and job; the nurse has input and some control over her future; the nurse knows the standard by which she will be judged; the nurse has knowledge of the supervisor's goals, priorities, and deadlines; there is increased understanding on the part of the staff nurse as to where she stands with her supervisor in relation to relative progress; there is a better basis for evaluation than an evaluation based on personality traits; MBO emphasizes the future, which can be changed, instead of the past; and it stimulates higher individual performance and morale.

Advantages for the supervisor include a reservoir of personnel data and performance information for updating personnel files, an indication of personnel development needs within the agency, a basis for promotion and compensation, a relationship with the staff that makes her a coach rather than a judge, and better supervisory planning and utilization of the employee.

MBO directs work activities toward organizational goals, facilitates planning, provides standards for control, provides objective appraisal criteria, reduces role conflict and ambiguity, and utilizes and motivates human resources.

MBO is limited because it is not an easy system to implement and requires hard work for maintenance; the process must be taught and reinforced in order for the supervisor to become and remain proficient in utilizing the principles of the system; the MBO system assumes that the staff nurse and her supervisor will define suitable standards that will serve the agency; it presumes that the supervisor understands her limitations; the supervisor is responsible for assessing actual results rather than activities that seem to indicate results; some supervisors are unable to manage by objectives; some staff nurses may not want to get involved in setting goals; the supervisor and staff may give lip service to MBO while the supervisor really sets the goals; the staff nurse may set her goals according to what she knows the supervisor expects; MBO stresses results but does not supply the methods for achieving them; nurses can become frustrated if they believe that increasingly higher goals will be expected of them; overlapping objectives are difficult to evaluate; MBO lends itself to quantitative assessment but may neglect qualitative factors; and MBO does not provide comparative data for promotions and salary increases.

Peer review. Peer review is a process whereby a group of practicing registered nurses evaluate the quality of another registered nurse's professional performance. Peer review provides a feedback mechanism for sharing ideas, comparing the consistency of the nurse's performance with standards, recognizing outstanding performance, and identifying areas that need further development. This process can increase personal and professional growth and job satisfaction because of the recognition from peers.

Once it has been decided that an institution will use peer review, appraisal tools must be developed. A review of the evaluation tools currently used and the literature on evaluation tools is in order. Various standards may also be reviewed. The tool developed may address technical competence, human relationship skills, communication skills, organizational skills, leadership skills, and others. The process must also be determined, and then staff must be oriented to the system.

The staff should be oriented to the components of the peer review before it is implemented and thereafter during orientation. It is appropriate to give them copies of the peer review process and forms used for peer review. Opportunities to learn how to fill out the forms, how the peer review committee uses the materials, and what questions are to be expected during the peer review interview should be provided.

The peer evaluation process typically includes a review of an employee's self-evaluation form (including short- and long-term goals), reference letters, committee work, special projects, additional education, and contributions to nursing; a performance evaluation by the immediate supervisor; a review of the nurse's past performance; care plans and charting done by the nurse; assessment; observation of the nurse; interviews with her patients; a summary of the findings; a presentation of the findings; and recommendations to the nurse. It is appropriate to allow the candidate some agency time to prepare her review folder. A leader is assigned to the nurse to help clarify policy and procedures and to check the documents for completeness.

Who will evaluate whom must be determined. A committee may be appointed, elected, or randomly selected, but it should represent a number of job titles and a wide variety of specialty areas. The members should be familiar with committee responsibilities. The committee's recommendations should be made by consensus, with dissenting opinions recorded.

Once the candidate has been evaluated, there should be a peer review interview for feedback. All feedback must be well documented in the review materials. Hearsay reports are not permitted. The review committee chairperson or designee is responsible for arranging the interview and helping the candidate feel welcome and comfortable. The interview may provide recognition of outstanding performance, identification of areas that need further development, recommendations regarding learning needs, and possibly a recommendation for classification.

Peer review can be threatening and time consuming. There is a risk of rating candidates too high or too low. However, nurses will be held accountable and responsible for their nursing performance when they are measured against realistic and attainable standards.

Appraisal interview

There are several kinds of appraisal interviews. They include tell and sell, tell and listen, problem solving, and goal setting. When using the tell-and-sell technique, the superior does most of the talking while the subordinate listens. The superior reports the results of the evaluation to the employee and tries to persuade the subordinate to improve. This assumes that the superior is qualified to evaluate the subordinate and that the subordinate will want to correct her weaknesses if she knows them. In this role of judge, the interviewer risks losing the loyalty of the employee and inhibiting independent judgment. Face-saving problems are created. The employee usually suppresses defensive behavior and attempts to cover her hostility to protect herself. The tell-and-sell method uses positive and negative extrinsic motivation and is most likely to be successful when the employee respects the interviewer. It tends to perpetuate existing values and practices. The tell-and-sell method works best with young or new employees or someone who is new to an assignment. These employees may want advice and assurance from an authority figure. Under these conditions, the superior is most likely to be respected because of her position, knowledge, and experience. Unfortunately, the tell-and-sell method fosters either dependent and docile or rebellious behavior. After a tell-and-sell style evaluation, the employee often feels like looking for another job.

When using the tell-and-listen method, the superior speaks for about half the time and lets the subordinate speak for the remainder of the time. The interviewer outlines the strong and weak points of the subordinate's job performance and then listens to the interviewee's response. Although still in the role of judge, the interviewer listens to disagreement and allows defensive behavior without attempting to refute any responses. This tends to remove defensive behavior. The employee expresses defensiveness and feels accepted while the interviewer listens, reflects, and summarizes. Thus resistance to change is reduced, and the subordinate develops a more favorable attitude toward the superior. Although this method fosters upward communication and allows the interviewer to learn and change her views, the need for change may not be developed in the employee. Tell and listen works best when there is a good relationship between the interviewer and interviewee. The interviewer can learn about the subordinate's needs and aspirations, but the latter may not know where she stands. There are no plans for personnel development.

With the problem-solving method, the interviewer assumes the role of helper to stimulate growth and development in the interviewee. It assumes that change can occur without correcting faults and that discussing problems can lead to improvements because the discussion develops new ideas and mutual interests. The subordinate does most of the talking while the interviewer listens, reflects ideas and feelings, asks exploratory questions, and summarizes. Intrinsic motivation is stimulated through increased freedom, increased responsibility, and problem-solving behavior; thus, change is facilitated. Both the superior and subordinate learn from each other. The subordinate may view her job in relation to others more accurately, and the superior gains insights into the subordinate's working conditions. Unfortunately, the employee may lack ideas, and change may be other than what the interviewer had planned. Although this method is excellent for problem solving and personnel development, it does not warn the subordinate or let her know where she stands, evaluate her for lateral transfers or promotional purposes, provide a rating or furnish an evaluation record, or supply top administration with an inventory of talent.

Goal setting is future oriented. It focuses attention on the employee's achievement and consequently stimulates accomplishment. The philosophy behind MBO is teamwork. Top administration sets the organization's objectives, and employees set individual objectives. This method integrates institutional and personal achievement goals. It clarifies objectives and, because it focuses on results and not methods, encourages the person closest to a job to decide how to do it. MBO involves participative management. An autocratic leader is likely to tell a subordinate what her goals are. Although that is not consistent with a participative management philosophy, it is better for the subordinate to know what is expected of her than not to know.

Which appraisal interview style is used is largely dependent on the purpose of the evaluation, the superior's philosophy of management, and institutional guidelines. The manager can create an atmosphere during the interview that is consistent with the appraisal interview style. To create an authoritative image for the tell-and-sell method, the manager should have the interview in her office and sit behind a desk, preferably looking down on the subordinate (p. 298).

To create an atmosphere of equality for the tell-and-listen, problem-solving, or goal-setting style, the interviewer and employee may sit at a corner table looking at each other.

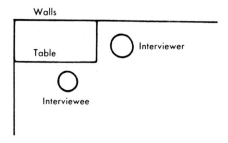

Sitting at a table helps create a working situation for problem solving and goal setting. Sitting either side by side or at the corner of the table helps create a sense of equality and a working relationship.

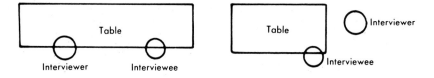

Nonverbal communication is important and should be consistent with verbal communication. Active listening can be expressed through eye contact, a responsive posture and facial expressions, and lets the interviewee know that the interviewer is trying to understand the employee's attitudes and feelings. Pauses give the employee time to think and respond. The interviewer may restate what the employee said. Although this helps the interviewee know the interviewer is listening, it does not guarantee that the meaning of the message was understood. Paraphrasing states the message in fewer and simpler words. If the interviewee says, "I don't understand! One minute she tells me to do it this way and the next minute she tells me to do it that way," the interviewer may paraphrase, "She confuses you." One should ask for clarification if the intent is not clear or say, for example, "Do you mean . . . ?" Reflection of feelings such as, "You sound proud of that" helps show understanding. Summarizing what has been said at the end of the interview is particularly important.

The supervisor's assessment of the staff nurse's performance should be continuous rather than once a year. This maximizes feedback for learning. The supervisor and staff nurse should have an appointment to do the appraisal interview when both are unhurried and should meet where they have privacy. Adequate time should be allowed and interruptions avoided. The purpose of the interview should be clear. Both should enter the interview ready to compare notes, knowing that the counseling notes will not become part of the personnel file. Emphasis should be on the growth of the nurse and on accomplishments related to specific targets. Actual, observed behavior rather than broad personality traits should be discussed during the exchange of ideas between the supervisor and the staff nurse. The staff nurse should be encouraged to take the initiative in setting goals for improving performance, with the supervisor supporting, guiding, and validating her plans.

If the supervisor finds it necessary to make unfavorable comments, she should insert them between favorable comments. It is important that the supervisor not create an atmosphere in which she appears to be sitting in judgment. When the supervisor enumerates improvement needs, the staff nurse's self-esteem is threatened and defensive behavior tends to result. The greater the threat to the self-image, the poorer the attitude toward evaluations will be, and less improvement in job performance results. If the staff nurse becomes defensive or aggressive, the supervisor should accept comments without a fight. Keeping quiet and not exposing alibis can help the staff nurse save face.

Before the interview is terminated, ways in which the supervisor can help the staff nurse accomplish goals should be explored. The staff nurse will probably approach her work with more enthusiasm and confidence if she feels she has the respect and support of her supervisor.

Appraisal reports

The appraisal report is to be written jointly by the supervisor and staff nurse. It should be reliable, valid, and accurate, showing progress made by the nurse and giving illustrations to substantiate value judgments. If both have kept notes that they have periodically assessed, and if the staff nurse believes the supervisor's intent is to help rather than to blame, the nurse will feel more free to be honest in an evaluation of her strengths and weaknesses. If the staff nurse has not been functioning satisfactorily, she will already be aware of it. If her performance has not improved adequately since previous interviews, the nurse should be informed that the weakness will be included in the report. Any improvements are to be noted, and the staff nurse should know exactly where she stands. It may be necessary to tell her she has to make certain improvements within a definite time period or she will be fired.

Permanent, cumulative evaluation records can be used to assess how the nurse can best be used in the agency. They can be used as a basis for pay increases and promotions or terminations. These records are frequently used as a source of information for letters of reference to be sent to other agencies.

PROBLEM EMPLOYEES

Substance abusers, angry or withdrawn workers, personnel with excessive absenteeism, and the terminating employee provide challenges to nurse managers. In each case, the manager must be alert to symptoms, help the employee solve the problem, and evaluate the results.

Substance abusers

Substance abuse is not uncommon among nurses. It affects all socioeconomic classes, cultures, and races. Only 5% or less of all alcoholics are skid-row bums. Among alcoholic nurses studied, most had been in the top third of their class, held advanced degrees, held responsible and demanding jobs, and had an excellent work history.

Nurses with alcohol or other drug addictions often exhibit psychosocial problems. Personality changes may be noted as the nurse becomes more irritable, withdrawn, and moody. Because of a decreased interest in outside activities, isolation increases. Related social changes include eating alone and avoiding social gatherings.

Changes in personal appearance become apparent. Changes in dress, an unkempt appearance, flushed complexion, red eyes, swollen face, and hand tremors are common. Mental status changes include forgetfulness, confusion, and decreased alertness.

General behavior changes too. Inappropriate responses and irritability occur more frequently. Excuses for behavior become more elaborate. Intolerance and suspicion of others and nervousness increase. Avoidance of others is noted. Work efficiency drops, there is a decline in the quality and quantity of work, and the work pace becomes uneven. Some assigned tasks are forgotten. Arriving late and leaving early and extended lunch hours and break times become patterns of behavior. Accidents increase.

When a nurse reports to work in a state of acute intoxication, the manager notes the signs objectively and gets a second person to validate the observations.

The odor of alcohol, slurred speech, unsteady gait, and errors in judgment are symptoms of intoxication. The intoxicated nurse is removed from the situation, confronted briefly and firmly about the behavior, and sent home to rest and recuperate. Then the incident is recorded. The manager describes the observation, states the action taken, indicates future plans, and has the employee sign and date the memo when she returns to work. Refusal to sign and date the memo should be noted by the manager and a witness.

Chronic performance problems are more common than acute intoxication. Each time performance problems are observed, they should be documented including date, time, who was observed by whom, and a description of the incident and circumstances. At a prearranged conference, the nurse is confronted with the observations and how they affect job performance and patient care. The nurse is allowed to give her explanation. Alternatives are explored, and a course of action is planned.

When substance abuse is identified as the problem, the offender is encouraged to take voluntary action. Self-help groups such as Alcoholics Anonymous or Narcotics Anonymous may be suggested. The manager refers the nurse to a local treatment facility and meets with the nurse periodically to monitor progress. The manager is not to serve the role of therapist.

When alcoholics or drug abusers refuse counseling or fail to follow the plan of care, they are told treatment is mandatory for continued employment. If the employee still refuses mandatory participation in the treatment, she is terminated in accordance with the hospital's policies.

Angry or withdrawn employees

Nurse managers often deal with angry or withdrawn employees. Anger and withdrawal are the fight and flight responses to anxiety. The angry nurse is more likely to be considered a troublemaker. The withdrawn person may be viewed as nice. However, both need help.

Anxiety occurs from the frustration of unmet expectations or loss of self-respect. The anxiety is transformed into feelings and/or actions and relief is felt. Angry, hostile, and destructive behavior is a primary response to frustration. It is intended to gain mastery over the situation. The angry employee may become hostile and use critical, sarcastic, and obscene language with others. Consequently, interpersonal relationships suffer, and productive work may be impaired. Anger can also be displaced to patients and others.

The withdrawn person does not invest emotional energy in others. Fear of self-disclosure or having others become attached to her is frightening. Withdrawal is a protective mechanism to avoid hurt. The withdrawn person sits through meetings without becoming involved. She is not assertive to protect her rights. She may be delegated more than her fair share of the work because she is so cooperative and polite. This leads to more feelings of use, abuse, and helplessness.

Nurse managers need to recognize aggressive and passive behaviors among employees, teach and display assertive behavior, and encourage problem solving. They should help personnel understand themselves and their job responsibilities, develop trust, and promote group harmony. Employees should be encouraged to express themselves without fear of reprisals. Managers should be sincere, firm, and fair. Job expectations need to be clear and personnel rewarded liberally and disciplined justly.

Decreased productivity

Decreased productivity is a side effect of personnel problems. Managers should make sure that desired performance is not being punished or undesirable behavior rewarded. Expectations are clarified. Employees are taught how to do what they are expected to do. If boredom is a problem, job rotation and special projects are considered.

Absenteeism

Absenteeism is also a side effect of personnel problems. Ineffective supervision, poor working relationships, boredom, lack of control over decisions affecting one's life, and overwork are contributing factors. Some workers are immature and lack the self-discipline to get themselves to work. Others stay away to avoid an unpleasant or boring job. Some are poorly motivated, do as little as possible to keep from getting fired, and do not see their job as a means toward an end. The hypochondriac uses absenteeism to get attention and sympathy from others. Abusive absenteeism may be used to get even with a supervisor. Some personnel are exhausted from overwork, have lost their enthusiasm for the job, or are burned out.

Managers should make sure that there are attendance policies, that the policies do not reward nonattendance, and that they are enforced consistently. Attendance records should be maintained, and grievance procedures should be in place.

Documented attendance policies greatly influence absence rates. Traditional sick leave policies have rewarded employees for absenteeism and have encouraged them to be dishonest to collect sick pay or be punished by losing it. Employees who receive sick pay are absent considerably more than those who do not. Some agencies have required a physician's excuse before an employee can receive sick pay to decrease the dishonest use of sick time. Because most people are only sick 1 or 2 days at a time, some hospitals do not compensate for the first 2 days of any sickness. The third and successive days are compensated.

Other agencies have gone to paid time off. Each employee receives a certain amount of paid time off inclusive of holiday, vacation, and sick leave with few restrictions as to its use. It is typically collected at a rate calculated by length of continuous service. It simplifies record keeping but provides incentive to use the days whether sick or not.

Absenteeism data need to be collected and analyzed to determine trends and patterns of individuals and personnel in general. Recording the date of absence, the reason and whether excused or unexcused, day of the week, preceding or following a day off, the employee's job classification, shift, tenure, age, sex, marital status, or any other information thought to be useful provides information to detect trends and pinpoint problems. Absenteeism often occurs more frequently in certain job classifications or departments, on specific days or shifts, or among a group working under a specific supervisor. Problems need to be identified so managers can develop control measures. Baseline data are also useful to determine the success of the control program.

A progressive discipline policy that imposes increasingly severe penalties is appropriate. Such a policy allows employees to know in advance the consequences of their behavior. Progressive discipline often starts with an oral reprimand that is documented and progresses through a written warning, pay deduction, suspension without pay, and dismissal.

Terminating employees

Working with a terminating employee (whether voluntary or involuntary) is also challenging for the nurse manager. The manager must help the employee deal with the related feelings. A sense of loss and grief are common. A period of shock or denial that is then followed by disorganization, anger, guilt, and loneliness is normal. This is followed by a deorientation period and a reestablishment phase.

The manager can help the terminating employee by providing an opportunity to talk about her feelings. Airing feelings about leaving, her self-image, not working anymore or filling another position, and other interests that may be pursued helps relieve the anxiety. Helping the employee plan for the future is also useful.

It is not uncommon for terminating employees to detach themselves from the job and do little for some time before the termination. The manager can assign tasks that are considered important that can either be finished or transferred to someone else at the time of the employee's termination.

Rituals such as best wishes cards and going away parties serve to acknowledge the termination and provide a rite of separation that facilitates the termination process.

Employee counseling

Counseling helps improve employees' mental health, thus enhancing understanding, self-control, self-confidence, and consequently their ability to work effectively. Counseling accomplishes several activities on a directive to nondirective scale. It provides an opportunity to give advice, offer reassurance, improve communication, release emotional tension, clarify thinking, and reorient.

When giving advice, a counselor tells the employee what the counselor thinks she should do. Unfortunately, it is almost impossible to understand another person's complicated problems, and consequently the advice may not be sound. Advice may foster feelings of inferiority and dependence on the counselor.

Reassurance provides courage to face a problem and confidence that one is handling the situation appropriately. False reassurance is dangerous. It may prevent the employee from getting the professional help needed. It offers little comfort when the counselee knows that the counselor cannot predict the outcome. Even if there is some comfort obtained, it tends to dissipate when the person faces the problem again.

Counseling improves both upward and downward communication. It allows employees to express their feelings to management. Although individual names must be kept confidential, feelings can be grouped into categories and interpreted to higher management. The counseling session allows the counselor to explain company policies and activities to the employee, thus achieving downward communication.

Catharsis or the release of emotional tension often occurs when people have the opportunity to talk about their frustrations. They become more relaxed, and their speech becomes more coherent and rational as they explain their problems to a sympathetic listener. Then, as emotional blocks to clear thinking are eliminated, thinking becomes more rational. People may realize that their emotions are not appropriate for the situation. This may help people recognize and accept their limitations and bring about a reorientation or change in values and goals. The manager should refer an employee to professional help when reorientation is needed.

Directive counseling occurs when the counselor listens to the employee's problems, decides how to solve the problems, and tells the employee what to do. The counselor predominately gives advice. This type of counseling does give some emotional release, can be reassuring, and fosters communication. Thinking may be clarified in a limited way. Reorientation seldom occurs.

Nondirective counseling is client centered. The counselor listens and encourages the employee to explain her problems, identify alternatives, explore the ramifications of each option, and determine the most appropriate solution. Emotional release occurs more frequently in nondirective than in directive counseling. Clear thinking and reorientation are fostered. Reassurance may be used, but advice should be limited. This approach can be very beneficial, but managers must be cautious not to neglect their normal directive leadership responsibilities.

Nondirective counseling is more time consuming and costly than directive counseling. To be effective, the employee must have the intelligence to identify problems and assess solutions and the emotional stability to deal with them. The nondirective counselor must be cautious not to allow the emotionally dependent employee to avoid her work responsibilities.

Cooperative counseling is a compromise between directive and nondirective counseling. It is the cooperative effort by the counselor and employee through an exchange of ideas to help solve the problem. The cooperative counselor starts by listening, as would a nondirective counselor. As the interview progresses, however, the cooperative counselor offers information and insight and is likely to discuss the problems with a broad knowledge of the organization's point of view. This may help change the employee's perspective. Cooperative counseling combines the advantages of both directive and nondirective counseling and avoids most of the disadvantages.

The manager usually provides cooperative counseling when employees have job-related emotional problems. Because of employees' rights to privacy, it is appropriate for the manager to refer an employee to professional help when personal problems are interfering with job performance or when a person needs reorientation.*

OUTPLACEMENT COUNSELING

Although not many registered nurses are fired, during economic recessions there is an increasing incidence in reduction in work forces. Outplacement counseling can be used to minimize the emotional and professional scarring that results from being dismissed from one's position.

Poor job performance, tardiness, absenteeism, substance abuse, inappropriate behavior, and staff reduction are the most common reasons for discharging nurses. A termination of this nature is usually a progressive process. However, for some offenses, nurses can be terminated immediately. These are likely to include abuse of patients and visitors, insubordination, intoxication, possession of drugs, theft, gambling, disorderly conduct, willful destruction of property, sleeping on duty, or falsification of records.

The termination procedures used must be consistent with the agency policies. Termination usually involves several steps, beginning with an oral warning. If

---

*Employee counseling is discussed in more detail in Davis, K.: Human behavior at work: organizational behavior, New York, 1981, McGraw-Hill Book Co., pp. 447-459.

the employee does not change her behavior in response to the oral warning, written warnings with corrective interviews are used. There need to be well-documented, sufficient grounds for termination. The nurse manager can use anecdotal notes to record both strong and weak attributes of the worker. They should contain factual information about who was observed by whom, where, and the background of the incident. There should be a sufficient number of observations to establish a pattern of behavior.

Written warnings used with corrective interviews should state the expected level of performance and the consequence if that standard is not met. Suspension is typically used before termination. The counseling note should be signed by both the nurse manager and the worker. If the worker refuses to sign, a witness can validate that the worker has read the counseling notes and refuses to sign them.

Poor job performance should be analyzed. Has the person ever been taught how to do what is expected of her? If not, she should be taught. Does she practice the skill often enough to keep her talents refined? If not, practice sessions could be made available. Specific, descriptive feedback should be given. Demonstrations and return demonstrations are appropriate. The feedback should be as close to the act as possible. Positive reinforcement for what was done well is as important as identifying weaknesses and making plans to overcome them. Follow-up by noting changes is also important.

A problem-solving approach can be used for tardiness and absenteeism. Why does the person think she is late or absent so often? If a person has difficulty getting children to a babysitter and to work by 7 AM, could her hours be changed to 8:00 AM to 4:30 PM so she can fulfill her maternal responsibilities and also help provide a smooth transition at the change of shift? If the person is a night owl who has difficulty getting up in the morning, could she be assigned the evening shift? Is the person working two jobs to make ends meet? Are financial assistance and counseling available? Are family problems interfering with attendance? Is the person hung over when she should be reporting to duty? The social services that are available for patients should also be used for staff, for example self-help groups such as Alcoholics Anonymous, Single Parents, and Shelters for Women. Social services, the chaplain, or family counseling are also useful.

Repeated failure to meet performance standards, lack of compliance with company policies, and staff reductions are just causes for termination. Each should be a progressive process. The employee should know what level of performance is expected to avoid termination and the risk of termination.

Support services are needed by people who are terminated. The agency should have termination policies regarding severance pay, terminal vacation, accrued holidays and sick time, and insurance. The person may need information about unemployment. This is an opportune time for a counselor in personnel to help the terminating employee to reassess her location and vocation. Where does the person want to live? What climate does she like? What type of work interests her and provides the most satisfaction? What do her educational background and skills prepare the person to do? What can she do to better prepare herself to reach her goals? How important are salary, fringe benefits, retirement plans, work hours, and opportunities for advancement?

Once the person decides what she wants to do and where, she may need assistance to locate job openings. Professional journals, employment agencies, and college placement services are sources of information. Recruiters are often present at professional meetings. Friends, relatives, and acquaintances may help locate positions, and employers can be contacted directly.

A terminating employee is likely to need help preparing résumés, writing marketing letters, and interviewing. She does not need to state the reason that she left the last job on this marketing letter, résumé, or job a application. However, she should be prepared to address the issue during an interview. She should be honest about the reason for termination, speak about the treatment she has had, if any, and focus on the knowledge and skills she has learned on the last job that she can transfer to the new one. She should not be critical of the last employer.

The sooner one accepts the fact that she has been fired, the sooner she can put the pieces back together and move on. The boss should be very clear about the reason. The termination should not come as a surprise. With the progressive process, the employee should know the consequences of not meeting the performance standards. Any reduction in work force should be done with fair warning and target dates. The employee should be informed of the grievance policy and procedure when reflecting if she has been fairly treated. The outplacement counseling can help the person know what questions to ask about pay and benefits, how to tell the family, how to solicit help from friends and acquaintances, and how to budget to protect securities until another job can be obtained. Career counseling and job placement counseling are useful.

Being fired initiates stress and can be quite devastating. Outplacement counseling can help reduce the related personal and professional scarring that inevitably results from being dismissed.

DISCIPLINE OF PERSONNEL

Need for discipline

Lack of knowledge about policies and procedures is a major cause of the need for disciplinary action. Management should provide orientation beginning on the first day of employment. A nurse cannot be expected to follow rules that are unknown to her, vague, or loosely enforced. Consequently, each new employee should be given an employee's handbook. The handbook itemizes the rules and procedures of the agency and specifies the type of discipline that will be imposed for infractions. New employees should be encouraged to read the handbook and ask questions about it.

During orientation, the supervisor should explain in detail the most frequently violated rules and discuss the significance of the rules and the rationale for them. It is recommended that the supervisor conduct regularly scheduled meetings with staff to discuss changes or to review policies. Rules and regulations also may be posted in a consistent and conspicuous manner.

Most employees are not disciplinary problems, but a minority does exist that requires more than positive stimuli. These few cases are potentially explosive. About half of the grievance cases appealed to an arbitrator by labor unions involve disciplinary action. In about half of those cases, management either reversed or modified its decision when the individual's appeal was upheld. Consequently, it is of utmost importance that disciplinary action be undertaken in a judicious manner. The disciplinary action program and grievance procedure must be uniform for all personnel of a specific grade or classification. A standard disciplinary action program with procedures outlined and forms provided should be available to managers.

Principles of disciplinary action

Positive attitude. The manager's attitude is very important in preventing or correcting undesirable behavior. If the staff nurse is treated as suspect, she is more likely to provide the trouble that the supervisor anticipates. People tend to do what is expected of them; therefore, it is the supervisor's duty to maintain a positive attitude by expecting the best from her staff.

Investigate carefully. The ramifications of disciplinary action are so serious that the manager must proceed with caution. She should collect the facts, check allegations, talk to witnesses, and ask the accused for her side of the story. She should accept the staff nurse's account until and unless the allegations are proven. The supervisor may wish to consult other supervisors or her superiors. If the situation is serious enough to require action before a full investigation can be conducted, it is better to suspend the staff nurse subject to reinstatement after investigation than to take more drastic action.

Be prompt. One should not be so expeditious that she neglects to be thorough in ascertaining the facts. If a staff nurse is disciplined unfairly or unnecessarily, the effects on the entire staff may be severe. However, if the discipline is delayed, the relationship between the punishment and the offense may become less clear.

Because of the distastefulness of disciplinary action, the supervisor may tend to postpone the punishment as long as possible. The longer the delay, the more the staff nurse forgets her actions, the more likely she is to feel that the discipline is not deserved, and the fewer are the positive educational effects for the future.

Protect privacy. Disciplinary action affects the ego of the staff nurse. Thus it is better to discuss the situation in private. By helping the nurse save face, there is less possibility of future resentment and a greater chance for future cooperation. However, a public reprimand may be necessary for the nurse who does not take private criticism seriously.

Focus on the act. When disciplining a staff nurse, the supervisor should emphasize that it was the act that was unacceptable, not the employee. If the employee is not acceptable, she should be fired.

Enforce rules consistently. Offending employees should be treated equally or consistently for similar transgressions. Equal treatment is based on rules with specific penalties for various acts and the number of offenses. Consistency reduces the possibility of favoritism, promotes predictability, and fosters acceptance of penalities.

Be flexible. Consistent implementation is complicated by the fact that individuals and circumstances are never the same. A penalty should be determined only after the entire record of the employee is reviewed. The supervisor should consider length of service, past accomplishments or problems, level of skill, and expendability to the organization. The intent of the staff nurse, the extenuating circumstances, and whether this situation constitutes a test case and will set precedent for the future should also be taken into consideration. If the supervisor enforces identical penalties for seemingly similar offenses, she may be excessively severe with one person and lenient with the other.

Advise the employee. The employee must be informed that her conduct is not acceptable. Personnel files containing anecdotal notes can be a useful supervisory tool, but they are of little value in upholding disciplinary action if the staff nurse is not informed of the contents promptly.

Take corrective, constructive action. The supervisor should be sure that the staff nurse understands that her behavior was contrary to the organization's requirements and should explain why such regulations are necessary. The staff nurse should be counseled as to what behavior is required and how she can avoid future disciplinary action.

Follow up. The supervisor should quietly investigate to determine if the staff nurse's behavior has changed. If the staff nurse continues to invite disciplinary action, the supervisor should re-evaluate the situation to try to determine the reason for the nurse's attitude. The supervisor must try to come to terms with the offender and the reasons for the transgression.

Penalties

Oral reprimand. For minor violations that have occurred for the first time, the manager may opt to give an oral warning in private. She might tactfully correct the deviation by telling the staff nurse the proper way to deal with the situation or by rebuking the nurse. An oral reprimand is of limited value beyond alerting the nurse in a relatively friendly way to a need for correction. Because nothing is in writing and the reprimand is done in private, it is difficult to prove that a warning was given. Over time the supervisor may become unsure and inexact about what was said to whom and under what conditions. When an oral warning is given, the supervisor is advised to make an anecdotal note of the time, place, occasion, and the gist of the reprimand. Oral comments may be easily forgotten, but too formal handling of initial minor offenses can be counterproductive.

Written reprimand. If the offense is more serious or repeated, the reprimand may be written. It is suggested that the superior and subordinate develop a written plan for improvement that defines what the subordinate will do to make her performance acceptable and what the superior will do to change the environmental situation if appropriate. A time limit should be set. Additional penalties may be defined in case the subordinate's behavior does not adequately improve during the allowed time period. The written notice should include the name of the worker, the name of the supervisor, the nature of the problem, the plan for correction, and the consequences of future repetition. It is recommended that the worker sign the report to indicate that she has read it, received a copy of it, or both. A copy should be given to the employee and one retained for the personnel file. If personnel believe that signing such a document would be considered an admission of guilt and hence refuse to sign, the supervisor may ask another managerial person to sign as witness to the fact that the document was discussed with the worker and that a copy was given to her. It is appropriate for higher management and the personnel department to review this report. At the end of the designated time, the supervisor and worker should have another conference to determine if the terms of the agreement have been met. It is hoped that the nurse can be complimented for her progress and no further action deemed necessary. However, if no change or inadequate change has occurred, the continuing nature of the problem should be identified and documented. Additional penalties will probably be necessary.

Other penalties. Fines may be charged for offenses such as tardiness. Loss of privileges might include transfer to a less desirable shift, loss of preference of assignment, placement at bottom of seniority list, or reduced holiday and vacation time.

Layoff, demotion, and discharge are the most serious penalties and need approval beyond the supervisor. Layoff may be appropriate in situations where it is best to remove the nurse while an investigation is conducted. The staff nurse may be reinstated with no loss of pay if cleared through the investigation or may be suspended if found guilty of a serious offense. Demotion is a questionable solution. It creates hard feelings, which may be contagious, and more than likely places the offender in a position for which she is overqualified. Termination becomes necessary as a last resort.

Components of a disciplinary action program

Codes of conduct. Employees must be informed of the nature and meaning of codes of conduct. Agency handbooks, policy manuals, and orientation programs may be used. The staff nurse must understand that the rules are reasonable and directly related to efficient, effective operation of the agency.

Authorized penalties. During disciplinary action, the personnel record should indicate that a fair investigation was made of charges before the assessment of guilt and determination of penalties. The agency's disciplinary action program should indicate that the current action is being administered without bias and is directly related to the offense.

Records of offenses and corrective measures. Records are of utmost importance when disciplinary action is appealed. The personnel record should clearly indicate the offense, management's efforts to correct the problem, and resulting penalties.

Right of appeal. Formal provision for the right of employee appeal is a part of each disciplinary action program. Appeal beyond the supervisor ensures equitable treatment and encourages more employee acceptance of the disciplinary process. At the same time, the fair supervisor need not fear a review of her actions by others.

MODIFICATION OF EMPLOYEE BEHAVIOR

Can an employee's behavior be changed by changing her manager's behavior? Is behavior that recurs in the presence of the manager being reinforced by her? Is it possible that doing nothing is doing something? In all three instances the answer is yes. Behavior leads to consequences, and the consequences that follow the behavior affect the probability of recurrence of that behavior. Because behavior is a function of the consequence, it is important for nurse managers to identify the contingency relationship.

Consequences may be favorable, punitive, absent, or insufficient. Positive consequences increase the probability of recurrence of the behavior that preceded them. Absence of consequences decreases the probability, and insufficient consequences have little effect. Punishing consequences have varied and unpredictable effects. Punishment is not the opposite of a favorable consequence. No consequence is.

Reinforcement

Positive reinforcement increases the probability of a recurrence of desired behavior. It is more effective the sooner it follows the desired behavior, and it should be clearly connected to the behavior that the manager wishes to increase. Positive reinforcement may be as subtle as a smile or a nod of the head when someone speaks. Whatever is being said when the manager smiles or nods is reinforced and will recur with increasing frequency. Recognition is a powerful reinforcer. "Mr. Jones must feel so much better now since you have completed his morning care" and "You collected a lot of valuable information during your interview with Mrs. Smith" are examples. "I'm glad to see you here today" reinforces attendance, while "I see you were absent again yesterday" gives attention to the absence.

The nurse manager can even stimulate new behavior by using verbal acknowledgment of the desired response. Words are used to describe the behavior the nurse manager wants to encourage. A comment such as "I really appreciate nurses attending in-services" is likely to increase attendance at in-services. A number of stimuli—such as feedback, attention, praise, avoidance of punishment, merit pay increases, special assignments, assistance with tuition, or tickets to a ball game or play—can be used to reinforce behavior. However, the nurse manager must consider that any stimulus can be reinforcing or aversive depending on the person and the situation, and so she should carefully select stimuli that are reinforcers for the individual in a given situation. For example, tickets to a ball game may be reinforcing to some and aversive to others. Recognition is one of the easiest, cheapest, and most universally effective reinforcers.

Shaping

Shaping is a behavior-modification technique used when the response does not meet the criteria. By systematically reinforcing successive approximations, the nurse manager can shape the responses into the desired behavior and get the nurse to do something new to her. The supervisor provides favorable consequences after any attempt at the desired behavior, then withholds consequences until improvement is made. When working with the staff nurse who is chronically absent or late, the supervisor may acknowledge that the nurse is at work: "I see you were only 30 minutes late today." Later, "I see you were only 15 minutes late today." Still later, "I noticed you were only 5 minutes late today." The supervisor may initially praise a new employee for attempting a new task and then note improvements in skill as they occur. Once the level of desired performance has been reached, it can be maintained by providing favorable consequences intermittently. Too many positive consequences cause satiation, and they lose their effect on the behavior. Performance that has been intermittently reinforced is most resistant to extinction.

Extinction

Withholding reinforcers will decrease the probability of the occurrence of the behavior and contribute to its extinction. Therefore, if the supervisor does not mention or otherwise reward undesirable behavior, the lack of action should contribute to extinction. Conversely, any reinforcer that is presented frequently, but not paired with another reinforcer, will lose its effectiveness. Promises of "raises" or "hiring more help and getting some relief" become meaningless if not paired with a pay increase or recruitment and selection of personnel. The supervisor who praises everyone for everything all of the time will find that her words lose their effectiveness as reinforcers. When the consequences are not worth the effort, the behavior will decrease also.

Punishment

The supervisor can decrease the probability of a response by pairing the behavior with an aversive stimulus. People who are late to work will not be paid for the time they are absent. There will be no overtime pay for people who did not complete their work on time. Employees who do not meet work standards will be fired. Firing a few workers who were not meeting standards can have an immediate impact on the remaining personnel who initially work harder to avoid being fired. However, if management does nothing to reinforce the more productive work behavior, avoidance behavior is likely to occur. Employees may cover up for each other, steal from the agency what they rationalize is theirs, or resign. By using aversive stimuli to control behavior, management pairs itself with those stimuli and becomes viewed as aversive.

Once the superior has started an aversive stimulus, she should not stop it until the behavior has been corrected or the cessation may act as a positive reinforcer. Absences, tardiness, excuse making, rationalizing, placing blame elsewhere, and other avoidance behaviors will increase if they successfully reduce the aversive stimuli. If the supervisor gruffly asks a nurse why some work has not been done (aversive stimulus), the staff nurse replies she thought someone else was doing it, and the supervisor backs off; blaming others is reinforced. Although punishment causes behavior to occur less frequently, it does not teach new behaviors and is likely to increase avoidance behaviors. Most motivation problems are caused by punishment, absence of consequences, or insufficient consequences.

313

Behavior modification for the employee with a performance problem

Besides being aware of the subtle ways that her behavior may reinforce, shape, or reduce behavior of others, the nurse manager may apply behavior modification to personnel with performance problems. First she must identify the performance problem and analyze the antecedent, behavior, and consequence. What happened before the behavior occurred? Each time nurse *A* was late to work, she had worked the evening shift the night before. Each time nurse *B* yelled at her staff, an emergency treatment was being performed. Head nurse *C* was condescending to her staff after a physician had scolded her. What happened after the behavior occurred? Someone had already done part of nurse *A*'s work by the time she got to the ward. Staff nurses responded quickly when nurse *B* yelled at them during an emergency procedure. Nurse *C*'s staff avoided her.

Once the performance problem has been identified, the baseline frequency is determined. The baseline measure is the frequency before any attempts to change it. If the nurse is interested in modifying her own behavior, she may collect the baseline data herself. The behavior must be precisely defined, observable, and consequently countable. Written records should be kept, preferably on a portable recording system that is present when the behavior occurs, so the nurse can record it immediately. A tailor-made tally sheet is useful because one can see data in relation to time (Fig. 5-1). If the behavior occurs daily, it should be recorded for 1 week. If there are large variations in the behavior from one day to the next, observations should be recorded for 2 weeks. A time-sampling technique can be used by a busy manager by randomly selecting short time periods to observe and tally behaviors. This is only effective for high-frequency behavior. She must consider if the period of data collection was rep-

Fig. 5-1. Tally sheet.

	M	T	W	Th	F	Sat	Sun
7:00	|||	||	||	|||	||		
8:00							
9:00	||						
10:00							
11:00							
12:00							
1:00							
2:00	||		||	||			
3:00	|||	||	|||	||	|||		

Fig. 5-2. Frequency graph.

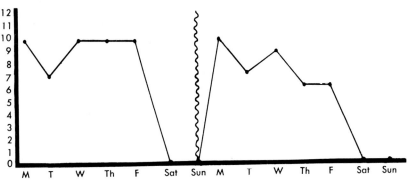

resentative of the normal situation and use a stable baseline rate as a clue to start the intervention.

If one transfers the information from the tally sheet to a graph that depicts frequency over time, it is easy to visualize the effect of the intervention strategy (Fig. 5-2). One can put a wavy vertical line on the graph to depict the point where intervention was started.

After identifying the relevant variables, the supervisor and nurse select appropriate reinforcement, extinction, punishment, or any combination of intervention strategies to decrease the frequency of the undesirable behavior. If the desired performance is punished, the punishment should be removed. Instead of making a fast worker finish everyone else's work, she can be allowed time to do what she chooses, such as read in the library or meditate in the chapel, receive a bonus day at a specified frequency, or be given a merit pay increase specifically for doing more than her share of the work. If undesirable behavior is rewarded, the reward should be removed. Instead of having the slow employee's work completed by others, the supervisor should inform the worker that she is responsible for so much work by herself, must have that work completed before going home, and will receive no overtime pay for completion of the normal work load.

If desired behavior has not been rewarded, the manager should arrange a consequence. This may be as simple as orally acknowledging a nurse's accomplishment occasionally. Nurses' accomplishments can be acknowledged in the agency's newsletter. Awards can be created to recognize desirable behavior.

If obstacles are identified, they should be removed. Nurses can be referred to professional counseling to help them work through situational crises that are interfering with their work performance. The manager can try to get the resources the nurse needs to do her job. The nurse should also have the necessary education to do what is expected of her. She may need formal education, on-the-job training, practice sessions, or simply feedback. The subordinate is the best source of information for what can serve as a positive reinforcer to her, for what may be desirable for the supervisor may be aversive to the subordinate.

Once the intervention strategy has been planned, it should be implemented and the response frequency recorded. The strategy should be evaluated for effectiveness. If it is not working, it should be analyzed and revised. Once the desired behavior is obtained, it should be maintained through intermittent reinforcement.

LABOR RELATIONS
Why employees join unions

Employees essentially join a union to increase their power to get certain responses from management. Management's actions or inactions have probably caused the employees to reach their limit of tolerance. Poor working conditions and job inequities in increments, promotion, and benefits cause distress. Poor quality of immediate supervision, arbitrary treatment from management, and poor communications between employer and employee are major reasons for unionization. Instead of quitting their jobs and giving up their seniority, security, and friends to move to another job, they form a union.

Labor law

In 1935 the National Labor Relations Act (NLRA), or the Wagner Act, was passed in an effort to end the depression. It prevented some employers from cutting wages in the hopes that higher worker incomes and increased spending would lessen the severity of the economic depression. Unfortunately, some employers went bankrupt because they could not reduce wages. Employers could not legally fire employees who sought unionization. The NLRA created the National Labor Relations Board to investigate and initiate administrative proceedings against employers who violated a law that listed employer violations only.

Because the NLRA was biased toward unions, it was amended in 1947 by the Taft-Hartley or Labor Management Relations Act. It listed union restrictions to restore equality between employers and employees. Nonprofit health care institutions, however, were exempted from the law. The unions developed public relations problems when some of them went on strike during the war and when unions were blamed for the postwar inflation.

In 1959 the laws were further modified by the Landrum-Griffin or Labor-Management Reporting and Disclosure Act to safeguard against corrupt financial and election procedures used by some unions. The Union Members' Bill of Rights resulted.

In 1974, Public Law 93-360, the Nonprofit Health Care Amendments to the Taft-Hartley Act, extended federal collective bargaining rights to private sector employees. It created notification procedures that must precede a strike and assured employees of the right to join, or refrain from joining, a union.

Unfair labor practices by management. The NLRA's section 8(a) prohibitions on management are known as the unfair labor practices. They include interference, 8(a)(1); domination, 8(a)(2); discrimination, 8(a)(3); discrimination, 8(a)(4); and refusal to bargain, 8(a)(5). Restraining or coercing or otherwise interfering with employees during the exercise of their right to organize is an unfair labor practice. Management may not contribute financial or other support or otherwise dominate or interfere during the development or administration of a labor organization. The employer may not discriminate in hiring or tenure or other terms of employment to encourage or discourage membership in a labor organization. Nor can the employer discriminate against an employee for filing charges or giving testimony. The employer is also forbidden to refuse to bargain with representatives of the employees.

Unfair labor practices by unions. Before 1935, management's power had few limitations. From 1935 to 1947 managers had to contend with unfair labor practice limitations, but no such unfair labor practices were defined for labor organizations. In 1947, the Labor Management Relations Act amended the NLRA and added restrictions for labor organizations. These include interference, 8(b)(1); induced discrimination, 8(b)(2); refusal to bargain, 8(b)(3); strikes and boycotts, 8(b)(4); initiation fee, 8(b)(5); featherbedding, 8(b)(6); and recognition picketing, 8(b)(7). Labor organizations may not restrain or coerce an employer in the selection of a representative for collective bargaining. The union may not cause an employer to discriminate against an employee who is not a member of the union. Nor can a union representative of the employees refuse to bargain with the employer. With adherence to required notification procedures, an employee organization may strike against the employer when negotiations have failed. A primary boycott is a strike action taken by union members against their employer. The illegal or protected status of strikes or boycotts depends on the union objectives and the tactics used. Labor unions may not force an employer to join any organization or cease using specific products or doing business with someone, thus making "hot cargo" clauses illegal. Hot cargo agreements are stipulations on the employer's use of products that give the union power over other organizations. A secondary boycott that is directed at a customer or supplier of the employer is also illegal. An employee group may not force an employer to bargain with them if the employees are represented by another bargaining agent. Labor organizations may not force "any employer to assign particular work to employees in a particular labor organization . . . rather than to employees in another labor organization," and they may not honor strike lines against other employers by refusing to cross the picket lines. Informational picketing is not barred, as it does not disrupt the employer's operation. Recognition picketing to get an employer to recognize an employee group is lawful except when the employer has recognized another labor organization, when it is within twelve months preceding a valid election, and when picketing has been conducted without a petition. The union may not charge discriminatory or excessive initiation fees or cause an employer to pay for services not performed, a practice called featherbedding.

Unionization

Organizing phase. To form a union, an organizer must establish internal contacts. In a hospital or other health agency the organizer needs at least one nurse on each shift to assist with unionization. The organizer should be known by a majority of the nurses, be knowledgeable about related laws, and be able to use free time for organizing. The organizers ascertain the level of interest informally by listening, asking questions, and supplying information. After an assessment period, the organizers meet, discuss the prevailing climate, identify the frustration level, enumerate the kinds and extent of employment problems, and assess the nurses' interest in unionization. If interest is minimal, further organizing efforts should be postponed. If nurses show interest in organizing, the campaign is planned.

There must be commitment from the nurses before a formal organization can be established. To achieve this, the organizers hold informational meetings. Coordination of efforts, development of unity, identification of problems and concerns, education about collective bargaining, and active participation of nurses are the tasks to be accomplished in the organizing meetings. The organizers should work in nonwork areas on their own time. The organizers contact the labor organization that they want to represent them for information and authorization cards. The labor organization can send a letter to the employer informing management that the nurses within that agency are organizing and that the activity is protected by law.

Recognition phase. The organizers must get at least 30% of the nurses to be represented to sign individual authorization cards before the labor organization can act on behalf of the group. Handing out authorization cards is solicitation and cannot be prohibited by management anywhere in the agency during nonworking time. Recognition of the labor organization by the employer is necessary before collective bargaining can begin. Some employers will recognize the labor organization on a voluntary basis when given proof of the majority representative status. However, employers often refuse to recognize the labor organization voluntarily on the basis of a good faith doubt of majority representation. Thus it becomes necessary to obtain certification from the National Labor Relations Board (NLRB).

The NLRB does not start an election until requested to do so by an employee organization. A petition for an election must be accompanied by designation cards signed by 30% of the employees in the bargaining group to indicate a substantial show of interest. Labor organizations usually obtain signatures from at least 50% of the potential members before they file a petition.

A preliminary hearing is held before an election is scheduled. This provides participants an opportunity to express their opinions. The regional director of the NLRB assesses that the employer is under the board's jurisdiction; determines that other criteria are met; determines the bargaining unit and voter eligibility; and sets the date, hours, and place for the election. The election usually takes place during working hours on the employer's premises about a month after the hearing. All employees in the bargaining unit who were on the employer's payroll during a given payroll period in the recent past are allowed to vote. This rule prevents hiring people to vote in the election.

The number of bargaining units within an agency is held to a minimum. Appropriate bargaining units include (1) technical employees, such as x-ray technicians, surgical technicians, and licensed practical nurses; (2) service and maintenance employees, such as employees doing kitchen work, laundry, and housekeeping; (3) business office clerical employees, such as receptionists, clerks, and switchboard operators; and (4) professional employees, such as nurses.

Spouses and children of the employers, temporary employees, and supervisory employees are not eligible to vote. People who have the authority to hire, fire, and direct others are considered supervisors. This may include nursing supervisors, head nurses, and charge nurses. As a member of management, the director of nursing is ineligible to vote.

During the pre-election period, the employer is required to post NLRB election notices stating the time, date, and place of the election. On election day the field examiner from the regional board sets up the election machinery and does not allow electioneering around the polling place. Eligible employees cast secret ballots. Ballots are counted in the regional office. The tabulation of votes is forwarded to the office of the General Counsel in Washington, D.C., and the General Counsel decides the election. If employees no longer want to be represented by the labor organization, they can initiate a decertification election with a requisite 30% show of interest. If a bargaining unit is denied because of the vote tabulation, the labor organization is not permitted to seek certification among the same people until after a 12-month moratorium, and the management group should rectify the problems identified during the organization. If a union wins the election, both parties prepare to negotiate.

Contract negotiation phase. The piecemeal, total, and combination approaches are used for contract negotiations. The piecemeal is a step-by-step approach that tries to settle the issues one by one. The total approach considers nothing settled until everything is settled. This allows for calculation of the effects of the interdependent variables on each other. The combination method uses both approaches. The step-by-step method is used to progress from the easy to the hard issues. The decisions are not irrevocable, trading takes place, and decisions are reworked until negotiations are acceptable to both parties. The union representatives present the solutions to the members for a ratification vote to accept or reject the offer. If the solutions are accepted, the employee and management representatives sign the agreement, and it becomes binding. If they are rejected, the representatives reassemble to continue negotiating the contract.

During contract negotiations, the union is on the offensive and management is on the defensive. The union makes most of the demands, while management defends itself against them and prepares for a strike. The threat of a strike strengthens the union negotiator's position.

Strikes in the health care field require more special and elaborate notification procedures than in other industries. This allows for the delay of new admissions or referral to other facilities. Alternative health care plans are made for ambulatory patients. Some hospitalized patients may be transferred to other agencies, and supervisory personnel are scheduled to care for the remaining patients.

The NLRB categorizes collective bargaining into three groups: illegal, voluntary, and mandatory. Illegal topics violate the NLRB and other laws. Voluntary subjects need not be negotiated unless both sides consent to do so. Voluntary issues include size of the bargaining team, union dues, management salaries, and patient charges. Mandatory subjects are related to conditions of employment, work hours, and remuneration.

Contracts often start with a preamble that states both parties' objectives and a pledge of cooperation. Near the beginning there is a statement of the employer's recognition of the union as the bargaining representative for specific employees with specification of employees who are excluded.

A union security clause requires new workers to join the union. Union security is protected by establishing a closed shop, union shop, agency shop, or maintenance-of-membership arrangement in the contract. The closed shop requires the employer to hire and retain only union members in good standing. However, this is prohibited by the Labor Management Relations Act of 1947 for employers and employees in industries affecting interstate commerce. A union shop requires all employees to become members of the union within a specific time after hiring (usually 30 to 60 days) and to maintain membership as a condition of employment. An agency shop requires all employees in the negotiating unit who do not join the union to pay a fixed amount equivalent to organization dues on a regular basis as a condition of employment. The money may go to the organization's welfare fund or to a charity. The maintenance-of-membership clause requires union members to maintain their membership during a specific period, such as the duration of the contract.

Financial remuneration—including wages and salaries, shift differentials, overtime rates, holiday pay, cost-of-living adjustment, longevity, and merit increases—receives considerable attention. Nonfinancial remuneration—including insurance, retirement plans, employee services such as free lunches and parking, vacations, holidays, leaves, and educational assistance—also receives considerable attention. The union usually strives to have rewards made on the basis of seniority. Guidelines for discipline, grievance procedures, and professional standards are also negotiated. After acceptance of the contract by the union members through a ratification vote, the contract is signed by employee and employer representatives and becomes binding.

Contract administration. Implementation of the agreement, the final phase of the unionization process, interprets and enforces the agreement developed during negotiations. When one of the parties involved does not abide by the terms of the contract, a grievance may result. Grievances are most commonly filed against management because management has a more active role than the union in the administration of the contract. The grievance procedure is usually addressed in the contract.

Underlying causes of grievances should be identified and corrected so that future grievances will be avoided. Different types of grievances require different reactions from managers and union leaders. A legitimate grievance results when one party violates the agreement between parties. Supervisors' ignorance of the agreement and lack of commitment are the major causes. It is not uncommon for first-line managers to function without having read the contract and with the attitude that labor relations are a chore. On the other hand, union stewards are more motivated to understand the agreement and must have an interest in labor relations to obtain their positions. Consequently, most legitimate grievances are against management. It is advisable to develop training programs to familiarize managers with the contract and to set labor relations objectives as priorities for managers.

Imagined grievances occur when a party incorrectly believes that there has been a violation. It is usually an employee who imagines a grievance because she does not understand her rights. The steward should correct the misunderstanding before it becomes a formal grievance.

Political grievances occur for reasons other than the concern itself. Management may want to appear supportive to subordinate managers and stewards to union members, so they do not adequately advise the complainant. A cooperative atmosphere between labor and management is the best way to avoid political grievances.

Harassment grievances are fabricated to distress the other side. They are most commonly used by unions in connection with negotiations. Management usually denies the grievances, forcing the union to drop the grievance or request arbitration. If the contract indicates that both sides share arbitration expenses, harassment grievances are usually dropped.

Organizations should have a grievance procedure even if they are not unionized. This allows employees access to management regarding issues of concern to them and conveys management's intent to be fair. Grievances should be handled quickly through the use of a grievance procedure. Grievances may be handled in a centralized or decentralized manner. In a decentralized process, the immediate supervisor tries to resolve as many problems as possible, and grievances rarely progress further. This encourages a close working relationship between superior and subordinates. Unfortunately, there may be inconsistent decisions because of the number of different people involved in the process. In a centralized grievance procedure, the immediate supervisor denies the validity of the grievance, and it is handled by the next level of supervision or by a personnel department. Thus, decisions are made consistently among units because of the few people involved in the decision making. Unfortunately, cooperation between the superior and subordinate is not fostered.

Arbitration. Most contracts allow either side to seek arbitration when a grievance is not satisfactorily resolved, but both parties must agree on the arbitrator. The American Arbitration Association and the Federal Mediation and Conciliation Service are primary sources for professional arbitrators. The payment of costs involved is specified in the contract. Commonly, both parties share the costs, but some contracts specify that the loser must pay.

In any case, arbitration is not automatic and must be requested by the dissatisfied party. Both sides select a representative, the grievance is reviewed, fact finding is done, and witnesses are interviewed. Preparation of one's case from the opponent's view encourages one to consider both sides and develop a stronger case. Presenting one's case to a friend who will act as an advocate helps further identify weaknesses in one's presentation and further strengthens the case. Documents should be prepared in triplicate for the hearing so that the arbitrator, opponent, and presenter can each have a copy. Witnesses may be used for the hearing. Their availability should be confirmed. Witnesses should be informed of where and when to attend the hearing and what will be expected of them.

A hearing is similar to courtroom proceedings. The arbitrator makes opening remarks, and the initiating party comments on the purpose of the hearing and outcomes desired. The responding side may respond then or wait until later. Witnesses are presented and cross-examined in an alternating pattern. First a witness testifies for the initiator, and then one for the responding party testifies and is cross-examined. The initiating party makes closing remarks followed by the responding party's closing statement, each pointing out evidence to support her side. The arbitrator studies the evidence and makes a decision. The arbitrator may issue a summary judgment shortly after the proceedings or a written decision to both parties within a month. The decision of the arbitrator is enforceable in court.

Decertification. When employees no longer want to be represented by their present union, they can request a decertification election. Management may also request an election if it is in good faith doubt that the union is representing the majority of employees. The decertification election is similar to the certification process. First a decertification petition must be signed by at least 30% of the bargaining unit to file a show of interest. In reality, more than 50% and probably closer to 75% need to show interest to guarantee a successful election. The petition is filed with the NLRB by the employer. It can be filed on the expiration date of a contract or ideally during the 30-day period before the 90-day period preceding expiration of the contract.

After receiving the decertification petition, the NLRB distributes a notice about it to the union, the petitioners, and the employer. The employer is asked to submit to the NLRB (1) names and addresses of other interested unions, (2) copies of current and recent contracts covering the employees petitioning for decertification, and (3) names and job classifications of all employees in the bargaining unit.

A pre-election hearing may be scheduled if there are questions regarding representation. If neither the union nor the employer requests a hearing, an election date and time are set. The selection of the date is extremely important to the success of the election. Campaigning is limited to 24 hours before the election so that the decertification process momentum is not disrupted by a weekend. Wednesday, Thursday, or Friday are preferable days for the election. A day that will ensure maximal turnout, such as payday, is desirable. The election should be held within three weeks of confirmation of the election by the NLRB.

Decertification campaigns are similar to certification efforts. Managers should have various meetings, including individual meetings, small group meetings, and entire unit meetings to assure personnel that they are in good hands with management and that they will be better off without a union. However, decertification cannot be accomplished just by holding meetings during the campaign. Management needs to have earned the confidence of the employees over time through the use of good management techniques.

The NLRB conducts the election on the specified date. If the union loses the election, management stops negotiating with the union. If not, the next contract is negotiated.

Nurse managers' role in collective bargaining

Nurse managers should evaluate their management skills and take continuing education courses to improve them. Motivational techniques are particularly important for the nurse administrator to possess because she works through others. She must listen carefully to staff concerns and represent subordinates' wishes to top management. Nurse administrators need to know about labor relations.

The director of nursing should not serve as the chief negotiator during collective bargaining because it would put her in an adversary role. The agency legal representative is usually the negotiator. During negotiations, the director of nursing defines what is best for the nursing care of patients. Once the contract has been negotiated, nurse managers must learn the terms of the contract and have copies of the contract available to them. Problems should be solved through problem-solving techniques as they arise.

Advantages and disadvantages of collective bargaining

There are advantages and disadvantages to collective bargaining. Some equalization of power between administrators and subordinates can be obtained because of the subordinates' strength in numbers. Grievance procedures become viable, and staffing for systematic and equitable distribution of work can be established. The quality of services can be influenced. Unfortunately, an adversary relationship may develop between administration and subordinates, and strikes may not be avoided. Unionization is considered unprofessional by many nurses. Leadership for unions may be difficult to obtain, because professional nurses have little experience in positions of authority. Women tend to view employment as a job instead of a career, minimizing interest in leadership positions, and if the bargaining unit and the professional association are the same, top administrators may have to drop membership in the professional organization, further depleting the leadership.

PROGRAM EVALUATION

Program evaluation is an essential part of effective administration. It is the evaluation of a set of activites designed to determine the value of the program or of the program elements. Evaluative research is the utilization of scientific research methods to make an evaluation. Program evaluation may be formative or summative. Formative evaluations provide information about the program during the developmental stages. Summative evaluations provide information for judging a developed program. Evaluation may be descriptive or comparative.

Programs are evaluated for any number of reasons. Federal, state, or local agencies may require program evaluation. Program evaluation can be used to improve programs systematically or to determine the state of the programs. It can be used to evaluate the effect of new technologies on programs and help determine if parts responsible for success in one program can be used in other parts of the system.

Once the program to be evaluated and the purpose for its evaluation have been decided, someone should be made accountable for the evaluation. Credibility is the major argument in favor of an external evaluator. A person who is part of the program may have difficulty in being objective about the program's strengths and weaknesses because of pride, loyalty, or job security. On the other hand, an internal evaluator may be as objective as an external one and has knowledge about the program, its history, and circumstances; such knowledge facilitates the evaluation.

Calendar of events

One of the first things the evaluator should do is develop a calendar of events that depicts the tasks to be done, the schedule, and organization of the project. A calendar of events for program evaluation itemizes activities to be done down the left-hand margin and projected dates across the top (Table 5). The projected date for each activity is estimated. This is a valuable tool for planning and judging the progress of the program evaluation.

Program evaluation model

The formulation of program goals is essential for program evaluation. The goals should be clear, specific, and measurable. The evaluator will need to develop indicators to measure the extent to which the goals are achieved. These program-outcome indicators are the dependent variables of the study. The standards set by accrediting agencies such as the American Nurses' Association, the National League for Nursing, and the Joint Commission on Accreditation for Hospitals can be used to determine goals and criteria.

Methods of data collection should be decided next. There are numerous sources for the collection of data, including questionnaires, interviews, observations, ratings, government statistics, instructional records, policy and procedure manuals, financial records, documents such as minutes of meetings or transcripts of trials, and tests.

Table 5. Calender of events for program evaluation

	Jan.-Feb.	March-April	May-June	July-Aug.	Sept.-Oct.	Nov.-Dec.
Inform personnel of purpose of the evaluation and who is responsible	X					
Define goals	X					
Determine criteria	X					
Develop instrument		X				
Train data collectors		X				
Pilot test			X			
Collect data			X			
Analyze data				X		
Report findings				X		
Correct deficiencies					X	
Reassess (follow up)						X

A model that depicts the program goals, the indicators to determine the extent to which the goals are achieved, and sources of the data helps direct the evaluation project. There are existing models, such as the Joint Commission on Accreditation of Hospitals self-assessment form. Others can be created. Table 6 is an example.

Sources of internal and external invalidity

When designing research, the evaluator gives careful consideration to sources of internal and external invalidity. Validity is the measurement of what is to be measured. Extraneous variables can confound the effects of the experimental variable and are therefore sources of internal invalidity. Factors that reduce the generalizability are sources of external invalidity.

There are several sources of internal invalidity. History is a problem when an event extraneous to the purpose of the study occurs between the pretest and posttest and confounds the effect of the experimental variable. It is a hidden treatment or a change-producing event that occurred in addition to the treatment. The problem of history is a more plausible explanation of the change the longer the time lapse between pretests and posttests. It can be controlled with experimental isolation, which can almost never be used when human subjects are involved. For example, a group-training technique to reduce racial prejudice against blacks has been developed. A group of prejudiced individuals is convened, pretested, trained, and posttested. If a black political leader is assassinated during that time, one would suspect that history confounded the experimental effect. The reduced prejudice can proba-

Table 6. Model for program evaluation

Goal	Standard	Observation
Nursing service has a current written organizational plan.	Organizational plan delineates the functional structure and the mechanism for cooperative planning and decision making.	Content analysis of the organizational plan.
Nursing service has goals.	Goals are written and made known to all personnel.	Locate written goals; interview management regarding how personnel are informed of goals; questionnaire to personnel.
Nursing committees are formally organized.	Purpose and function of each standing committee are defined; nursing is represented on committees concerned with nursing service.	Content analysis of documents for purpose and function of standing committees; content analysis of committee composition; interviews; questionaires.

bly be attributed to sympathy for the assassinated black politician rather than to the therapy.

Maturation is another internal invalidity problem. It is a systematic change over time in a person's biological or psychological condition, including growing older or becoming tired or hungry. Prescribed plan activities to promote walking for 12- to 15-month-olds or bladder control for 2- to 3-year-olds would be questionable because children normally learn those skills during those times.

Testing is a practice effect or the effect on the scores of the posttest of taking the pretest. The practice effect is larger for the same test than for an alternative form of the test. A form of test wiseness, the practice effect lasts about 3 months. People taking an achievement, intelligence, or personality test for a second time within a 3-month period will usually do better than people taking them for the first time, although it is unlikely that they have become brighter or better adjusted.

Instrumentation becomes a problem when there are changes in the measuring instrument over time. Changes in tests, judges, measuring devices, or calibrations cause instrumentation problems. Results from one test cannot usually be compared with results of a different test. Instrument decay or the fatiguing of spring scales causes invalidity problems. Observations produce instrumentation problems. There are intrahuman differences of the observer through fatiguing, the process of learning, the process of increased skill with practice, and learning to establish rapport. There are differences in observations by the same person at different times. One may be more lenient at one time than at another. One becomes more skillful with experience. There are also interhuman differences, such as knowledge and skill. A researcher observing disruptive behavior in psychiatric patients before and after a treatment may become more aware of disruptive behavior by the second observation and record more behaviors, or she may record fewer minor disruptions the second time because of the high level of disruptive behavior she had observed. In either case, the treatment effect is difficult to determine.

Statistical regression becomes a problem when groups have been selected because of their extreme scores. The phenomenon of regression toward the mean is the inevitable tendency of persons whose scores are extreme (far above or below the norm) on the first test to be less extreme on the second test. Patients chosen for a therapy group because of their high anxiety would show less anxiety on a second test regardless of the treatment.

Selection is a problem when the experimental group differs from the control group. For example, we may have a selection problem if we try to compare a control ward with an experimental ward because patients were assigned as a function of systematic characteristics, such as presenting symptoms or histories. Randomization is a control for selection. This problem often occurs when the subjects are already formed into groups for reasons other than the study.

Experimental mortality is a differential loss of subjects from comparison groups. It includes lost cases, cases on which only partial data are available, and cases who refuse to participate. The experimental group may appear stronger or more intelligent only because the weak and stupid dropped out of it. Heavy smokers and drinkers are likely to be the first to drop out of therapy groups to reduce smoking and drinking, leaving the clients who appear most successful with the therapy.

Researchers must also be aware of external invalidity problems that complicate the generalizability of the findings. Subjects who are available to the experimenter may not represent the population, and consequently the results of the research are not generalizable. Random sampling solves this problem. The independent variable needs to be operationally defined so that replication of the research is possible. Multiple-treatment interference, Hawthorne effect, novelty effect, and experimenter effect are considered. When two or more treatments are given consecutively to the same subjects, it is difficult, if not impossible, to know the cause of the results, and multiple-treatment interference occurs. When a person knows she is a subject, she may change her behavior, not because of the treatment, but because she knows she is being observed. This is the Hawthorne effect. The subject may react either positively or negatively because of the newness of the treatment, thus producing the novelty effect. The experimenter effect occurs when the subject is influenced by the experimenter. Such subtle behavior as smiling and nodding one's head during an interview may unintentionally influence the subject.

Pretest sensitization is the same as the testing internal validity problem except as it relates to generalizability of the results, which makes it an external validity problem. Identification of the dependent variables and selection of instruments to measure those variables are necessary for external validity. One must also consider if the effect will be lasting or if one is likely to get different results at different times. In the situation where the black political leader was assassinated, thereby reducing prejudice against blacks among those in group therapy, we had a history internal validity problem. Now we have an interaction-of-treatment-with-time external validity problem. The racial prejudice may have been temporarily reduced as a result of the assassination but will probably not be maintained for long. Treatments to reduce smoking may appear most successful right after a cancer scare but not as successful later. One must have internal validity to obtain external validity, which is the ability to generalize the research results. With program evaluation there may be little intent to generalize the results.

Research designs

Next, the evaluator should design the evaluation. Will the evaluation be one shot only or a continuous process? Will a program be assessed, or will programs be compared? Will an experimental or a quasi-experimental design be used? The pretest-posttest control group, posttest-only control group, Solomon four group, and factoral are experimental designs.

Experimental designs

Pretest-posttest control group. In the pretest-posttest control group, experimental subjects are randomly divided into two comparison groups as follows:

$$R \quad O \quad X \quad O$$
$$R \quad O \quad \quad O$$

R = Randomly assigned individuals
O = Observation
X = Experimental treatment

The control and experimental groups are randomly assigned. The two groups are considered equivalent during initial observation. During final observation, the difference between groups should be the result of a variable being applied to one group but not to the other. The pretest-posttest control group true experimental design controls for history, maturation, testing, instrumentation, regression, selection, and mortality. One should consider the Hawthorne and novelty effects, as the interaction of the testing and the experiment are not controlled.

Posttest-only control group. In the posttest-only control group, experimental subjects are randomly divided into two groups to be compared as follows:

$$R \quad X \quad O$$
$$R \qquad O$$

The control and experimental groups are randomly assigned. A pretest is not administered. A treatment is applied to one group only. Because of the random selection, it is assumed that the groups are equivalent before the treatment is administered to one group and that the difference noted on the posttest is due to the treatment. This design controls for history, maturation, testing, instrumentation, regression, selection, mortality, and the interaction of the testing and the experiment. It is superior to the pretest-posttest control design unless there is a question about the randomness. This design is appropriate when a pretest is awkward and is convenient for maintaining anonymity. The Solomon four group design is a better design but may not be worth more than double the effort.

Solomon four group. The Solomon four group design uses four randomly selected groups. It combines the pretest-posttest control group and the posttest-only control group designs as follows:

$$R \quad O \quad X \quad O$$
$$R \quad O \qquad O$$
$$R \qquad X \quad O$$
$$R \qquad\qquad O$$

It is considered the most desirable of the experimental designs because it allows the investigator to examine the effects of the treatment in four independent comparisons. The Solomon four group design controls for history, maturation, testing, instrumentation, regression, selection, mortality, and the interaction of testing and the experiment. However, it may not be worth the effort.

Factoral design. Factoral design allows for observation of some subjects at all levels of all experimental variables and can be used when the situation is under the complete control of the experimenter, which is rarely the situation.

Quasi-experimental designs. The evaluator usually cannot control the time and subjects to whom experimental variables are applied. However, the evaluator may be able to select the time and persons on whom observations will be made and can consequently gain some control through the use of quasi-experimental designs.

Time series. A time series involves a series of measurements over a period of time with an experimental variable introduced at some point in the sequence as follows:

$$O \quad O \quad O \quad O \quad X \quad O \quad O \quad O \quad O$$

Maturation is controlled because it is not likely to cause the difference between each of the observations. Testing, regression, and selection are controlled. History is the most probable problem, and the longer the time over which the observations are made, the more probable the problem. Instrumentation is also a potential problem. It is important not to change the instruments or their calibration. It is best if this design is repeated by several researchers in separate situations.

Equivalent-time-samples design. When the equivalent-time-samples design is used, the time available for making the observations is divided into equal time periods as follows:

$$XO \quad XO \quad XO \quad XO \quad XO$$

The times to make observations are randomly selected. This design controls for history, maturation, testing, instrumentation, regression, selection, and mortality. The multiple-treatment effect is a problem, and generalization of the findings is limited to similar populations.

Nonequivalent control group. The broken line (---) means the groups are not equivalent samples:

$$O \quad X \quad O$$
$$------$$
$$O \qquad O$$

For this design, a control and an experimental group are both given a pretest and posttest. However, the groups are not randomly selected and do not have sampling equivalence. It is better than a one-group pretest-posttest design because it controls for history, maturation, testing, and instrumentation. Regression, mortality, and interaction between selection and maturation need to be considered as potential problems.

Counterbalanced designs. The counterbalanced designs are sometimes called

Latin square, switchover designs, crossover designs, and rotation experiments. The following is an example:

$$X_1O \quad X_2O \quad X_3O \quad X_4O$$
$$X_2O \quad X_4O \quad X_1O \quad X_3O$$
$$X_3O \quad X_1O \quad X_4O \quad X_2O$$
$$X_4O \quad X_3O \quad X_2O \quad X_1O$$

Four experimental treatments are applied in a random manner in turn to four individuals or groups. Counterbalanced designs control for history, maturation, testing, instrumentation, regression, selection, and mortality. Multiple-treatment interference is a problem. Strength can be obtained through replication.

Separate-sample pretest-posttest design. For separate-sample pretest-posttest design, a pretest is given on one group and a posttest on another as follows:

$$R \quad O \quad (X)$$
$$R \quad \quad X \quad O$$

This simulated before-and-after design is weak, but it is better than a single-group pretest-posttest design because it controls for testing, regression, and selection. History, maturation, and mortality are not controlled, and the instrumentation needs to be questioned.

Separate-sample pretest-posttest control group. For the separate-sample pretest-posttest control group, two groups are pretested, one receives the experiment, and two are posttested. This excellent design controls for history, maturation, testing, instrumentation, regression, selection, and mortality. Because it is an expensive design, it has probably never been used.

$$R \quad O \quad (X)$$
$$R \quad \quad X \quad O$$
$$R \quad O$$
$$R \quad \quad \quad O$$

Multiple time-series design. For the multiple time-series design, a series of measurements is taken over a period of time on two separate groups with an experimental variable introduced at some point in the sequence of one of the groups as follows:

$$O \quad O \quad O \quad X \quad O \quad O \quad O$$
$$\text{------------------------}$$
$$O \quad O \quad O \quad \quad O \quad O \quad O$$

This excellent design can be used to compare one agency with a similar one. Controlling for history, maturation, testing, instrumentation, regression, selection, and mortality, it is the best of the more feasible designs. Power is increased through repeated measures.

Recurrent institutional cycle design. The recurrent institutional cycle design (see below) is a patched-up design that starts with an inadequate design and adds features to control for sources of invalidity. It becomes an accumulation of precautionary checks that approaches experimentation.

$$X \quad O$$
$$- - - - - - - -$$
$$O \quad X \quad O$$

Regression-discontinuity analysis design. The solid line (—) means the groups are not equivalent (see below). They differ by known amounts along a variable. The treatment is applied to individuals or groups that exceed a certain level of a variable rather than randomly. This design controls for history, maturation, testing, regression, and selection. Instrumentation and mortality would need to be questioned.

$$\frac{X \quad O}{}$$
$$\frac{X \quad O}{}$$
$$\frac{X \quad O}{}$$
$$\frac{O}{}$$
$$\frac{O}{}$$
$$\frac{O}{}$$

As with other research, data must be collected and analyzed. It is particularly important to communicate the results to appropriate people so that corrective actions can be taken, to do follow-up reassessments to make sure the corrections were made, and to check the results.

QUALITY ASSURANCE

In October 1972, the Ninety-second Congress passed Public Health Law 92-603, an amendment to the Social Security Act that mandated the establishment of Professional Standards Review Organizations (PSRO) to review the quality and cost of care received by clients of Medicare, Medicaid, and Maternal Child

Health programs. Health facilities were to develop quality control programs by 1976 or the government would do it for them. Consequently, quality assurance has received considerable attention. The American Nurses' Association developed guidelines for standards of nursing practice under the PSRO system; the American Hospital Association and the Joint Commission on Accreditation of Hospitals developed a retrospective review of care. Individuals and agencies developed criteria and processes for the measurement of quality of care.

Committee selection and functions

Each agency needs a quality assurance committee to establish criteria and a process for quality assurance and to evaluate care, make recommendations, and do follow-up. A chairperson with enthusiasm and attention to detail helps assure a successful program. Members also need to be interested in quality assurance and knowledgeable about channels of communication, hospital resources, patient population, and nursing needs. Representation of staff nurses, head nurses, clinical specialists, and in-service instructors from various nursing units helps produce a wide variety of ideas. Preset meeting times allow for staffing to accommodate attendance, and large committee membership supplies manpower to do the work.

Conceptual framework

Structure, process, and outcome or any combination of these are the common approaches to evaluation. The structure approach focuses on the delivery system by which nursing care is implemented. Quality assurance committee members evaluate policies, procedures, job descriptions, orientation schedules, in-service schedules, and charting. The process approach measures what the nurse does while delivering patient care. Both nurse and patient may be interviewed to collect evidence of professional judgment and functions. The outcome approach measures the results of the care administered to the patient and evaluates whether the goals were reached, by considering clinical manifestations, patient knowledge, and the client's self-care.

Audits may be concurrent or retrospective. Concurrent audits evaluate care as it is being administered and may include observation of staff; inspection of patient; open-chart auditing; staff and patient interviews; and group conferences including participation from the client, family, and staff. Retrospective audits judge care after it has been delivered through the study of patient charts or care plans after the patient has been discharged, postcare questionnaires, patient interviews, or all of these.

334

Review of the literature

A review of the literature locates instruments, criteria, and standards that have been developed and allows committee members to benefit from others' accomplishments and mistakes. Some of the major contributions follow. A more exhaustive listing is available in the bibliography.

The Standards of Nursing Practice outlined by the American Nurses' Association are process oriented and include the following:

I. The collection of data about the health status of the client/patient is systematic and continuous. The data are accessible, communicated, and recorded.
II. Nursing diagnoses are derived from health status data.
III. The plan of nursing care includes goals derived from the nursing diagnoses.
IV. The plan of nursing care includes priorities and the prescribed nursing approaches or measures to achieve the goals derived from the nursing diagnoses.
V. Nursing actions provide for client/patient participation in health promotion, maintenance and restoration.
VI. Nursing actions assist the client/patient to maximize his health capabilities.
VII. The client's/patient's progress or lack of progress toward goal achievement is determined by the client/patient and the nurse.
VIII. The client's/patient's progress or lack of progress toward goal achievement directs reassessment, reordering of priorities, new goal setting, and revision of the plan of nursing care.

The quality assurance program recommended by the Joint Commission on Accreditation of Hospitals is a retrospective review of patient care through a closed-chart audit that focuses on patient-care outcomes.

Maria C. Phaneuf also recommends a retrospective review of the records of discharged patients. She developed fifty components and descriptive statements for the seven dependent and independent nursing functions identified by M.J. Lesnik and Bernice E. Anderson in *Nursing Practice and the Law*. These functions are (1) application and execution of the physician's orders, (2) observation of symptoms and reactions, (3) supervision of the patient, (4) supervision of care givers, (5) reporting and recording, (6) execution of nursing procedures and techniques, and (7) promotion of health by direction and teaching. Phaneuf's instrument focuses on the patient and his care rather than on the nurse and her activities for appraising the content and process of the care. Care is rated on a graded scale as excellent, good, incomplete, poor, or unsafe.

The Slater Scale, originally constructed by Doris Slater Stewart, contains 84 items—18 actions directed toward meeting individual psychosocial needs, 13 actions related to group psychosocial needs, 13 activities to satisfy physical needs, 16 operations to meet general needs, 7 communication items, and 17 behaviors reflecting professional expectations. A cue sheet listing several examples to illustrate each of the items is also included. The nurse is rated for each action as best, average, or poor. The cue sheet contains additional columns for not applicable and not observed. The quality of care expected from first-level staff nurses is the standard of measurement. Unlike Phaneuf's work, the Slater Scale focuses on the nurse instead of the patient and measures the nurse's competencies as care is being provided. It yields both numerical and descriptive information of the nurse's strengths and weaknesses. The Slater Scale can be used to improve the nurse's performance.

Qualpacs, the Quality Patient Care Scale, is a revision of the Slater Nursing Performance Rating Scale. It lists 68 items under the same subsections used in the Slater Scale—individual psychosocial, group psychosocial, physical, general, communication, and professional implications. A cue sheet lists examples to illustrate each item. The care is rated according to best, average, or poorest care, with not applicable and not observed options. The care expected of a first-level staff nurse is the standard of measurement. This is a concurrent process-oriented approach.

Sharon Van Sell Davidson and peers have identified concurrent and retrospective review criteria for numerous health conditions in *Nursing Care Evaluation* (1977). Susan Martin Tucker and others (1975) outline observations, immediate care, ongoing care, patient teaching, and discharge planning for numerous medical-surgical, obstetrical, and pediatric conditions. Other books and articles about quality assurance are plentiful and contain material that can be adopted or modified.

Instrument development

An operational definition of quality of care gives direction to instrument development. Instruments may be general and appropriate for all patients or structures or applicable only to a specific process or to a homogeneous group in which differences in scores are due to variations in the concept being evaluated rather than to other factors. Medical diagnosis, symptom, acuity, age, and health care settings often are used to determine homogeneity. A taxonomy of nursing diagnoses is being developed. Identification of homogeneous patient groups for the development and application of instruments necessitates the development of numerous tools.

Once the patient group or specific process has been identified, selection of goals, criteria, and items is the priority. The goal is a statement of the end that one strives to attain. Criteria are the standards or scales against which judgments are made. Criteria describe what is implied in the goal in concise, measurable statements of desired structure, process, or outcome. They are written for a specific condition and are understandable, clinically sound, and achievable.

Brainstorming is a common approach for identifying items. Actual problems—those that patients generally experience—and potential problems—those with a high risk of occurring—are identified, and the structure, process, or outcome to resolve or prevent them is determined. The generation of as many ideas as possible without immediate evaluation is recommended initially. Later, items can be eliminated, checked for comprehensiveness, put into a uniform format, precisely defined, and quantified. A pilot study to collect data with the instrument can clarify which items should be retained, discarded, or rewritten.

Scales and measurements must be developed. A checklist to determine whether a characteristic is present; ratings to give each item a measure of worth such as good, average, or poor; and ranking by comparison, such as more or less than the standard, are common measurements. Scales are either nominal, ordinal, interval, or ratio. The simplest type is the nominal. Its categories are collectively exhaustive, and each is mutually exclusive, meaning that there is a category for all the observations and that each observation can fit only one category. Sex, marital status, and the presence or absence of a condition are examples. Ordinal scales classify observations into a specific order of more or less, such as good, average, or poor. Interval scales are ordered with equal measurement between each class, but the unit of measurement is determined arbitrarily. Examples are the thermometer and sphygmomanometer. Ratio scales contain the properties of the other scales plus an absolute-zero point. Multiplication and division are possible because each number has a relationship to any other number. Currency systems are examples.

Validity and reliability

Establishment of validity and reliability is important. Validity is the measurement of what is supposed to be measured and is difficult to establish. Face validity is an analysis of the instrument's appearance as valid. Someone simply looks at an instrument and decides if it has face validity. It is the easiest assessment of validity but is a questionable criterion because of its high degree of subjectivity. Content validity is a judgment that the content of the instrument is appropriate and closely related to what is to be measured. It is best determined by a jury of experts. Construct validity is particularly important when phenomena or concepts that are not directly observable, such as intellectual skills, human characteristics, and personal adjustment, are involved. The construct is a hypothetical definition that clearly defines observable phenomena. Construct validity is theory oriented. An instrument contains predictive validity to the extent that it predicts future behavior. It can be determined by checking the prediction after a period of time. Concurrent validity reveals the behavior that is being demonstrated presently and is particularly important for concurrent audits.

337

Reliability is repeatability and is easier to determine than validity. Scores obtained by different raters' observations of the same event at the same time or by the same rater at different times can be compared. The test-retest method involves administration of the same test again after a period of time with the hope that the results will be consistent. The fact that people may remember items from the first administration or that people change over time are problems. This method is appropriate for stable characteristics but is problematic for unstable traits. The split-half method compares halves of the test to determine internal consistency. Reliability is suggested when the results of both halves are similar. To use the split-half method, both halves need to contain enough items to be reliable. Statistical methods to check reliability include the Kuder-Richardson test for internal consistency and the Spearman-Brown formula for a coefficient for the total test.

Methods of data collection

Observation, interviews, questionnaires, and content analysis of charts and care plans are the most common methods for data collection. When observation is used, the quality assurance committee determines what to observe, develops observational procedures, and trains observers. Observations should be planned and recorded systemically and subjected to controls. Observation is suitable for concurrent audits. Behavior is observed and recorded as it occurs, and the process can be noted. Because observation does not demand participation of the observed, it is relatively independent of the subject's willingness to cooperate and therefore makes subjects readily available. Observation is a comparatively inexpensive method that lends itself to simple data-gathering instruments and recording equipment. Although it can be stopped at any time, it is limited to the length of the occurrence. The timing of an event may be difficult to predict, and consequently the observer may waste time waiting for something to happen. The presence of an observer also may influence the subject's behavior. Observations may be difficult to record, are subject to observer bias, and may vary between observers. Consequently, observers need training. Specifications of observer tasks; detailed instructions; sharp, measurable categories; immediate, detailed recording; observation averaging; and the use of recording equipment such as cameras and tape recorders help overcome observer bias and variability.

Interviews of both clients and staff may be used to evaluate care. Interviews may be (1) nondirective—the subject talks about whatever she desires; (2) focused—the subject speaks to a list of topics; (3) nonstandardized—the interviewer makes up her own questions; (4) semistandardized—the interviewer asks a specific number of questions and probes; and (5) standardized—the interviewer conducts each interview in exactly the same manner using the same wording without probing. The interviewer can minimize misunderstanding by probing, clarifying, pursuing topics in depth, and observing nonverbal communication. Subjects do not need to be literate. Interviewing provides more flexibility and a greater response rate than questionnaires. However, it is an expensive method because it requires so much time. The subject may be nervous or may attempt to please the interviewer, and the recording of answers is problematic.

Questionnaires are less time consuming and consequently less expensive than interviews. They are particularly useful when subjects are dispersed over a large geographical area. Less skill is needed to administer a questionnaire than to conduct an interview. Questionnaires put less pressure on the subject for immediate response, standardize instructions and questions, and offer anonymity. The participants, however, must be literate. Unfortunately, often only a small percentage of questionnaires are returned, and the effect of nonrespondents is difficult to evaluate. Items may be omitted or misunderstood. A forced choice may not be an actual choice, and probing is not possible.

When preparing a questionnaire, the subjects' frame of reference and information level and the social acceptability of the item need to be considered. Language should be gauged to the level of the subjects. Lengthy or leading questions and double negatives are to be avoided, and each question should contain only a single idea. Questions are arranged from general to specific. A pretest is helpful for identifying problems with the instrument. A high proportion of omissions, "other," "don't know," or all-or-none responses suggests poor questions. Added qualifications and comments and variation in answers when questions are reordered also suggest problems.

The percentage of returns of the questionnaires is influenced by a personal cover letter requesting cooperation, sponsorship by the health agency, attractive format, short length, ease of filling out and returning, and inducements for replying. The best response is from people interested in the topic.

Content analysis of charts and care plans is a common method of data collection. It is a method of observation and measurement that is systematic, objective, and quantitative. Frequency of occurrences usually is noted on a checkoff list. Descriptive statements can then be given about frequency of occurrences and changes in conditions. Unfortunately, it can take a long time to review records; classification systems may be too ambiguous for a phenomenon to fit a category; the chart chosen may not represent the phenomenon; and prejudices in the scoring method can bias the results.

Sampling

Sampling is a technique of selecting a sample from the whole population being studied. The evaluator wants to be able to generalize her conclusions concerning the quality of care given the total population. Adequacy of sample size is important, especially with small samples, if the quality assurance committee members are to have confidence in their inferences. The more homogeneous the population, the smaller the sample size necessary to be representative. Budgetary and time restrictions greatly influence sample size.

The best sampling technique is random sampling, which allows each patient an equal chance to be included in the sample. A table of random numbers that can be located at the back of most statistics books is frequently used. To use this method, patient records are numbered. The evaluator closes her eyes and points to a number on the table to start the selection. She then systematically progresses by row or column until the appropriate number of records is selected. A roulette wheel can be used. The wheel is spun, and the patients' charts whose numbers are chosen by the pointer are selected for review. The wheel is repeatedly spun until the desired sample size has been reached. A third possibility is to put pieces of paper with a chart number or patient name on each into a large container. The evaluator draws a piece of paper, rotates the papers, and draws another until the desired sample size is reached.

Systematic sampling consists of selecting every-nth patient. Selection can be according to admission, discharge, or an alphabetical listing. The evaluator makes a random start and then selects systematically. The size of the interval is determined by the percentage of the population desired in the sample size. For example, if one wants the sample to be 10% of the population, the evaluator chooses every tenth patient.

Stratified sampling divides the population into sections and then takes a random sample from each section to ensure that important variables are represented. For instance, patients may be classified according to body systems by the major diagnosis. If 30% of hospital admissions are classified as cardiovascular cases, 30% of the sample would be drawn from those cases.

Cluster sampling uses small samples from various sections of the population. A certain number of audits may be selected from each hospital unit. Instead of randomly selecting 100 patient charts, 10 charts may be randomly selected from each of 10 hospital units.

Multistage sampling randomly selects some percentage of the population and then randomly samples smaller subunits. For instance, in a large hospital system, the evaluator would randomly select which hospitals are to be audited. Next, the specialty area to audit within the selected hospitals is randomly selected. Finally, the specific units within those specialty areas and the specific patients on those units are randomly chosen.

Incidental or convenience sampling utilizes readily available subjects. The families of patients who happen to be in the coffee shop at a particular time or patients who happen to be in their rooms at a particular time may be interviewed.

The sample mean is not truly representative of the total population average.

It is an attempt to approximate it. The difference between the mean or average of the sample and the total population is the sampling error.

Analysis of data

Simple scoring is preferred and can be subjected to descriptive measures. Frequency distribution indicates how many times observations were assigned to specific categories. Measures of central tendency can be calculated from the frequencies. The mean is the average. It is calculated by adding all the scores and dividing that sum by the total number of scores. The mode is the most frequently occurring score, and the median is the score in the middle with half the number values above it and half below it.

Expected level of performance

The quality assurance committee must determine the level of expected performance below which they will take corrective action. Staff should know what criteria are being used to evaluate the quality of care and should have an opportunity to review reports of audits. The committee identifies performance discrepancy and completes problem analysis. Once they identify the problem, they can recommend corrective measures. The corrective action recommended, time schedule for completion, and responsible person are documented and shared with appropriate people. A reaudit determines if the corrective action was implemented successfully.

Sharing favorable audits and evidence of improvement in care provides recognition for good work and increases morale. Research regarding the cost and effects of audits is still needed.

TOOLS FOR CONTROL

Statistics, reports, and observations

Statistical analysis of data may be of a historical or forecast nature and may be presented in tabular or chart form. The use of charts makes it easier for the manager to visualize trends and relationships and to make predictions. Special reports with analysis in addition to the statistical analysis are helpful in problem areas. Recommendations for corrective actions may be included in the report. A manager can also collect considerable data by walking through the institution, doing site visits, and visiting with personnel.

Audits

External audits are usually done by a public accountant's firm to determine if the agency's records of financial transactions accurately represent the agency's financial condition. The external audit verifies the accuracy of records by spot checking financial transactions, thus encouraging honesty from employees. If the internal control system is considered effective, the auditor's sample will be smaller and less expensive than if the internal control is deemed weak.

Internal audits are done by agency staff to determine the effectiveness of other controls. Internal audits may check accounting controls to safeguard assets and to ensure reliability of information generated by the accounting process. They may also be used to check administrative controls for efficiency and for compliance with policies. Internal audits protect the interests of the agency by assessing the accuracy of accounting and statistical data; the safety of the agency's assets; and compliance with policies, procedures, and plans. They further the interest of the organization by assessing the organizational structure, lines of authority, policies, procedures, practices, and performance. Internal auditing should be continuous and constructive.

Inventory control

The manager needs to determine the most economical level of inventory, as supplies represent a significant cost factor. The purchasing, order, storage, and costs of long and short stock must all be considered to determine the most economical level of inventory. The purchasing cost is the price paid per item. Cost may be related to the size of the order with cost per item decreasing as the size of the order increases. Purchasing cost equals PD, with P being the cost or price per unit and D being the number of units purchased.

The order costs involve writing specifications, soliciting and analyzing bids, writing orders, receiving the supplies, accounting for the materials, and paying the bills. The order cost may be relatively large the first time an item is purchased or relatively small for routine purchasing processes. The order cost varies with the number of orders placed. The more orders per year, the greater the annual costs will be. Annual order cost equals $(D/Q)O$ when D is the number of units purchased, Q is the order size, and O is the average cost of placing a single order.

The carrying cost is the expense involved with holding inventories. It involves expenses such as storage, insurance, and security. To keep carrying costs down, small orders should be placed frequently; this approach is in direct conflict with keeping the purchasing and order costs low. Carrying cost equals $HQ + IPQ/2$ when H is the cost of storage per item and Q is the order size. $IPQ/2$ is the opportunity cost element, with I representing the highest obtainable rate of return at the current interest rate, P being price per unit, and Q being the order size.

The short or stock-out costs involved with holding an insufficient amount of inventory must be considered. The manager considers the consequences of running out of stock. Not only is a sale lost, but client satisfaction may suffer. Although this expense is difficult to measure, it is a real cost.

Total cost is expressed as follows:

$$TC = PD + \frac{DO}{Q} + \left(HQ + \frac{IPQ}{2}\right) + L + S$$

TC = Total cost

PD = Purchase cost

$\frac{DO}{Q}$ = Order cost

$HQ + \frac{IPQ}{2}$ = Carrying cost

L = Overstocked cost

S = Stock-out cost

The economical order quantity is expressed as follows:

$$EOQ = \sqrt{\frac{2DP}{C}}$$

EOQ = Economical order quantity

D = Usage in units or demand

P = Order cost

C = Annual cost of carrying one unit in inventory

A large order size is merited when there is a large demand, high order cost, and low carrying cost. However, a smaller order size is desired when there is little demand for the item, the order cost is small, and the carrying cost is high.

A high inventory turnover is desired. Low inventory turnover may be caused by poor purchasing policies, overstocking, and a decrease in demand for the item. The inventory turnover can be calculated as follows:

$$\text{Inventory turnover} = \frac{\text{Total cost of supplies}}{\text{Inventories}}$$

To determine when to reorder, the manager needs to know the average daily usage and the lead time required to receive the supplies. A manager needs to keep the average daily usage multiplied by the number of days it takes to receive the goods in order not to run out of stock.

Some managers use the *ABC* method for maintaining inventories. *A* refers to a small number of items that account for a large percentage of the budget and are carefully monitored; *B* refers to moderate cost items that receive some monitoring; and *C* refers to a bulk of inexpensive, expendable items, such as rubber bands, that receive little monitoring.

Fig. 5-3.   Variable costs.

Fig. 5-4.   Fixed costs.

Fig. 5-5.   Semifixed costs.

Fig. 5-6.   Semivariable costs.

Fig. 5-7.   Break-even costs.

Fig. 5-3

Fig. 5-4

Fig. 5-5

Fig. 5-6

Fig. 5-7

Break-even calculations

Full costs equal all direct costs that can be traced to a source plus indirect costs such as maintenance, administration, and the building that are allocated to the source. Cost finding is an attempt to find the full cost and to allocate indirect costs. Indirect costs allocated may include housekeeping calculated by square feet, utilities by square feet, laboratory by number of tests, and dietary services by number of meals served.

The cost-volume-profit relationships can be visualized on a break-even chart. The manager considers variable, fixed, semifixed, and semivariable costs when doing a break-even analysis. Variable costs vary in direct proportion to volume (Fig. 5-3). Two disposable syringes probably cost twice as much as one. Fixed costs are relatively fixed in total regardless of changes in volume (Fig. 5-4). A nurse receives a certain salary regardless of the number of injections she gives. Semifixed costs are fixed within a range of activity (Fig. 5-5). One nurse can give just so many injections per shift, and beyond that a second nurse will need to be hired. Semivariable costs are fixed at zero output and increase with volume (Fig. 5-6). The break-even point is depicted on a break-even chart where revenues equal expenditures (Fig. 5-7). The formula for break-even analysis is

$$R = FC + VC + P$$
$$R = \text{Total revenue}$$
$$FC = \text{Fixed cost}$$
$$VC = \text{Variable cost}$$
$$P = \text{Profit}$$

STRESS MANAGEMENT

Source of stress

Adjustment to change is stressful. Many events in life produce individual stress reactions. Death of a spouse or close family member, divorce, marital separation, marriage or remarriage, and personal injury or illness are highly stressful events. Change in the health of a family member, pregnancy, gain of a new family member, marital reconciliation, increased arguing with spouse, sexual difficulties, changes in financial state, mortgages, trouble with in-laws, a son or daughter leaving home, and the death of a close friend are stressful. Changes in living conditions and personal habits such as changes in work, residence, school, recreation, church activities, social activities, sleeping habits, and eating habits cause stress. Even personal achievements, vacations, and holidays are stressful. These personal stressors can affect one's job performance.

In addition to the personal stressors, there are many sources of stress at work. Dismissal and retirement are highly stressful. Business readjustments such as changing jobs or responsibilities, changes in working hours or conditions, and problems with the boss are stressful. Even outstanding achievement is stressful. Poor physical working conditions; physical danger; work overload; time pressures; responsibility for people; role ambiguity and conflict; conflicts with superiors, peers, and subordinates; restrictions; little participation in decision making; over- or under-promotion; and lack of job security are stressors common to jobs.

Nurses face stress with life and death situations; heavy work loads involving physical and mental strain; knowing how to use numerous pieces of equipment and knowledge of the consequences of equipment failure; reporting to numerous bosses; communication problems among staff members, physicians, families, and other departments; and knowledge of the serious consequences of mistakes. A hospital is one of the most stressful work environments.

People often needlessly increase their own stress. The difference between demands people place on themselves or perceive from others and the resources they perceive as available to meet the demands is a threat or stress. Individuals are typed by the demands they place on themselves. Type A people set high standards, are competitive, and put themselves under constant time pressure. They are even very demanding of themselves in leisure and recreation activities. Type B people are more easygoing and relaxed. They are less competitive and more likely to accept situations than fight them.

Stress response

Stress is impossible to avoid. It is a nonspecific response of the body to any demand. There are two types of stress: (1) eustress, a positive force that adds excitement and challenge to life and provides a sense of well-being, and (2) distress, a negative force caused by unrelieved tension that threatens effectiveness. Whether one will experience eustress or distress is largely dependent on the person's perceptions, physical activity or inactivity, mental activity or inactivity, sound nutrition, and meaningful relationships.

A stressor is anything an individual perceives as a threat. Stressors produce a state of stress by disrupting homeostasis. There are three stages in the stress response. First, the alarm reaction is the mobilization of resources to confront the threat. Second, in the resistance stage, there is a large increase in energy consumption. Once the reserve energy has been used, the body needs time to recover and to replenish the supply. When stress continues for long periods of time, the energy is used but not replaced and the third stage, exhaustion, results.

Consequently, unrelieved stress interferes with one's physical and mental well-being. After the stress event, the body returns to a state of equilibrium. Stable periods for bodies to restore adaptive energy allow one to meet new stressful situations.

Symptoms of stress

Numerous symptoms indicate that stress is becoming distress. These include but are not limited to:

Fatigue	Lack of concentration
Depression	Tendency to be demanding
Tearfulness	Loss of appetite or overeating
Restlessness	Indigestion
Nervousness	Constipation or diarrhea
Withdrawal or sudden	Nausea
gregariousness	Coughing

Irritability
Anger
A feeling of being unloved
Insecurity
A feeling of vague anxiety
Pessimism
Self-criticism
Frequent frustration
Loss of interest in going out
Loss of interest in people and
    things
Decrease in self-care
Disorganization
Inability to relax or rest
Nightmares
Early morning waking
Feeling of not being able to get any-
    thing done
Feeling that everything is too much
Forgetfulness

Headaches
High blood pressure
Rapid pulse
Heart palpitation
Perspiration
Aching neck and shoulder
    muscles
Low back pain
Allergy problems
Accidents
Arthritis
Asthma
Colds
Colitis attacks
Dermatitis
Influenza
Hives
Menstrual distress
Ulcers

High stress levels accumulated over several months are likely to result in physical and psychological reactions. The amount of stress necessary before one manifests symptoms varies, depending on factors such as heredity, habits, personality, past illnesses, and previous crises and coping mechanisms. Well-educated, intelligent, creative people in management are at high risk for burnout. They may become workaholics but get little accomplished, experience chronic fatigue, feel they do not want to go to work, take increasing amounts of sick time, become negative, blame and criticize others, engage in backbiting, and talk behind others' backs.

Stress control

The nurse manager can prevent and control burnout by setting personal and professional goals, establishing priorities, practicing good health habits and relaxation techniques, improving her self-esteem by obtaining the skills she needs, and using support systems.

Values' clarification. Values' clarification is a useful activity. Values should be chosen freely from alternatives with thoughtful consideration to the consequences of each alternative. They should be cherished and shared with others. The value should be integrated into one's life-style, and actions should be consistent with the values. To help clarify one's values, one may assign priorities to a list of values such as:

Affection	Pleasure
Duty	Power
Expertise	Prestige
Health	Security
Independence	Self-realization
Leadership	Service
Parenthood	Wealth

One can also list in order or priority characteristics such as:

Ambitiousness	Honesty
Broadmindedness	Imagination
Cheerfulness	Independence
Cleanliness	Logic
Courage	Lovingness
Forgiveness	Responsibility
Helpfulness	

Goal setting. Goals should be consistent with one's values, and one should consider goal alternatives. To do this, one considers why a goal is desired. One may want a promotion for recognition or for economic reasons. If the promotion is not forthcoming, one may receive recognition through community service. Money might be generated through wise investments or fees for community services. The achievement of desired outcomes through different approaches increases flexibility and decreases stress caused by unmet goals.

Stress avoidance and regulation. When reappraising situations, one should avoid troublesome transactions. The frequency of stress-inducing situations should be minimized. Every change takes energy. Therefore during periods of high stress, routines and habits should be maintained as much as possible. One should be cautious about moving and starting a new job at the same time one is getting a divorce. That would be a particularly poor time to try to stop smoking or lose weight. Unnecessary changes should be avoided during periods of high stress. Deliberately postponing some changes helps one deal with unavoidable change constructively and reduces the need for multiple adjustments at one time. However, increasing positive sources of tension that foster growth such as learning a sport can help offset the deleterious effect of negative tension.

Time blocking. Time blocking is the setting aside of specific time for adaptation to a stressor. To reduce the stress from having been promoted to a management position, one could set aside time for reading about management or for observing a manager. This helps ensure that concerns are addressed and tasks accomplished. It decreases anxiety, time urgency, and feelings of frustration.

Time management. Time management helps control stress. Much time can be conserved when one knows her value system and acts consistently with it, sets goals, and plans strategies for accomplishment of those goals. One can also use organizers such as to-do lists and calendars to plan good use of one's time.

Assertiveness. When one asserts oneself, one increases self-esteem and reduces anxiety, thus reducing stress. As with time management, assertiveness involves thinking through goals and acting consistently with one's values through the use of effective work habits and by setting limits on other's attempts to block one's goals. It involves stating what one wants and how one feels, making requests, taking compliments, handling put-downs, and setting limits. An assertive person makes eye contact with others, stands straight, sits in an open, listening posture, and speaks in a clear voice. Assertive people choose for themselves and achieve desired goals through self-enhancing behavior that reduces stress.

Feeling pauses. Feeling pauses are useful. One should take time to identify a feeling, label it, distinguish between thinking and feeling, and accept the feeling for what it is rather than talking oneself into what it should be. One should be aware if she is feeling the following:

Amusement	Happiness
Calmness	Joy
Care	Love
Compassion	Passion
Elation	Relaxation
Excitement	Thrill
Forgiveness	Satisfaction
Hope	

She should also acknowledge negative feelings such as:

Anger	Fear
Anxiousness	Frustration
Confusion	Hurt
Depression	Jealousy
Embarrassment	Restlessness
Envy	Terror

Then one should determine if the feeling is appropriate for the situation and decide how to give expression to the feeling in a safe and appropriate way. Feelings can be expressed in "I feel" messages rather than "You" messages that blame or attack others. Feelings can be talked about with an uninvolved person. One can fantasize about how one would like to handle the situation better the next time. Negative feelings may be acted out symbolically by punching a pillow, drawing a picture, or writing a poem. One may set aside negative feelings by getting involved in something pleasant such as exercise, hobbies, music, television, or talking to a friend. Feelings can also be experienced vicariously by getting involved in another's experience through reading a book, watching a movie, or listening to someone.

Inner shouting. Inner shouting is the process of shouting "I feel . . . " inside one's head; the person blurts the feeling out spontaneously rather than say it quietly. Anger should be viewed as a symptom. Pains should be focused on to help one take responsibility for feelings of hurt and humiliation.

Anchoring. Anchors are associated feelings that are initiated either by an event or by the memory of that event. Anchors may be sounds, sights, smells, tastes, or touches that stimulate positive or negative feelings. Birds chirping may remind one of happy lazy mornings with the family. One may recall an awful accident at the sight of blood. One might remember fall walks through the woods with a lover at the smell of dry leaves. A taste may revive memories of grandma's home cooking. A light touch to the face may remind one of earlier loving moments and cause one to experience a sense of well-being. Our lives are filled with anchors that cause associations. We can use anchoring in a useful way to experience desired feelings. Because touch can be inconspicuous and easy to replicate, one can associate a positive feeling with a familiar touch to the body. This may be so simple as clasping one's hands and being reminded of soft music, beautiful colored glass, and the peaceful sanctuary of church. Exact pressure at a very specific spot makes the anchor work most accurately and should be done when one desires to bring back a pleasurable feeling.

Sorting. Sorting is choosing the interpretation of an event. One can have an optimistic or pessimistic interpretation of events. Is the glass half full or half empty? We become what we think and therefore can make ourselves happy or miserable. To be more happy and fun loving, one should sort for the positive aspects of situations.

Thought stopping. Thought stopping helps get rid of negative thinking. Excessive rehearsals in our minds of negative past events are unhelpful thoughts that waste time, reduce our self-esteem, and encourage maladaptive behavior patterns. To prepare for thought stopping, one should think of beautiful pleasant experiences: a sunrise, a waterfall, a flower, a pet, favorite music, baking bread, holding hands. One should also identify not so helpful thoughts: I'm stupid; I'm fat; Nobody likes me. One should identify the negative thoughts that are most bothersome. In private, one can think about a negative thought momentarily and suddenly yell, "Stop!" while clasping one's hands or hitting one's head or leg. One startles herself, and the thought escapes. Immediately one should insert a pleasant thought. If the negative thought returns, the procedure can be repeated. It is reinforced when the negative thoughts are stopped. Thoughts lead to feelings that lead to behaviors, so by changing the way one thinks, she can change the way she is. Thought stopping should not be used, however, when physical or emotional safety and grieving are involved.

Compartmentalization. Compartmentalization of thought is the deliberate decision to think negative thoughts at specified times of the day. During the alloted time, one thinks about her worry, guilt, or jealousy. One does not allow herself to think these thoughts at other times of the day.

Environmental changes. Environmental changes can be designed to reduce stress. This may be as extreme as changing jobs or residence or as minor as painting a room a favorite color or adding a picture, candle, or basket. The short time inconvenience of remodeling may be worth the long-term stress reduction. Temporary changes in jobs can add variety and stimulation.

Humor. Humor related to an attitude toward life is most likely to reduce stress. There is a cluster of qualities that characterize this frame of mind including flexibility, spontaneity, unconventionality, shrewdness, playfulness, humility, and irony. These are qualities that can be developed. Flexibility is the ability to examine all sides of the issues. One should try to look at a situation from several different viewpoints: the boss's, the subordinate's, the client's. Spontaneity is the ability to swing from one mood to another quickly. One might practice the body language of several emotions including fear, anger, sadness, and love. One can free herself from current values, places, and occupations through unconventionality and imagine living a day as a favorite animal, a famous historical person, an Eskimo, an Indian on a reservation, or a spaceman. Shrewdness is refusal to believe that people or things are what they appear to be. One can think of a list of people and things and give an example of how each is not what they seem to be. Playfulness is the ability to see life as a fun game. One can visualize life as a game and give the game a name. One should identify times of various emotions—fun, enjoyment, fear, anger, sadness—and chart wins and losses. Humility is a willingness to question the importance of one's values, ideas, achievements, and existence. One must consider the meaning of one's life and consider how difficult situations have brought happiness and how happy relationships have included suffering. Irony is the ability to see that situations are not black or white.

Centering. Centering helps reduce stress by bringing the mind and body back into balance. One is to put her tongue on the centering button, which is about a quarter of an inch behind the upper front teeth. This spot apparently stimulates the thymus gland, weakens the effect of stress, and balances the cerebral hemispheres. With left-sided dominance, intuitive, esthetic, and creative functions are reduced under stress. Other activities that seem to balance the two hemispheres of the brain include reading a poem in a rhythmic fashion; listening to a person with a soothing voice; listening to classical music; listening to natural sounds such as cats purring, birds chirping, or a babbling brook or waterfall; looking at pictures of pleasant landscapes or smiling people making caring gestures; swinging one's arms during a vigorous walk; and taking a shower. Good posture is also beneficial.

Nutrition. Good nutrition helps maintain the body for full functioning. Eating a balanced diet, taking vitamin supplements, and drinking plenty of water are important. In general, Americans need to reduce fat and cholesterol, sugar, salt, and food additives consumption. American diets contain high levels of fat and cholesterol that are abundant in red meats, eggs, cheese, and prepared foods. Excessive consumption of fat is associated with cardiovascular diseases. Americans are obtaining an increasing proportion of their calories from sugar that is associated with obesity, tooth decay, diabetes, and heart disease. There is a growing concern that additives and pollutants are related to cancer. These food additives include preservatives, coloring, flavoring, and stabilizers that extend shelf life and make processed food taste better. In addition, pesticides and other chemical pollutants are health hazards.

The increasing consumption of saturated fats and sugar coupled with a decrease in activity levels contributes to a widespread occurrence of obesity. In general, Americans need to increase exercise while decreasing caloric intake particularly from fats and sugars. At the same time, the percentage of calories from foods containing fiber, such as fresh fruits, vegetables, and whole grains should be increased. Canned, frozen, and prepared foods are usually devoid of their original fiber content but often have sugar and salt added. The grains we eat have often been refined to white flour and rice, thereby losing much of the roughage. Although improving eating habits may not prevent stress, it is one way to maintain the level of fitness needed to fight stress.

Exercise. Regular, vigorous exercise can also help one withstand chronic stress. Aerobic exercise elevates the heart rate during and for a period after the exercise. The range of elevation necessary to produce an aerobic effect is from 60% to 80% of the maximal heart rate the person can achieve, which is calculated at 220 minus the person's age in years. Jogging, cycling, and swimming are particularly good aerobic exercises. Dance allows one to stretch and strengthen muscles and to reduce tension.

Regular exercise develops greater capacities in several areas of function. It increases the strength of cardiac contractions, the size of the coronary arteries, the blood supply to the heart, the size of the heart muscle, and the blood volume per heart beat. It decreases the heart rate at rest and with exertion and reduces vulnerability to cardiac arrhythmias. It increases the blood oxygen content, blood volume, and efficiency of peripheral blood distribution and return. Exercise increases the blood supply to the lungs and the functional capacity during exercise. It increases lean muscle mass and functional capacity during exercise.

Exercise also reduces strain and nervous tension resulting from psychological stress and reduces the tendency for depression.

Sleep. Sleep is also important for dealing with stress. Sleep needs decrease with age, and people may awaken several times during the night as they grow older. This should not be confused with insomnia, which is a prolonged inability to sleep. There are three types of insomnia: (1) initial, when it takes more than 15 minutes to fall asleep, (2) intermittent, with awakening during the night and difficulty returning to sleep, and (3) terminal, with early morning awakening and inability to go back to sleep.

Physical, emotional, and nutritional factors may contribute to insomnia. A lack of physical exercise, digestive problems, heart trouble, and high blood pressure interfere with sleep. Disturbing emotional states such as anger, fear, guilt, depression, and anxiety create tension that interferes with sleep. An unbalanced diet, alcohol, caffeine consumption, and a large meal shortly before bedtime can interfere with sleep.

To foster a good night's sleep, the day's activities should be tapered off before getting ready for bed. Regular exercise promotes deep sleep but should not be done for a couple of hours before bedtime. Likewise, biofeedback and meditation have stress-reducing properties that foster sleep but should not be done before bedtime because they boost energy and alertness. Chocolate, cola, coffee, and tea should be restricted particularly in the evening. Overeating, particularly heavy foods at night, should also be avoided. The bed should be associated with sleep, and the room should be dark and quiet.

Relaxation

Abdominal breathing. There are numerous techniques that can be used to foster relaxation. Abdominal breathing is a quick method. When stressed, people tend to breathe in short, shallow breaths. Consequently, the lungs do not fill up completely. The remaining air is stale, and oxidation of tissues is incomplete. Muscle tension results. Without being conspicuous, one can take a few abdominal breaths almost anywhere at anytime. It is best to do abdominal breathing for 5 to 10 minutes once or twice a day while sitting upright. It may be done during normally low times or to reverse the stress response when it has been triggered. To do abdominal breathing, one should inhale slowly through the nose while keeping the back straight. First the abdomen expands, then the chest, and finally the shoulders. Then one should exhale slowly and hold the breath for a second or two before starting another inhalation.

Massage. Massage can relieve tension, provide a passive form of exercise, and foster tactile communication. It stimulates relaxation and flexibility. Self-massage can be done from a chair. It can be done as a full-body massage or to a part of the body that is particularly tense. To do a full-body massage, one may start by placing both hands on the top of the head and moving them in slow circular motions down the back of the head, neck, and shoulder area. The neck and shoulder are common sites for tension. They may be most easily massaged by crossing hands over so that the right hand massages the left shoulder and the left hand massages the right shoulder. Then the hands are returned to the top of the head and moved forward in circular motions over the forehead, face, neck, and chest. To relax the right arm, one grasps the fingertips of the right hand with the left hand and moves up the hand and arm to the shoulder in circular motions with the fingers on top and the thumb on the underside. Then one massages down the right side of the chest. The procedure is repeated up the left arm and down the left side. Then hands are placed on the lower abdomen with fingertips touching. Circular motions are used up to the chest.

The low back is another area that is commonly tense, particularly from sedentary work. One places the hands on the lower back with fingertips touching at the coccyx. The fingertips then massage up as high as one can reach. A foot should be massaged with the massage continuing up the foot, over the ankle, and up the calf and thigh. Then the massage should be repeated on the other foot and leg. This full-body massage can be done after a warm bath at bedtime to foster sleep.

Progressive relaxation. Progressive relaxation may also be used to foster sleep. It is the conscious contraction and relaxation of muscles. By deliberately tensing muscles, one can learn to identify what muscles are tight and learn to relax them. It can be used before, during, or after an anxious situation. If done routinely once or twice a day, it can help keep one's level of anxiety down.

Progressive relaxation can be done in a standing, sitting, or lying position. There is greater likelihood of falling asleep in a lying position. In a sitting position, one should keep the head squarely on the shoulders, back against the chair, feet on the floor, legs uncrossed, and hands on the lap in a relaxed position. During progressive relaxation, one tenses specific muscles to a maximal degree and notices how the tight muscles feel for about 5 seconds. Then the muscle is relaxed, and the pleasant feeling of relaxation is enjoyed for about 10 seconds. For a head-to-toe progression, one starts by wrinkling up the forehead and noticing where it feels particularly tense. Then one relaxes that part slowly, identifies the muscles that are relaxing, notices the difference between tension and relaxation, and enjoys the relaxed feeling. Abbreviated instructions for other body parts are:

Close eyes tightly
Wrinkle nose
Place teeth together and press lips against teeth into a forced smile
Press tongue hard against the roof of the mouth
Clench teeth

Pucker lips

Pull chin toward chest

Put head back as far as it will go

Press head to right shoulder

Press head to left shoulder

Hold arm out straight, make a fist, and tighten the whole arm or pull elbow
tightly into side

Repeat with the other arm

Push shoulder blades toward each other

Pull chest in

Pull stomach in

Tighten muscles in lower abdomen, buttocks, and thighs and raise self in
the chair

Push foot against the floor, then point toes toward the head and repeat with
the other leg and foot

With experience in progressive relaxation, one can also learn to relax without
tension. One first concentrates on relaxing each body part and then on generalized relaxation with deep breathing. One takes a deep breath, holds it, and
then exhales slowly while relaxing the entire body from head to toe, saying
"relax" so that the "x" is said as the focus reaches the toes.

Biofeedback. Biofeedback uses mechanical devices to gain self-regulation to
control autonomic responses. The Galvanic Skin Response uses electrodes attached to the fingertips to measure skin resistance, which is moisture of the skin
that indicates nervousness. Arteries contract under stress and dilate with relaxation. A thermistor on the finger detects changes in peripheral skin temperature
that are associated with activity of the smooth muscles in peripheral arteries.
This skin temperature is particularly useful for control of migraine headaches.
The electroencephalograph uses electrodes attached to the scalp to detect electrical activity on the brain's cortex. Different brain wave patterns are associated
with different states of mind. The electromyograph uses electrodes attached to
the forehead or forearm to measure muscle tension from electrical impulses
generated by muscles. People with migraine and tension headaches, hypertension, and gastrointestinal problems have responded well to biofeedback. Because
the instruments convert skin resistance, skin temperature, brain waves, and
muscle tension into readily observable signs, people can tell if they are controlling
their body responses or not. They can also learn to read and interpret body
signals without the use of instruments to modify their responses.

Autogenic training–self-hypnosis. Autogenic training produces deep relaxation
through self-hypnosis. These regular but brief sessions of passive concentration
on physiologically adapted stimuli reduce other extraneous stimuli and have

helped people with asthma, arthritis, constipation, hypertension, migraine head-aches, and sleep disturbances.

To do self-hypnosis, one should lie down with eyes closed in a quiet room, and take a few deep breaths. Each autogenic training session should last 2 to 20 minutes, preferably 20 minutes two or three times a day. There are six phrases. When learning autogenic training, only one phrase should be added at a time once a week.

The first phrase focuses on heaviness, the next on warmth, then on heartbeat, breath, the solar plexus, and the forehead. Supporting phrases such as "I am relaxing" or "I am at peace" are interspersed between induction phrases. For the heaviness induction, one systematically concentrates on thinking that each part of the body feels heavy: "My face is heavy. I am relaxing. My neck is heavy. I am at peace. My shoulders are heavy. I am resting. My chest is heavy. I am quiet." For the warmth induction phrase, one substitutes "warm" for "heavy" in the previous phrases. The heart induction phrase is, "My heartbeat is calm and regular." Then one concentrates on, "My breathing is relaxed and com-fortable." Next one puts her hands on her abdomen to create warmth and re-peats, "My solar plexus is warm." Lastly, one thinks, "My forehead is cool." To return to an alert state, one takes a few deep breaths and thinks, "I will arise refreshed and alert," then moves her arms and legs, opens her eyes, and slowly gets up.

Meditation. Meditation focuses attention on an experience, helps one become aware of one's response, and facilitates the integration of the physical, mental, emotional, and spiritual aspects of one's life. There are many methods for medi-tating. One may focus on an object such as a candle, chant, listen to music, or meditate on one's own breath. To meditate on one's breath, one can count while breathing: one on inhalation, two on exhalation, three on inhalation, and four on exhalation. That process can be repeated until the allotted time for meditation is over. Usually people experience an inner calm and sense of well-being from meditation.

Visualization and mental imagery. Visualization and mental imagery can be used to relax. One starts in a relaxed position and visualizes pleasant thoughts. One can meditate on a visualized colored object, such as a blue sky, white cloud, green tree, red apple, or pink flower. One can imagine being in a favorite place, such as a sandy beach, in the mountains, or in front of a fireplace in a favorite room listening to music. One can concentrate on the sights, sounds, smells, tastes, and feelings of the pleasant thoughts.

Poetry. Poetry reading or writing is useful for reducing tension, particularly if one is depressed and movement and verbalizing have not worked sufficiently. Poems are chosen for their rhythm, mood, and the feelings expressed. Poems can be read in a one-to-one or group meeting. Discussions about the meaning can help verbalize feelings.

Music. Soft, classical music can help release feelings and emotions and bring about relaxation.

Baths. Water is a relaxant. One should fill the bathtub with water that is body temperature and immerse herself up to her neck for about 15 minutes.

Enhancing self-esteem. Positive affirmations can be used to enhance one's self-esteem. A person can become more comfortable with positive thoughts about herself and decrease the amount of self-devaluation. Several methods can be used. One might imagine positive scenes and see herself as she wants to be. One can repeat positive affirmations such as, "I am happy," "I am healthy," or "I am beautiful." One can also write positive affirmations on cards, put them in conspicuous places, and read them often. People may take turns making positive comments about each other.

Support groups. Support systems are synergistic. One can accomplish more through support groups than alone. Support groups provide a feeling of being accepted, valued, loved, esteemed, and a sense of belonging. In addition to providing emotional support, support systems help provide a social identity and are a source of information, services, and material aid.

There are several types of support systems. Usually, the family is the natural support system that constitutes the primary support group. Peer support groups are also important. They are composed of people who have had similar experiences, have adjusted, and want to share their insight. A head nurse may receive support from other head nurses or a jogger from other joggers. Religious organizations provide a congregation that sets guidelines for living, shares values, and provides traditions. Voluntary service groups and self-help groups provide support for specific purposes such as to lose weight, to stop drinking alcohol, to quit smoking, or to adjust to a mastectomy or a stoma. Family, friends, and peers are usually sought out before professional support systems, but the helping professions are available when support from others is inadequate.

It is extremely important that managers take excellent care of their own well-being. They can function at their best if they are healthy. They need considerable energy to be supportive of others and will not have strength to share if they are hurting. Likewise, staff nurses need a sense of health and well-being to provide the best nursing care. Managers are responsible for providing care to the caregivers.

The manager should help protect personnel from undue stress. Personnel may be taught identification of stress symptoms and stress management. Annual physical examinations could be required. Vacations are provided and encouraged. Counseling and referral services can be provided as support systems.

Nutrition, educational, and health promotional programs are presented, and nutritious food is served in the cafeteria. Exercise programs can be provided and encouraged. Managers should monitor stress levels and intervene when necessary.

LEARNING ACTIVITIES

1

Practice force-field analysis. Identify a problem and its driving and restraining forces. Weigh the forces. Plan strategies to strengthen the driving forces and weaken the restraining forces.

2

Evaluate an evaluation tool and share your assessment with a classmate.

3

Practice an appraisal interview with a classmate. Evaluate classroom participation by the appraisal interview style of your choice. Discuss how it felt to appraise and be appraised in that manner.

4

Identify a behavior that you would like to change. Determine your baseline behavior. Graph the frequency. Plan reinforcement and extinction strategies.

5

Interview a union member about the pros and cons of unions.

6

Evaluate the research design of a research report related to management.

7

Identify your major stressors. Identify where you feel stress in your body. Plan how you will control that stress. Practice stress management.

BIBLIOGRAPHY

Books

Anderson, R.A.: Stress power! New York, 1981, Human Sciences Press, Inc.

Beal, E.F., Wickersham, E.D., and Kienast, P.: The practice of collective bargaining, Homewood, Ill., 1972, Richard D. Irwin, Inc.

Bean, J.J., and Laliberty, R.: Understanding hospital labor relations, Reading, Mass., 1977, Addison-Wesley Publishing Co., Inc.

Bennis, W.G., Benne, K., and Chin, R., editors: The planning of change, ed. 4, New York, 1985, Holt, Rinehart & Winston, Inc.

Benson, H.: The relaxation response, New York, 1975, Avon Books.

Berger, M.S., et al., editors: Management for nurses, ed. 2, St. Louis, 1980, The C. V. Mosby Co.

Berman, H.J., and Weeks, L.E.: The financial management of hospitals, ed. 5, Ann Arbor, Mich., 1982, Health Administration Press.

Boyer, J.M., Westerhaus, C.L., and Coggeshall, J.H.: Employee relations and collective bargaining in health care facilities, St. Louis, 1975, The C. V. Mosby Co.

Brook, R.H.: Quality of care assessment: a comparison of five methods of peer review, Washington, D.C., 1973, United States Department of Health, Education and Welfare.

Brooten, D.A.: Managerial leadership in nursing, Philadelphia, 1984, J.B. Lippincott Co.

Campbell, D.T., and Stanley, J.C.: Experimental and quasi-experimental designs for research, Chicago, 1966, Houghton Mifflin Co.

Carter, J.H., et al.: Standards of nursing care: a guide for evaluation, New York, 1976, Springer Publishing Co., Inc.

Cautela, J.R., and Groden, J.: Relaxation, Champaign, Ill., 1978, Research Press.

Christian, W.P., and Hannah, G.T.: Effective management in human services, Englewood Cliffs, N.J., 1983, Prentice-Hall, Inc.

Clark, C.C.: Enhancing wellness: a guide for self-care, New York, 1981, Springer Publishing Co., Inc.

Clark, C.C., and Shea, C.A.: Management in nursing: a vital link in the health care system, New York, 1979, McGraw-Hill Book Co.

Claus, K.E., and Bailey, J.T., editors: Living with stress and promoting well-being: a handbook for nurses, St. Louis, 1980, The C. V. Mosby Co.

Connor, P.E.: Dimensions in modern management, ed. 3, Boston, 1982, Houghton Mifflin Co.

Cummings, L.L., and Schwab, D.P.: Performance in organizations: determinants and appraisal, Glenview, Ill., 1973, Scott, Foresman & Co.

Davidson, S.V.S.: PSRO: Utilization and audit in patient care, St. Louis, 1976, The C. V. Mosby Co.

Davidson, S.V.S., et al.: Nursing care evaluation, St. Louis, 1977, The C. V. Mosby Co.

Davis, K.: Human behavior at work: organizational behavior, ed. 7, New York, 1985, McGraw-Hill Book Co.

Deegan, A.X.: Management by objectives for hospitals, Germantown, Md., 1977, Aspen Systems Corp.

DiVincente, M.: Administering nursing service, ed. 2, Boston, 1977, Little, Brown & Co.

Doughty, D.B., and Mash, N.J.: Nursing audit, Philadelphia, 1977, F.A. Davis Co.

Drew, C.: Introduction to designing research and evaluation, St. Louis, 1976, The C. V. Mosby Co.

Duke University Hospital Nursing Services: Guidelines for nursing care: Process and Outcomes, Philadelphia, 1983, J.B. Lippincott Co.

Epstein, C.: The nurse leader: philosophy and practice, Norwalk, Conn., 1982, Appleton & Lange.

The Federal Mediation and Conciliation Service: Its role in the health care industry: ℞ for labor peace, Washington D.C., 1975, U.S. Government Printing Office.

Feldman, D.C., and Arnold, H.J.: Managing individual and group behavior in organizations, New York, 1983, McGraw-Hill Book Co.

Fessler, D.R.: Facilitating community change: a basic guide, La Jolla, Calif., 1976, University Associates, Inc.

Festinger, L., and Katz, D.: Research methods in the behavioral sciences, New York, 1966, Holt, Rinehart & Winston, Inc.

Flippo, E.B.: Management: a behavioral approach, Boston, 1970, Allyn & Bacon, Inc.

Franklin, J.L., and Thrasher, J.H.: An introduction to program evaluation, New York, 1976, R.E. Krieger Publishing Co., Inc.

French, W.L.: The personnel management process, ed. 5, Boston, 1982, Houghton Mifflin Co.

Froebe, D.J., and Bain, R.J.: Quality assurance

programs and controls in nursing, St. Louis, 1976, The C. V. Mosby Co.

Ganong, J.M., and Ganong, W.L.: Nursing management, Germantown, Md., 1976, Aspen Systems Corp.

Ganong, J.M., and Ganong, W.L.: Cases in nursing management, Germantown, Md., 1979, Aspen Systems Corp.

Ganong, J.M., and Ganong, W.L.: Nursing management, ed. 2, Rockville, Md., 1980, Aspen Systems Corp.

Ganong, J.M., and Ganong, W.L.: Performance appraisal for productivity, Rockville, Md., 1983, Aspen Systems Corp.

Gibson, J.L., Ivancevich, J.M., and Donnelly, J.H.: Organizations: behavior, structure, processes, Plano, Tex., 1985, Business Publications, Inc.

Gillies, D.A.: Nursing management: a systems approach, Philadelphia, 1982, W.B. Saunders Co.

Girdano, D., and Everly, G.: Controlling stress and tension, ed. 2, Englewood Cliffs, N.J., 1986, Prentice-Hall, Inc.

Goldberg, P.: Executive health, New York, 1979, McGraw-Hill Book Co.

Goode, W.J., and Hatt, K: Methods in social research, New York, 1952, McGraw-Hill Book Co.

Gray, J.: The psychology of fear and stress, New York, 1971, McGraw-Hill Book Co.

Hampton, D.R., Summer, C.E., and Webber, R.A.: Organizational behavior and the practice of management, Glenview, Ill., 1982, Scott, Foresman & Co.

Hamrie, A.B., and Spross, J.: The clinical nurse specialist in theory and practice, ed. 5, Orlando, 1986, Harcourt, Brace, Jovanovich, Inc.

Hand, L.: Nursing supervision, Norwalk, Conn., 1981, Appleton & Lange.

Helmstadter, G.C.: Research concepts in human behavior, New York, 1970, Appleton-Century-Crofts.

Hemelt, M.D., and Mackert, M.E.: Dynamics of law in nursing and health care, Norwalk, Conn., 1978, Appleton & Lange.

Hill, L., and Smith, N.: Self-care nursing: promotion of health, Norwalk, Conn., 1985, Appleton & Lange.

Humble, J.W.: Management by objectives in action, New York, 1970, McGraw-Hill Book Co.

Jernigan, D.K., and Young, A.P.: Standards, job descriptions, and performance evaluations for nursing practice, Norwalk, Conn., 1983, Appleton-Century-Crofts.

Johnson, R.J., Steimetz, L.L., and Allen, A.D.: Labor law, Tustin, Calif., 1967, Media Masters, Inc.

Kalisch, B.J., and Kalisch, P.A.: Politics of nursing, Philadelphia, 1982, J.B. Lippincott Co.

Kaluzny, A.D., et al.: Management of health services, Englewood Cliffs, N.J., 1982, Prentice-Hall, Inc.

Keane, C.B.: Management essentials in nursing, Philadelphia, 1981, J.B. Lippincott Co.

Kerlinger, F.N.: Foundations of behavioral research, New York, 1967, Holt, Rinehart & Winston, Inc.

Kirk, R.K.: Nursing management tools, Boston, 1981, Little, Brown & Co.

Kjervik, D.K., and Martinson, I.M.: Women in stress: a nursing perspective, New York, 1979, Appleton-Century-Crofts.

Knowles, R.D.: A guide to self-management strategies for nurses, New York, 1984, Springer Publishing Co., Inc.

Koontz, H., and O'Donnell, C.: Principles of management: an analysis of managerial functions, New York, 1972, McGraw-Hill Book Co.

Lachman, V.D.: Stress management: a manual for nurses, New York, 1983, Grune & Stratton.

Langford, T.L.: Managing and being managed, Norwalk, Conn., 1981, Appleton & Lange.

Lefton, R.E., et al.: Effective motivation through performance appraisal, Cambridge, Mass., 1977, Ballinger Publishing Co.

Lippitt, G.: Visualizing change: model building and the change process, La Jolla, Calif., 1973, University Associates, Inc.

Lippitt, R., Watson, J., and Westley, B.: The dynamics of planned change, New York, 1958, Harcourt, Brace & World, Inc.

Litterer, J.A.: The analysis of organizations, New York, 1973, John Wiley & Sons, Inc.

Longest, B.B.: Management practices for the health professional, ed. 3, Norwalk, Conn., 1984, Appleton & Lange.

Luce, G.G.: Body time, New York, 1971, Bantam Books.

Luthans, F., and Kreitner, R.: Organizational behavior modification, ed. 2, Glenview, Ill., 1984, Scott, Foresman & Co.

Lynch, E.A.: Evaluation: principles and processes, New York, 1978, National League for Nursing.

Mager, R.F., and Pipe, P.: Analyzing performance problems of "you really oughta wanna," Belmont, Calif., 1970, Fearon Publishers.

Maier, N.R.F.: The appraisal interview: three basic approaches, La Jolia, Calif., 1976, University Associates, Inc.

Marriner, A.: Contemporary nursing management: issues and practice, St. Louis, 1982, The C. V. Mosby Co.

Mayers, M.G., Norby, R.B., and Watson, A.B.: Quality assurance for patient care: nursing perspectives, New York, 1977, Appleton-Century-Crofts.

McConnell, C.R.: The effective health care supervisor, Rockville, Md., 1982, Aspen Systems Corp.

McConnell, E.A.: Burnout: in the nursing profession, St. Louis, 1982, The C. V. Mosby Co.

Meisenheimer, C.C.: Quality assurance: a programming guide to effective programs, Rockville, Md., 1985, Aspen Systems Corp.

Moursund, J.P.: Evaluation: an introduction to research design, Monterey, Calif., 1973, Brooks/Cole Publishing Co.

Neale, J.M., and Liebert, R.M.: Science and behavior: an introduction to methods of research, ed. 3, Englewood Cliffs, N.J., 1986, Prentice-Hall, Inc.

Nicholls, M.E., and Wessells, V.G., editors: Nursing standards and nursing process, Rockville, Md., 1977, Aspen Publishers, Inc.

Odiorne, G.S.: Management by objectives: a system of managerial leadership, Belmont, Calif., 1965, Pitman Publishing Corp.

Ornstein, R.E.: The psychology of consciousness, ed. 2, New York, 1977, Harcourt, Brace, Jovanovich, Inc.

Peale, N.V.: The power of positive thinking, New York, 1978, Fawcett Crest.

Pender, N.: Health promotion in nursing practice, Norwalk, Conn., 1982, Appleton-Century-Crofts.

Raia, A.P.: Managing by objectives, Glenview, Ill., 1974, Scott, Foresman & Co.

Rezler, A.G., and Stevens, B.J.: The nurse evaluator in education and service, New York, 1978, McGraw-Hill Book Co.

Rossi, P.H., and Freeman, H.E.: Evaluation: a systematic approach, ed. 2, Beverly Hills, 1982, Sage Publications.

Rowland, H.S., and Rowland, B.L.: Nursing administration handbook, ed. 2, Germantown, Md., 1985, Aspen Systems Corp.

Rubin, I.M., Fry, R.E., and Plomick, M.S.: Managing human resources in health care organizations: an applied approach, Reston, Va., 1978, Reston Publishing Co., Inc.

Scanlan, B.K.: Principles of management and organizational behavior, New York, 1973, John Wiley & Sons, Inc.

Schulz, R., and Johnson, A.C.: Management of hospitals, New York, 1976, McGraw-Hill Book Co.

Schweiger, J.L.: The nurse as manager, New York, 1980, John Wiley & Sons, Inc.

Seawell, L.V.: Hospital financial accounting theory and practice, Chicago, 1975, Hospital Financial Management Association.

Sellitz, C., et al.: Research methods in social relations, New York, 1959, Holt, Rinehart & Winston, Inc.

Selye, H.: The stress of life, ed. 2, New York, 1978, McGraw-Hill Book Co.

Selye, H.: Stress without distress, New York, New American Library.

Sheridan, R.S., Bronstein, J.E., and Walker, D.D.: The new nurse manager: a guide to management development, Rockville, Md., 1984, Aspen Systems Corp.

Shortell, S.M., and Richardson, W.C.: Health program evaluation, St. Louis, 1978, The C. V. Mosby Co.

Simms, L.M., Price, S.A., and Ervin, N.E.: The professional practice of nursing administration, New York, 1985, John Wiley & Sons, Inc.

Sisk, H.L.: Management and organization, Cincinnati, 1973, South-Western Publishing Co.

Smith, H.P., and Brouwer, P.J.: Performance appraisal and human development, Reading, Mass., 1977, Addison-Wesley Publishing Co.

Stevens, B.J.: The nurse as executive, ed. 2, Rockville, Md., Aspen Publishers, Inc.

Stevens, W.F.: Management and leadership in nursing, New York, 1978, McGraw-Hill Book Co.

Stewart, C.J., and Cash, W.B.: Interviewing: principles and practice, ed. 4, Dubuque, Iowa, 1985, William C. Brown Co., Publishers.

Strauss, G., and Sayles, L.R.: Personnel: the human problems of management, Englewood Cliffs, N.J., 1972, Prentice-Hall, Inc.

Sullivan, E.J., and Decker, P.J.: Effective management in nursing, Reading, Mass., 1985, Addison-Wesley Publishing Co.

Sutterley, D.C., and Donnelly, G.F.: Coping

with stress: a nursing perspective, Rockville, Md., 1982, Aspen Systems Corp.

Tasto, D.L., and Skjei, E.W.: Spare the couch: self-change for self-improvement, Englewood Cliffs, N.J., 1979, Prentice-Hall, Inc.

Thompson, D.W.: Managing people: influencing behavior, St. Louis, 1978, The C. V. Mosby Co.

Treece, E., and Treece, J., Jr.: Elements of research in nursing, St. Louis, 1977, The C. V. Mosby Co.

Tucker, S.M., et al.: Patient care standards, ed. 4, St. Louis, 1988, The C. V. Mosby Co.

Vash, C.L.: The burnt-out administrator, ed. 3, New York, 1983, Spring Publishing Co.

Veninga, R.L.: The human side of health administration, Englewood Cliffs, N.J., 1982, Prentice-Hall, Inc.

Wandelt, M.A., and Ager, J.W.: Quality patient care scale, New York City, 1974, Appleton-Century-Crofts.

Wandelt, M.A., and Stewart, D.: Slater Nursing Competencies Rating Scale, New York, 1975, Appleton-Century-Crofts.

Warner-Reitz, A.: Healthy lifestyle for seniors, New York, 1981, Meals for Millions Freedom from Hunger Foundation.

Watson, D.L. and Tharp, R.G.: Self-directed behavior: self-modification for personal adjustment, ed. 4, Monterey, Calif., 1985, Brooks/Cole Publishing Co.

Weiss, C.H.: Evaluation research, Englewood Cliffs, N.J., 1972, Prentice-Hall, Inc.

Werther, W.B.: Unions do not happen, they are caused, New York, 1978, National League for Nursing.

Werther, W.B., and Lockhart, C.A.: Labor relations in the health professions, Boston, 1976, Little, Brown & Co.

White, J., and Fadiman, J., editors: Relax, New York City, 1976, The Confucian Press, Inc.

Journals

Planned change

Asprec, E.S.: The process of change, Supervisor Nurse 6:15-24, October 1975.

Beckhard, R.: Helping a group with planned change: a case study, J. Social Issues 15:13-19, 1959.

Beckhard, R.: Strategies for large system change, Sloan Management Rev. 16:43-55, Winter 1975.

Beyers, M.: Getting on top of organizational change. I. Process and development, J. Nurs. Adm. 14:32-39, October 1984.

Beyers, M.: Getting on top of organizational change. II. Trends in nursing service, J. Nurs. Adm. 14:31-37, November 1984.

Beyers, M.: Getting on top of organizational change. III. The corporate nurse executive, J. Nurs. Adm. 14:32-37, December 1984.

Billings, C. V., et al.: Growth and change: a nursing organization case study, Nurs. Management 17:68-75, August 1986.

Brosnan, J., and Johnston, M.: Stressed but satisfied: organizational change in ambulatory care, J. Nurs. Adm. 10:43-48, November 1980.

Claus, K.E., and Bailey, J.T.: Facilitating change: a problem-solving/decision-making tool, Nurs. Leadership 2:32-39, June 1979.

Deal, J.: The timing of change, Supervisor Nurse 8:73-79, September 1977.

deLodzia, G., and Greenhalgh, L.: Recognizing change and conflict in a nursing environment, Supervisor Nurse 4:14-25, June 1973.

DeVries, R.A.: Multi-hospital arrangements offer hospitals options in meeting change, J. Nurs. Adm. 8:43-46, December 1978.

Dietrich, B.: Effective change in nursing service is sometimes difficult to achieve because of a peculiar "two-headed" authority structure, Hosp. Management 108:44-50, December 1969.

Dugan, A.B.: Problems in leader initiated change studies, J. Psychiatr. Nurs. 8:17-20, May-June 1970.

Fenn, M.F.: Consultation: the road to change, Nurs. Mirror 135:40-41, August 11, 1972.

Fragmented process of change in nursing services wastes time, money, Can. Hosp. 47:5, June 1970.

Golembiewski, R.T.: The laboratory approach to organization change: "confrontation design," Acad. Management J. 11:199-210, 1968.

Goren, S., and Ottaway, R.: Why health-care teams don't change: chronicity and collusion, J. Nurs. Adm. 15:9-16, July-August 1985.

Greiner, L.E.: Patterns of organization change, Harvard Business Rev. 45:119-128, May-June 1967.

Greiner, L.E.: Evolution and revolution as organizations grow, Harvard Business Rev. 50:37-46, July-August 1972.

Haffer, A.: Facilitating change: choosing the appropriate strategy, J. Nurs. Adm. **16**:18-22, April 1986.

Heineken, J., and Nussbaumer, B.: Survival for nurses initiating change, Supervisor Nurse **7**:52-57, October 1976.

Hoffman, F.M.: A finger on the pulse of change, J. Nurs. Adm. **15**:24-26, April 1985.

Hofing, A.L., McGugin, M.B., and Merkel, S.I.: The importance of maintenance in implementing change: an experience with problem-oriented recording, J. Nurs. Adm. **9**:43-48, December 1979.

Kleiner, B.H.: A manager's guide to organizational change, Personnel **56**:31-38, March-April 1979.

Kriegel, J.: People are not resistant to change, Supervisor Nurse **2**:35-41, November 1971.

Labovitz, G.H.: How to improve your management effectiveness in coping with change, Hosp. Top. **52**:24-41, July-August 1974.

Lawrence, P.R.: How to deal with resistance to change, Harvard Business Rev. **47**:4-12 +, January-February 1969.

Levenstein, A.: Effective change requires change agent, J. Nurs. Adm. **9**:12-15, June 1979.

Luke, R.A., et al.: A structural approach to organizational change, J. Appl. Behavioral Sci. **9**:611-635, September-October 1973.

Marriner, A.: Behavioral aspects of planned change: reorganization, Supervisor Nurse **8**: 36-40, December 1977.

Marriner, A.: Planned change as a leadership strategy, Nurs. Leadership **2**:11-14, June 1979.

Nehls, D., et al.: Planned change: a quest for nursing autonomy, J. Nurs. Adm. **4**:23-27, January-February 1974.

New, J.R., and Couillard, N.A.: Guidelines for introducing change, J. Nurs. Adm. **11**:17-21, March 1981.

Niland, D.: Managing change: same staff, same unit—new role, Nurs. Management **16**:31-32, December 1985.

Nyberg, J.: Probing the change process, Supervisor Nurse **11**:31-33, May 1980.

O'Connor, P.A.: Poor communication: a barrier to change, Supervisor Nurse **10**:64-66, November 1979.

Olsen, E.M.: Strategies and techniques for the nurse change agent, Nurs. Clin. North Am. **14**:323-336, June 1979.

Ottaway, R.N., and Cooper, C.L.: Moving to-
ward a taxonomy of change agents, Int. Stud. Management Organization **8**:7-21, Summer 1978.

Pierik, M.M.: Experiment to effect change, Supervisor Nurse **2**:69-75, April 1971.

Porter, K.: Change . . . for patients' sake, J. Nurs. Adm. **3**:37-42, March-April 1973.

Poulin, M.A.: Nursing service: change or managerial obsolescence, J. Nurs. Adm. **4**:40-43, July-August 1974.

Rodgers, J.A.: Theoretical considerations involved in the process of change, Nurs. Forum **12**:160-174, Spring 1973.

Rosenman, H., and Jenkins, M.: A nursing staff designs its own system, Nurs. Management **17**:32-34, February 1986.

Rubin, I., Plovnick, M., and Fry, R.: Initiating planned change in health care systems, J. Appl. Behavioral Sci. **10**:107-124, January-February-March 1974.

Schlotfeldt, R.M., and MacPhail, J.: An experiment in nursing: rationale and characteristics, Am. J. Nurs. **69**:1018-1023, May 1969.

Schlotfeldt, R.M., and MacPhail, J.: An experiment in nursing: introducing planned change, Am. J. Nurs. **69**:1247-1251, June 1969.

Schlotfeldt, R.M., and MacPhail, J.: Experiment in nursing: implementing planned change, Am. J. Nurs. **69**:1475-1480, July 1969.

Schwier, M.E., and Gardella, F.A.: Identifying the need for change in nursing service, Nurs. Outlook **10**:56-62, April 1970.

Singleton, E.K., and Nail, F.C.: Guidelines for establishing a new service, J. Nurs. Adm. **15**:22-26, October 1985.

Spradley, B.W.: Managing change creatively, J. Nurs. Adm. **10**:32-37, May 1980.

Stevens, B.J.: Effecting change, J. Nurs. Adm. **5**:23-26, February 1975.

Taking the chance on change (editorial), Hosp. Forum **12**:13, November 1969.

Ward, M.J., and Moran, S.G.: Resistance to change: recognize, respond, overcome, Nurs. Management **15**:30-33, January 1984.

Watkin, B.: Management topics: change, Nurs. Mirror **139**:54, August 1974.

Welch, L.B.: Planned change in nursing: the theory, Nurs. Clin. North Am. **14**:307-321, June 1979.

Wiley L.: The safe way to introduce changes or do you like running headfirst into a brick wall? Nurs. 76 **6**:65-68, December 1976.

Zimmerman, B.M.: Changes of the second order, Nurs. Outlook **27**:199-201, March 1979.

Evaluation of personnel

Aiken, L., and Aiken, J.L.: A systematic approach to the evaluation of interpersonal relationships, Am. J. Nurs. **73**:863-867, May 1973.

Aime, D.B.: Employee evaluations: what's the difference, Supervisor Nurse **10**:52-60, June 1979.

Albrecht, S.: Reappraisal of conventional performance appraisal systems, J. Nurs. Adm. **2**:29-35, March-April 1972.

Anderson, M.: Activity contracting, Supervisor Nurse **10**:55-59, November 1979.

Behrend, B.J., et al.: Articulating professional nursing practice behaviors, J. Nurs. Adm. **16**:20-24, February 1986.

Blenkinsop, D.: Nursing staff appraisal in the Durham group of hospitals, Nurs. Times **69**:105-108, July 5, 1973.

Breeden, S.A.: Participative employee evaluation, J. Nurs. Adm. **8**:13-19, May 1978.

Brief, A.P.: Developing a usable performance appraisal system, J. Nurs. Adm. **9**:7-10, October 1979.

Clark, M.D.: Performance appraisal, Nurs. Management **13**:27-29, October 1982.

Cochran, T.C., and Hansen, P.J.: Developing an evaluation tool by group action, Am. J. Nurs. **62**:94-97, March 1962.

Colby, J.D., and Wallace, R.L.: Performance appraisal: help or hindrance to employee productivity? Personnel Adm. **26**:37-39, 1975.

del Bueno, D.J.: Performance evaluation: when all is said and done, more is said than done, J. Nurs. Adm. **7**:21-23, December 1977.

del Bueno, D.J.: Implementing a performance evaluation system, Supervisor Nurse **10**:48-52, February 1979.

Dracup, K.: Improving clinical evaluation, Supervisor Nurse **10**:24-27, June 1979.

Dunn, M.A.: Development of an instrument to measure nursing performance, Nurs. Res. **19**:502 +, November-December 1970.

Durham, R.C.: How to evaluate nursing performance, Hosp. Management **109**:24-32, May 1970.

Dyer, E.D., et al.: Can job performance be predicted from biographical, personality, and administrative climate inventories? Nurs. Res. **21**:294-304, July-August 1972.

Eigsti, D.G., and Vallone, B.B.: Ambulatory care nursing, Nurs. Management **14**:57-59, April 1983.

Engle, J., and Barkauskas, V.: The evolution of a public health nursing performance evaluation tool, J. Nurs. Adm. **10**:8-16, April 1979.

Goldstein, S.G.: On the process of evaluation, Supervisor Nurse **2**:22-23 +, July 1971.

Goodykoontz, L.: Performance evaluation of staff nurses, Supervisor Nurse **12**:39-43, August 1981.

Gordon, P.: Evaluation: a tool in nursing service, Am. J. Nurs. **60**:364-366, March 1960.

Haar, L.P., and Hicks, J.R.: Performance appraisal: derivation of effective assessment tools, J. Nurs. Adm. **6**:20-29, September 1976.

Hamric, A.B., Gresham, M.L., and Eccard, M.: Staff evaluation of clinical leaders, J. Nurs. Adm. **8**:18-26, January 1978.

Kabot, L.B.: Objective evaluation for clinical performance, Supervisor Nurse **8**:16-18, November 1977.

Kelly, R.L.: Evaluation is more than measurement, Am. J. Nurs. **73**:114-116, January 1973.

Kimball, S.J., Pardee, G., and Larson, E.: Evaluation of staff performance, Am. J. Nurs. **71**:1744-1746, September 1971.

Krumme, U.S.: The case for criterion-referenced measurement, Nurs. Outlook **23**:764-770, December 1975.

Lawson, B.N.: Evaluation: a sorry procedure, Supervisor Nurse **9**:32-33, October 1978.

Levenstein A.: The art and science of supervision: the challenge of personal growth, Supervisor Nurse **8**:66-67, November 1977.

Locher, A.H., and Teel, K.: Performance appraisal: a survey of current practices, Personnel J. **56**:245 +, May 1977.

Loraine, K.: Work evaluations: are they effective? Nurs. Management **13**:44-46, April 1982.

Lunde-Flatley, K., and Lafferty-Durbin, E.: Evaluating clinical competency in nursing, Nurs. Management **17**:47-50, August 1986.

Margerison, C.: A constructive approach to appraisal, Personnel Management **8**:30-33, 1976.

Marram, G.D.: Patients' evaluation of their care: importance to the nurse, Nurs. Outlook **21**:322-324, May 1973.

Marriner, A.: Evaluation of personnel, Supervisor Nurse **7**:36-39, May 1976.

McCoy, R.C.: Performance review: confronting the poor performer, Supervisory Management 21:12-16, 1976.

McGregor, D.: An uneasy look at performance appraisal, J. Nurs. Adm. 5:27-31, September 1975.

Medearis, N.D.: Conformity or creativity in performance evaluation, AORN J. 14:53-56, September 1971.

Meyer, H.H.: The annual performance review discussion: making it constructive, Personnel J. 56:508-511, 1977.

Milnar, R.F.: Performance analysis: a how to, Supervisor Nurse 12:14-15, February 1981.

Murphy, E.C.: Practical management course: module 6: performance evaluation, Nurs. Management 14:59-61, November 1983.

Norman, J.: The clinical specialist as performance appraiser, Supervisor Nurse 9:61-64, July 1978.

Nursing service problem: incompetent personnel, Regan Rep. Nurs. Law 15:4, August 1974.

Oberg, W.: Make performance appraisal relevant, Harvard Business Rev. 50:61-67, January-February 1972.

O'Brien, M.J.: Evaluation: a positive, constructive approach to the development of potential, Supervisor Nurse 2:24-39, April 1971.

O'Donovan, T.R.: Performance evaluation of subordinates, Supervisor Nurse 2:48-57, November 1971.

Olsen, L.O., and Bennett, A.C.: Performance appraisal: management technique or social process? I. Management Technique, Management Rev. 64:18-23, December 1975.

Patz, A.: Performance appraisal: useful but still resisted, Harvard Business Rev. 53:74-80, May-June 1975.

Riley, M.: Employee performance reviews that work, J. Nurs. Adm. 13:32-33, October 1983.

Rosen, A.: Performance appraisal interviewing evaluated by proximal observers, Nurs. Res. 16:32-37, Winter 1967.

Rosen, H., and Marella, M.: Basic quantitative thinking, J. Nurs. Adm. 11:6-10, May-June 1977.

Rowe, L.: Employee evaluation technics for supervisors, AORN J. 14:61-65, November 1971.

Schaefer, H.: Self-evaluation first, Training Business Industry 11:26-27, 1974.

Smith, J.: Managing employee performance, Nurs. Management 13:14-16, August 1982.

South, J.C.: The performance profile: a technique for using appraisals effectively, J. Nurs. Adm. 8:27-31, January 1978.

Stalker, M.Z., et al.: Measurement technology applications in performance appraisal, J. Nurs. Adm. 16:12-17, April 1986.

Stevens, B.J.: Performance appraisal: what the nurse executive expects from it, J. Nurs. Adm. 6:26-31, October 1976.

Stull, M.K.: Staff nurse performance: effects of goal-setting and performance feedback, J. Nurs. Adm. 16:26-30, July-August 1986.

Tavernier, G.: Public servants rate their own performance, Int. Management 32:19-21, 1977.

Teel, K.S.: Self-appraisal revisited, Personnel J. 57:364-367, July 1978.

Thomas, E.A.: Evaluating ancillary staff of a health center, Nurs. Management 12:52-54, September 1981.

Thompson, P.H., and Dalton, G.W.: Performance appraisal: manager beware, Harvard Business Rev. 48:149-157, January-February 1970.

Vengroski, S.M., and Saarmann, L.: Peer review in quality assurance, Am. J. Nurs. 78:2094-2096, December 1978.

Verralls, S.: Understanding staff appraisal, Nurs. Times 68:1424-1429, November 9, 1972.

Villareal, M.J.: Improving managerial performance, Personnel J. 56:86-96, February 1977.

Watkin, B.: Management topics: self appraisal, Nurs. Mirror 138:53, May 31, 1974.

Waxmann, H.: Adding to the performance appraisal, Supervisor Nurse 2:44-47, November 1971.

West, N., Sudbury, J., and Ayers, M.: An objective appraisal instrument for registered nurses, Supervisor Nurse 10:32-38, March 1979.

Wexler, K., Singh, J.P., and Yukl, G.A.: Subordinate personality as a moderator of the effects of participation in three types of appraisal interviews, J. Appl. Psychol. 58(1):54-59, 1973.

Winstanley, N.B.: Performance appraisal: another pollution problem, Conference Board Record 9:59-63, 1972.

Yura, H., and Walsh, M.: Guidelines for evaluation: who, what, when, where, and how? Supervisor Nurse 3:33-34+, February 1972.

Zawacki, R.A., and Taylor, R.L.: A view of performance appraisal from organizations using it, Personnel J. 55:290-299, 1976.

Zion, C., and Richter, S.: Selecting the right criteria for evaluation, Jr. College J. **43**:22, November 1973.

Management by objectives

Badawy, M.K.: Applying MBO to the public sector, Bureaucrat **6**:3-18, Fall 1977.

Bell, M.L.: Management by objectives, J. Nurs. Adm. **10**:19-26, May 1980.

Brady, R.H.: MBO goes to work in public sector, J. Nurs. Adm. **3**:44-52, July-August 1973.

Bucalo, J.: Personnel directors . . . what you should know before recommending MBO, Personnel J. **56**:176-202, April 1977.

Cain, C., and Luchsinger, V.: Management by objectives: applications to nursing, J. Nurs. Adm. **13**:35-38, January 1978.

Covaleski, M.A., and Dirsmith, M.W.: MBO and goal directedness in a hospital context, Acad. Management Rev. **6**:409-418, July 1981.

Dickens, S., and Stansbie, P.: Management by objectives in nursing, Nurs. Mirror **136**:28-30, June 8, 1973.

Golightly, C.: MBO and performance appraisal, J. Nurs. Adm. **9**:11-20, September 1979.

Hand, H.H., and Hollingsworth, A.T.: Tailoring MBO to hospitals, Business Horizons **18**:45-52, February 1975.

Holle, M.L.: How to make sure that things get done, RN **43**:127-128, September 1980.

Levinson, H., and La Monica, E.L.: Management by whose objectives? J. Nurs. Adm. **10**:22-30, September 1980.

McConkey, D.D.: MBO: twenty years later, where do we stand? Business Horizons **16**:25-36, August 1973.

Morrisey, G.L.: Without control, MBO is a waste of time, Management Rev. **64**:11-17, February 1975.

Odiorne, G.S.: Management by objectives: antidote to future shock, J. Nurs. Adm. **5**:27-30, February 1975.

Palmer, J.: Management by objectives, J. Nurs. Adm. **1**:17-23, January-February 1971.

Perrow, C.: The analyses of goals in complex organizations, Am. Sociol. Rev. **26**:854-865, 1981.

Pollok, C.S.: Adapting management by objectives to nursing, Nurs. Clin. North Am. **18**:481-490, September 1983.

Skarupa, J.A.: Management by objectives: a systematic way to manage change, J. Nurs. Adm. **1**:52-56, March-April 1971.

Tosi, H.L., and Carroll, S.: Some factors affecting the success of "management by objectives," J. Management Stud. **7**:209-223, May 1970.

Peer review

Dickson, B.: Maintaining anonymity in peer evaluation, Supervisor Nurse **10**:21-29, May 1979.

Mullins, A.C., Colavecchio, R.E., and Tescher, B.E.: Peer review: a model for professional accountability, J. Nurs. Adm. **9**:25-30, December 1979.

O'Loughlin, E.L., and Kaulbach, D.: Peer review: a perspective for performance appraisal, J. Nurs. Adm. **11**:22-27, September 1981.

Savage, J.: PSRO: the hospital manager's role, Nurs. Management **13**:20-24, June 1982.

Problem employees

Blose, I.L.: Confronting the alcoholic employee, AORN J. **25**:1159-1166, May 1977.

Durald, M.M.: Relating to the angry and withdrawn employee, Supervisor Nurse **11**:33-35, December 1980.

Eichhorn E.: Managing maladaptive attitudes among nursing personnel, Supervisor Nurse **12**:25-30, February 1981.

Elliott, B., and Williams, E.: Help for the helper: an employee assistance program, Am. J. Nurs. **82**:586-587, April 1982.

Flaherty, M.J.: Perspectives in nursing: how do we help incompetent colleagues? Nurs. Management **13**:11-13, July 1982.

Fulton, K.: Drug abuse among nurses: what nursing management can do! Supervisor Nurse **12**:18-20, January 1981.

Jefferson, L.V., and Ensor, B.E.: Help for the helper: confronting a chemically-impaired colleague, Am. J. Nurs. **82**:574-577, April 1982.

Kabb, G.M.: Chemical dependency: helping your staff, J. Nurs. Adm. **14**:18-23, November 1984.

Kibbee, P.: Working with the terminating employee, Supervisor Nurse **10**:34-35, December 1979.

Levenstein, A.: The art and science of supervision: alcohol and tension, Supervisor Nurse **11**:46-47, March 1980.

Marriner, A.: Problem employees . . . , Nurs. Management **17**:58-60, June 1986.

McDonald, J.M., and Shaver, A.V.: An absenteeism control program, J. Nurs. Adm. **11**:13-18, May 1981.

Mercer, M.: How to help an alcoholic without

making matters worse, Good Housekeeping pp. 50-56, November 1982.

Mercier, D.K.: Professional death sentence: why state government fires so few incompetents, Calif. J. 420-421, December 1977.

Monaghan, J., and Perro, K.: Objective management of attendance problems, Supervisor Nurse 12:44-46, August 1981.

Nursing service problem: incompetent personnel, Regan Rep. Nurs. Law 15:4, August 1974.

Samaras, J.T.: What do you do with an unproductive worker? Supervisor Nurse 10:36-37, October 1979.

Schniederjans, M.J., and Stoeberl, P.A.: Coping with ineffective subordinates, Nurs. Management 16:51-55, November 1985.

Tebbitt, B.V., and Pisani, S.H.: Staff counseling specialist: responding sensitively to workers, J. Nurs. Adm. 14:22-26, September 1984.

Discipline of personnel

Beletz, E.E.: Discipline: establishing just cause for correction, Nurs. Management 17:63-67, August 1986.

Chaska, N.L.: The "cooling out" process in a complex organization, J. Nurs. Adm. 9:22-28, January 1979.

Davis, L.A.: How do you follow up? J. Nurs. Adm. 10:25-30, February 1980.

Fair, E.W.: Cracking the whip, Supervisor Nurse 2:26-27, February 1971.

Feldman, J., and Daly-Gawenda, D.: Retrenchment: how nurse executives cope, J. Nurs. Adm. 15:31-37, June 1985.

Fleishman, R.: Disciplinary action: friend or foe? Supervisor Nurse 2:19+, May 1971.

Kjervik, D.K.: Progressive discipline in nursing: arbitrators' decisions, J. Nurs. Adm. 14:34-37, April 1984.

Marriner, A.: Discipline of personnel, Supervisor Nurse 7:15-17, November 1976.

Murphy, E.C.: Practical management course: module 2: discipline: who owns the responsibility? Nurs. Management 14:58-60, July 1983.

Murphy, E.C.: Practical management course: module 11: managing defiance, Nurs. Management 15:67-69, May 1984.

Rutkowski, B.C., and Rutkowski, A.D.: Employee discharge: it depends . . . , Nurs. Management 15:39-42, December 1984.

Smoyak, S.A.: The confrontation process, Am. J. Nurs. 74:1632-1635, September 1974.

Steines, P.A.: Employee discipline: be positive not punitive, Nurs. Management 13:29-32, March 1982.

Outplacement counseling

Borg, J.H., and Jensen, D.L.: Managing layoffs: a comprehensive approach, Nurs. Management 16:31-37, August 1985.

Dunham, B.: you can prevent it: how to tell if you're losing your job, Supervision, 7-9, September 1980.

Kangery, R., and Freund, C.M.: Outplacement service for the nurse executive, J. Nurs. Adm. 14:11-15, July-August 1984.

Murphy, E.C.: Practical management course: module 10: the counseling conundrum, Nurs. Management 15:75-77, March 1984.

Schwarz, T.H.: What to do if the boss says: you're fired! Advertising Age, February 1, 1982.

Werth, J.Z.: Wield the ax with care: you're fired! Supervision, 3-5, September 1980.

Behavior modification

Luthans, F., and Lyman, D.: Training supervisors to use organizational behavior modification, Personnel J. 50:38-44, September-October 1973.

Luthans, F., and White, D.D.: Behavior modification: application to manpower management, Personnel Adm. 35:41-47, July-August 1971.

Nord, W.R.: Beyond the teaching machine: the neglected area of operant conditioning in the theory and practice of management, Organizational Behav. Hum. Perform. 4:375-401, February 1969.

Labor relations

Adler, J.: When a nursing staff organizes: management rights and collective bargaining, Am. J. Nurs. 78:1-12, April 1978.

Amundson, N.E.: Labor relations and the nursing leader, J. Nurs. Adm. 2:10-11+, May-June 1972.

Atkinson, P.J., and Goodwin, L.: The role of the nursing administrator in collective bargaining, Nurs. Clin. North Am. 13:111-117, March 1978.

Beletz, E.E.: Some pointers for grievance handlers, Supervisor Nurse 8:12-14, August 1977.

Beletz, E.E.: Nurses' participation in bargaining

units, Nurs. Management **13**:48-57, October 1982.

Bond, G.E., and Del Togno-Armanasco, V.: Public Law 93-360, Nurs. Management **12**:27-30, November 1981.

Brown, M.L.: Effective management during labor disputes, Supervisor Nurse **11**:47-48, September 1980.

Bryant, Y.: Labor relations in health care institutions: an analysis of Public Law 93-360, J. Nurs. Adm. **8**:28-39, March 1978.

Cannon, P.: Administering the contract, J. Nurs. Adm. **10**:13-19, October 1980.

Castrey, B.G., and Castrey, R.T.: Mediation: what it is, what it does, J. Nurs. Adm. **10**:24-28, November 1980.

Claus, R.C.: The ins and outs of collective bargaining, J. Nurs. Adm. **10**:18-21, September 1980.

Cleland, R.: Grievance procedures: outlet for employee, insight for management, Hospitals **63**:58-60, August 1, 1967.

Cleland, V.S.: The supervisor in collective bargaining, J. Nurs. Adm. **4**:33-35, September-October 1974.

Cleland, V.S.: Shared governance in a professional model of collective bargaining, J. Nurs. Adm. **8**:39-43, May 1978.

Cleland, V.S.: Taft-Hartley amended: implications for nursing—the professional model, J. Nurs. Adm. **11**:17-21, July 1981.

Colangelo, M.: The professional association and collective bargaining, Supervisor Nurse **11**:27-32, September 1980.

Connelly, C., et al.: To strike or not to strike, Supervisor Nurse **10**:52-59, January 1979.

Coulton, M.R.: Labor disputes: a challenge for nurse staffing, J. Nurs. Adm. **7**:36-41, May 1976.

Creighton, H.: Law for the nurse supervisor: supervisor membership in ANA, Supervisor Nurse **7**:48-53, July 1976.

Curtin, L.L.: Negotiating for a change (editorial), Supervisor Nurse **11**:7, September 1980.

Emerson, W.L.: Appropriate bargaining units for health care professional employees, J. Nurs. Adm. **9**:10-15, September 1978.

Epstein, R.L., and Stickler, K.B.: The nurse as a professional and as a unionist, Hospitals **50**:44-48, January 16, 1976.

Erickson, E.H.: Collective bargaining: an inappropriate technique for professionals, J. Nurs. Adm. **3**:54-58, March-April 1973.

Fleishman, R.: Living with a contract, Hospitals **47**:51-54, November 16, 1973.

Fralic, M.F.: The nursing director prepares for labor negotiations, J. Nurs. Adm. **7**:4-8, July-August 1977.

Fulmer, W.E.: When employees want to oust their union, Harvard Business Rev. **56**:163-170, March-April 1978.

Goodfellow, M.: If you aren't listening to your employees, you may be asking for a union, Mod. Hosp. **113**:88-90, October 1969.

Hopping, B.: Professionalism and unionism: conflicting ideologies, Nurs. Forum **15**:372-383, 1976.

Hush, H.: Collective bargaining in voluntary agencies, J. Nurs. Adm. **1**:55-58, November-December 1971.

Imberman, A.A.: Communications: an effective weapon against unionization, Hosp. Prog. **54**:54-57, December 1973.

Jacox, A.: Conflicting loyalties in collective bargaining: an empirical illustration, J. Nurs. Adm. **1**:19-24, September-October 1971.

Jacox, A.: Collective action: the basis for professionalism, Supervisor Nurse **11**:22-24, September 1980.

Joiner, C.L.: Attitudes of primary care physicians in the state of Alabama: a preliminary report, Alabama J. Med. Sci. **2**:363-365, October 1974.

Joiner, C.L., and Blayney, K.D.: Career mobility and allied health manpower utilization, J. Allied Health **3**:157-162, Fall 1974.

Korn, R.: Nurses united! one staff's decision to strike, Am. J. Nurs. **80**:2218-2221, December 1980.

Levenstein, A.: The art and science of supervision: caught in a bind, Supervisor Nurse **11**:63-64, September 1980.

Lewis, H.L.: Wave of union organizing will follow break in the Taft-Hartley dam, Mod. Health Care **1**:25-32, May 1974.

Matlack, D.R.: Goals and trends in the unionization of health professionals, Hosp. Prog. **53**:40-43, February 1972.

Matlack, D.R.: Coping with the unionization of health professionals, Hosp. Prog. **53**:32-33+, March 1972.

Metzger, N.: Labor relations, Hospitals **44**:80-84, March 16, 1970.

Metzger, N.: The arbitration procedure. I. Hospitals **48**:47-49, April 16, 1974.

Metzger, N.: The arbitration procedure. II. Hospitals **48**:45-47, May 1, 1974.

Mignerey, D.: Report from economic and general welfare council, Colorado Nurse **77**:4-6, July 1977; 16-18, August; 3-4, September; 18, December; **78**:17-18, February 1978; 13, May.

Miller, M.: Nurses' right to strike, J. Nurs. Adm. **5**:35-39, February 1975.

Morgan, D.M.: The role of the director of nursing in collective bargaining, Can. Hosp. **50**:44-48, January 1973.

Munger, M.D.: Nursing supervision and labor laws, Supervisor Nurse **3**:15-28, September 1972.

Murphy, J.F., and Sandling, R.: Due process for student grievances, J. Nurs. Adm. **8**:39-43, November 1978.

Newstead, M.E.: Industrial relations act and nurse administrators, Nurs. Times **67**:1640-1641, December 30, 1971.

Nursing quality control: hospitals or unions, Regan Rep. Nurs. Law **16**:1, November 1975.

Phillips, D.F.: Taft-Hartley: what to expect, Hospitals **48**:18a-18d, July 1, 1974.

Phillips, D.F.: New demands for nurses. I. Hospitals **48**:31-34, August 16, 1974.

Quality not negotiable, Hospitals **48**:43, October 16, 1974.

Questions and answers about effects of Taft-Hartley amendments, Colorado Nurse **76**:15-16, June 1976.

Reece, D.A.: Union decertification and the salaried approach: a workable alternative, J. Nurs. Adm. **7**:20-24, July-August 1977.

Roach, D.L., et al.: Hospitals stand firm, ensure care in lengthy, areawide nurses' strike, Hospitals **51**:49-51, August 1, 1977.

The role of the director of an organized nursing service in collective bargaining, Am. J. Nurs. **70**:551-556, March 1970.

Rosasco, L.C.: Collective bargaining: what's a director of nursing to do? Hospitals **48**:79-113, September 16, 1974.

Rosmann, J.: One year under Taft-Hartley, Hospitals **49**:64-68, December 16, 1975.

Rotkovitch, R.: Do labor union activities decrease professionalism? Supervisor Nurse **11**:16-18, September 1980.

Sain, T.R.: Effects of unionization, Nurs. Management **15**:43-45, January 1984.

Samaras, J.T.: Administrative attitudes on collective bargaining in hospitals, Supervisor Nurse **9**:56-59, January 1978.

Sargis, N.M.: Will nursing directors' attitudes affect future collective bargaining? J. Nurs. Adm. **8**:21-26, December 1978.

Sargis, N.M.: Collective bargaining: serving the common good in a crisis, Nurs. Management **16**:23-27, February 1985.

Shaffer, F.A.: A 70-day strike by professional nurses, Supervisor Nurse **11**:49-53, September 1980.

Shaffer, F.A.: The decertification process, Supervisor Nurse **11**:55-57, September 1980.

Stevens, W.L.: Arbitrability and the Illinois courts, Arbitration J. **31**:1-25, March 1976.

Swanberg, G.: Nursing/labor relations, Hospitals **44**:54-56, August 1, 1970.

Taylor, V.E.: The dynamics of a strike, Supervisor Nurse **12**:51-52, July 1981.

Tice, K.S.: The director of nursing and collective bargaining, Supervisor Nurse **11**:34-38, September 1980.

Usery, W.J., Jr.: An interview with the director of the Federal Mediation and Conciliation Service, Hospitals **48**:45-48, September 16, 1974.

Veglahn, P.H.: Making the grievance procedure work, Personnel J. **56**:122-150, March 1977.

Werther, W.B., Jr., and Lockhart, C.A.: Collective action and cooperation in the health professions, J. Nurs. Adm. **7**:13-19, July-August 1977.

Zebrowski, D.: Collective bargaining and the director of nursing, Supervisor Nurse **5**:16-21, June 1974.

Quality assurance

Anderson, M.I.: Development of outcome criteria for the patient with congestive heart failure, Nurs. Clin. North Am. **9**:349-358, June 1974.

Anderson, N.: Audit of care processes and patient outcome: one facet of QA, Nurs. Adm. Q. **1**:117-128, Spring 1977.

Bailit, H., et al.: Assessing the quality of care, Nurs. Outlook **23**:153-158, March 1975.

Barba, M., Bennett, B., and Shaw, W.J.: The evaluation of patient care through use of ANA's standards of nursing practice, Supervisor Nurse **9**:42-54, January 1978.

Barney, M.: Measuring quality of patient care: a computerized approach, Supervisor Nurse **12**:40-44, May 1981.

Benedikter, H.: Assessing the status of a nursing audit process, Nurs. Adm. Q. **1**:129-137, Spring 1977.

Benson, C., Schmeling, P., and Bruins, G.: A systems approach to evaluation of nursing performance, Nurs. Adm. Q. **1**:67-75, Spring 1977.

Berg, H.V.: Nursing audit and outcome criteria, Nurs. Clin. North Am. **8**:331-335, June 1974.

Bille, D.A., and Jurkovic, J.: Nursing process audit: the style is individual, Nurs. Adm. Q. **1**:85-90, Spring 1977.

Blake, B.L.K.: Quality assurance: an ethical responsibility, Supervisor Nurse **12**:32-38, February 1981.

Bloch, D.: Evaluation of nursing care in terms of process and outcome: issues in research and quality assurance, Nurs. Res. **24(1)**:256-263, July-August 1975.

Bloch, D.: Criteria, standards, norms—crucial terms in quality assurance, J. Nurs. Adm. **7**:20-30, September 1977.

Brosnan, J.: Development of audit criteria for ambulatory nursing, Supervisor Nurse **12**:52-54, August 1981.

Bulman, T.: Ambulatory care: a practical way to quality assurance, Nurs. Management **16**:19-23, December 1985.

Burkey, S.L.: An audit outcome, home going instructions, Supervisor Nurse **10**:36-43, May 1979.

Byrd, J.M.: Peer review for quality charting, Supervisor Nurse **8**:25-27, July 1977.

Ceglarek, J.E., and Rife, J.K.: Developing a public health nursing audit, J. Nurs. Adm. **12**:37-43, December 1977.

Clinton, J.F., et al.: Developing criterion measures of nursing care: case study of a process, J. Nurse. Adm. **7**:41-45, September 1977.

Corn, F., and Magill, K.: The nursing care audit: a tool for peer review, Supervisor Nurse **5**:20-28, February 1974.

Correlates of the quality of nursing care, J. Nurs. Adm. **6**:22-27, November 1976.

Costanzo, G.A., and Vertinsky, I.: Measuring the quality of health care: a decision oriented typology, Med. Care **13**:417-431, May 1975.

Crockett, D., and Sutcliffe, S.: Staff participation in nursing quality assurance, Nurs. Management **17**:41-42, October 1986.

Curtis, B.J., and Simpson, L.J.: Auditing: a method for evaluating quality of care, **15**:14-21, October 1985.

Daubert, E.A.: A system to evaluate home health care services, Nurs. Outlook **25**:168-171, March 1977.

Davidson, G.E.: Collaborating with the medical staff in developing standards of care, Nurs. Clin. North Am. **8**:219-225, June 1973.

Davis, A.I.: Measuring quality: development of a blueprint for a quality assurance program, Supervisor Nurse **8**:17-26. February 1977.

Davis, D.S., et al.: Evaluating advance practice nurses, Nurs. Management **15**:44-47, March 1984.

Debski-Himberger, A.: A quality assurance program for psychiatric nursing, Supervisor Nurse **11**:25-26, November 1980.

Decker, C.M.: Quality assurance: accent on monitoring, Nurs. Management **16**:20-24, November 1985.

Decker, F., et al.: Using patient outcomes to evaluate community health nursing, Nurs. Outlook **27**:278-282, April 1979.

Devet, C. (Reezie): Monitoring: controlling the QA agenda, Nurs. Management **17**:52-56, November 1986.

Diddie, P.J.: Quality assurance: a general hospital meets the challenge, J. Nurs. Adm. **6**:6-16, July-August 1976.

Donabedian, A.: Some issues in evaluating the quality of nursing care. II. Am. J. Public Health **59**:1833-1836, October 1969.

Dorsey, B., and Hussa, R.K.: Evaluating ambulatory care: three approaches, J. Nurs. Adm. **9**:34-43, January 1979.

Dunham, G.W.: A quality of patient care project, Supervisor Nurse **7**:34-38, April 1976.

Dyer, E.E., Monson, M.A., and Cope, M.J.: Increasing the quality of patient care through performance counseling and written goal setting, Nurs. Res. **24**:138-144, March-April 1975.

Eddy, L., and Westbrook, L.: Multidisciplinary retrospective patient care audit, Am. J. Nurs. **75**:961-963, June 1975.

Edwardson, S.R., and Anderson, D.I.: Hospital nurses' valuation of quality assurance, J. Nurs. Adm. **13**:33-39, July-August 1983.

Eichorn, M.L., and Frevert, E.I.: Evaluation of a primary nursing system using the quality patient care scale, J. Nurs. Adm. **9**:11-15, October 1979.

Estes, M.D.: Introducing the nursing audit, Am. J. Nurs. **64**:91-92, September 1964.

Ethridge, P.E., and Packard, R.W.: An innovative approach to measurement of quality through utilization of nursing care plans, J. Nurs. Adm. **6**:25-31, January 1976.

Evenson, B.O.: Teaching quality assurance, Nurse Educator 5:8-12, March-April 1980.

Falls, M.E.: Collaboration for quality as seen by the nurse, Supervisor Nurse 7:49-52, November 1976.

Felton, G., et al.: Pathway to accountability: implementation of a quality assurance program, J. Nurs. Adm. 6:20-24, January 1976.

Ferguson, D.L., and Brunner, N.A.: Balancing priorities to attain quality care, Nurs. Management 13:67-69, October 1982.

Ferguson, G., and Ferguson, F.F.: As patients see us . . . , Nurs. Management 14:20-21, August 1983.

Fine, R.B.: Conceptual perspectives on the organization design task and the quality assurance function, Nurs. Health Care 7:101-104, February 1986.

Finkelman, A.W.: The standards of nursing practice and the supervisor, Supervisor Nurse 7:31-34, May 1976.

Flynn, B.C., and Ray, D.W.: Quality assurance in community health nursing, Nurs. Outlook 27:650-653, October 1979.

Fuller, M.E.: A nursing director looks at quality control, Supervisor Nurse 4:56-59, April 1973.

Gallant, B.W., and McLane, A.M.: Outcome criteria: a process for validation at the unit level, J. Nurs. Adm. 9:14-21, January 1979.

Gamberg, D., Hushower, G., and Smith, N.: Outcome charting, Nurs. Management 12:36-38, October 1981.

Gassett, H.: Q for q: quest for quality assurance, Supervisor Nurse 8:29-35, February 1977.

Gay, P.: Get it in writing, Nurs. Management 14:32-35, March 1983.

Glasson, P.L.: The struggle for total quality, Supervisor Nurse 8:36-40, February 1977.

Greenough, K.: Determining standards for nursing care, Am. J. Nurs. 68:2153-2157, October 1968.

Griffith, E.I.: A rational approach to patient service review, Nurs. Outlook 17:49-51, April 1969.

Gruendemann, B.: Evaluating nursing care: an interim AORN report, AORN J. 20:232-236, August 1974.

Hanna, K.L.: Nursing audit at a community hospital, Nurs. Outlook 24:33-37, January 1976.

Hatton, J.: Performance evaluation in relation to psychosocial needs, Supervisor Nurse 8:30-35, July 1977.

Hegedus, K.S.: A patient outcome criterion measure, Supervisor Nurse 10:40-45, January 1979.

Hegyvary, S.T., and Haussmann, R.K.D.: Monitoring nursing care quality, J. Nurs. Adm. 5:17-26, June 1975.

Hilger, E.E.: Developing nursing outcome criteria, Nurs. Clin. North Am. 9:323-330, June 1974.

Hill, B.S.: The missing ingredient in quality assistance programs, Supervisor Nurse 10:19-22, November 1979.

Holle, M.L.: Retrospective nursing audit: is it enough? Supervisor Nurse 7:23-29, July 1976.

Hover, J., and Zimmer, M.J.: Nursing quality assurance: the Wisconsin system, Nurs. Outlook 26:242-248, April 1978.

Howard-Purgatorio, K.: Improving a quality assurance program, Nurs. Management 17:38-42, April 1986.

Huang, S.H., Dasher, L.A., and Varner, C.F.: Performance appraisal for CCU nurses, Nurs. Management 12:50-55, October 1981.

Huckabay, L.: The significance of administrative control in quality assurance, Nurs. Adm. Q. 1:51-55, Spring 1977.

Hunter, A.R.: Nursing audit pinpoints needs, AORN J. 20:241-244, August 1974.

Jenkinson, V.M.: Select the right yardstick to measure nursing quality, Dimen. Health Serv. 52:40-41, May 1975.

Joyce, A.: Systematic review: you can afford it, Supervisor Nurse 8:13-18, September 1977.

Kirchoff, K.T.: Let's ask the patient: consumer input can improve patient care, J. Nurs. Adm. 6:36-40, December 1976.

Krekeler, Sister K.: Then: education control. Now: control of practice, Supervisor Nurse 7:25-27, May 1976.

Langford, T.: The evaluation of nursing: necessary and possible, Supervisor Nurse 2:65-66+, November 1971.

Laros, J.: Deriving outcome criteria from a conceptual model, Nurs. Outlook 25:333-336, May 1977.

Lewis, W.R.: Health behavior and quality assurance, Nurs. Clin. North Am. 9:359-366, June 1974.

Lindeman, C.A.: Measuring quality of nursing care. I. J. Nurs. Adm. 6:7-9, June 1976.

Lindeman, C.A.: Measuring quality of nursing care. II. J. Nurs.Adm. 6:17-19, September 1976.

Lohmann, G.: A statewide system of record audit, Nurs. Outlook **25**:330-332, May 1977.

Maciorowski, L.F., Larson, E., Keane, A.: Quality assurance: evaluate thyself, J. Nurs. Adm. **15**:38-42, June 1985.

MacKinnon, H.A., and Eriksen, L.: C.A.R.E.: a four track professional nurse classification and performance evaluation system, J. Nurs. Adm. **7**:42-44, April 1977.

Management audit for the nursing services. I. Nurs. Times **69**:49-52, March 29, 1973.

Management audit for the nursing services. II. Nurs. Times **69**:53-55, April 5, 1973.

Marriner, A.: The research process in quality assurance, Am. J. Nurs. **79**:2158-2161, December 1979.

McClure, M.L.: ANA standards for nursing services: considerations in evaluation, Supervisor Nurse **7**:27-31, August 1976.

McGuire, R.L.: Bedside nursing audit, Am. J. Nurs. **68**:2146-2148, October 1968.

McMorrow, G.: An emergency room audit for a small hospital, Supervisor Nurse **9**:33-35, August 1978.

McNally, F.: Nursing audit: evolution without pain, Supervisor Nurse **8**:40-46, June 1977.

Minniear, W.A., et al.: On the scene: the Duke University Hospital experience in Q.A., Nurs. Adm. Q. **1**:7-50, Spring 1977.

Moore, K.: Closing the audit cycle, Nurs. Management **12**:32-34, October 1981.

Moore, K.: Quality assurance and nursing audit: are they effective? Nurs. Management **13**:18-22, February 1982.

Moore, K.R.: What nurses learn from nursing audit, Nurs. Outlook **27**:254-258, April 1979.

Moore, M.A.: The Joint Commission on Accreditation of Hospitals Standards for Nursing Services, J. Nurs. Adm. **2**:12-17, March-April 1972.

Munley, M.J.: An evaluation of nursing care by direct observation, Supervisor Nurse **4**:28-34, April 1973.

Nadler, G., and Sahney, V.: A descriptive model of nursing care, Am. J. Nurs. **69**:336-341, February 1969.

Nehring, V., and Geach, B.: Patients' evaluation of their care: why they don't complain, Nurs. Outlook **21**:317-321, May 1973.

Nodal, M.R.: Facets of retrospective chart audit, Supervisor Nurse **9**:58-63, May 1978.

Nursing professional review, J. Nurs. Adm. **6**:6-12, November 1976.

O'Neal, E.A.: A framework for ambulatory care evaluation, J. Nurs. Adm. **8**:15-20, July 1978.

Pardee, G., et al.: Patient care evaluation, Am. J. Nurs. **71**:1958-1960, October 1971.

Paulen, A., and Rapp, C.: Person-centered caring, Nurs. Management **12**:17-21, September 1981.

Perkins, D.J.: Setting standards for care, Nurs. Homes **19**:22-31, March 1970.

Phaneuf, M.C.: A nursing audit method, Nurs. Outlook **12**:42-45, May 1964.

Phaneuf, M.C.: The nursing audit for evaluation of patient care, Nurs. Outlook **14**:51-54, June 1966.

Phaneuf, M.C.: Analysis of a nursing audit, Nurs. Outlook **16**:57-60, January 1968.

Phaneuf, M.C.: Quality of care: problems of measurements. I. How one public health nursing agency is using the nursing audit, Am. J. Public Health **59**:1827-1832, October 1969.

Phaneuf, M.C., and Wandelt, M.M.: Quality assurance in nursing, Nurs. Forum **13**:328-345, 1974.

Porter, S.F.: JCAH nursing standard IV, Supervisor Nurse **10**:32-38, November 1979.

Pridham, K.F.: Assessing the quality of well child care, Nurs. Clin. North Am. **9**:367-379, June 1974.

Ramey, I.G.: Setting nursing standards and evaluating care, J. Nurs. Adm. **3**:27-35, May-June 1973.

Ramirez, M.S.: Auditing of nursing care plans, Supervisor Nurse **6**:29-38, June 1975.

The relationship of nursing process and patient outcomes, J. Nurs. Adm. **6**:18-31, November 1976.

Rinaldi, L.: Managing a hospital audit committee, Supervisor Nurse **8**:60-62, June 1977.

Rinaldi, L.A.: Quality assurance '81: satisfying JCAH, Nurs. Management **12**:23-24, September 1981.

Rotkovitch, R.: The heartbeat of nursing services: standard IV, J. Nurs. Adm. **6**:32-35, May 1976.

Rosen, H., and Marella, M.: Basic quantitative thinking for nurse managers, J. Nurs. Adm. **7**:6-10, May 1977.

Routhier, R.W.: Tool for the evaluation of patient care, Supervisor Nurse **3**:15-27, January 1972.

Rubin, C.R., Rinaldi, L.A., and Dietz, R.R.: Nursing audit: nurses evaluating nursing, Am. J. Nurs. **72**:916-921, May 1972.

Rubin, C., Wallace, C., and Hill, R.: Auditing

the P.O.M.R. system, Supervisor Nurse **6**:23-31, September 1975.

Schick, D.: Steps for evaluating patient care, AORN J. **2**:237-239, August 1974.

Schwartz, D.R.: Toward more precise evaluation, Nurs. Outlook **13**:42-44, May 1965.

Selvaggi, L.M., et al.: Implementing a quality assurance program in nursing, J. Nurs. Adm. **6**:37-43, September 1976.

Singh, A.J., and May, P.R.A.: Acceptance of operations research/systems analysis in the health care field, Interfaces **7**:79-86, August 1977.

Smeltzer, C.H.: Organizing the search for excellence, Nurs. Management **14**:19-21, June 1983.

Smeltzer, C.H., Feltman, B., and Rajki, K.: Nursing quality assurance: a process, not a tool, J. Nurs. Adm. **13**:5-9, January 1983.

Spicer, J.G., and Lewis, E.M.: Intensive care staff nurses develop peer review criteria, Nurs. Adm. Q. **1**:57-61, Spring 1977.

Stevens, B.J.: Analysis of trends in nursing care management, J. Nurs. Adm. **2**:12-17, November-December 1972.

Stevens, B.J.: ANA's standards of nursing practice: what they tell us about the state of the art, J. Nurs. Adm. **4**:16-18, September-October 1974.

Strauss, M.B.: Quality assurance and nursing education, Nurse Educator **3**:19-21, March-April 1978.

Swansburg, R.C.: The consumer's perception of nursing care, Supervisor Nurse **12**:30-33, May 1981.

Taylor, J.W.: Measuring the outcomes of nursing care, Nurs. Clin. North Am. **9**:337-348, June 1974.

Thomas, Sister M.: Implementing the criteria for evaluating a hospital department of nursing, Nurs. Res. **16**:49-51, February 1968.

Trussell, P.M., and Strand, N.: A comparison of concurrent and retrospective audits on the same patients, J. Nurs. Adm. **8**:33-38, May 1978.

Wallace, R.F., and Donnelly, M.: Computing quality assurance costs, Hosp. Prog. **56**:53-57, May 1975.

Wandelt, M.A., and Phaneuf, M.C.: Three instruments for measuring the quality of nursing care, Hosp. Top. **50**:20-29, August 1972.

Watson, A., and Mayers, M.: Evaluating the quality of patient care through retrospective chart review, J. Nurs. Adm. **6**:17-21, March-April 1976.

Weinstein, E.L.: Developing a measure of the quality of nursing care, J. Nurs. Adm. **6**:1-3, July-August 1976.

Wiggins, A., and Carter, J.H.: Evaluation of nursing assessment and intervention in the surgical ICU, Nurs. Clin. North Am. **10**:121-144, March 1975.

Wiseman, J.: A nursing audit of basic care, or nursing A.B.C. II. Nurs. Times **72**:173-174, December 9, 1976.

Wolfe, H.: Can nonnurses make qualitative observations of nursing care? Nurs. Outlook **13**:52-53, February 1965.

Woolley, A.S.: The long and tortured history of clinical evaluation, Nurs. Outlook **5**:308-315, May 1977.

Wright, C., and Wheeler, P.: Auditing community health nursing, Nurs. Management **15**:40-42, March 1984.

Zimmer, M.J.: Guidelines for development of outcome criteria, Nurs. Clin. North Am. **9**:317-321, June 1974.

Zimmer, M.J.: Quality assurance for outcomes of patient care, Nurs. Clin. North Am. **9**:305-313, June 1974.

Control of stress

Armstrong, M., King, M., and Miller, B.: Avoiding orientation burnout, Nurs. Management **13**:24-27, July 1982.

Baldonado, A.: Routine role induced stress, Nurs. Management **13**:42-43, May 1982.

Baldwin, J.E.: Never jump out of a perfectly good airplane, Am. J. Nurs. **80**:916-917, May 1980.

Blainey, C.G.: Six steps to personal fulfillment in nursing, Nurs. Management **16**:37-38, February 1985.

Blau, B.: Understanding midcareer stress, Management Rev. **67**:57-62, August 1978.

Bowen, D., and Hall, D.: Career planning for employee development: a primer for managers, Calif. Management Rev. **20**:23-35, Winter 1977.

Brewer, J., et al.: A new dimension in employee development: a system for career planning and guidance, Personnel J. **54**:228-231, April 1975.

Cameron, M.: The moral and ethical component of nurse-burnout, Nurs. Management **17**:42B-42E, April 1986.

Campbell-Perry, R.: Does management style affect burnout? Nurs. Management **17**:38A-38H, March 1986.

Clark, C.: Burnout: assessment and intervention, J. Nurs. Adm. **10**:39-43, September 1980.

Clark, C.: Inner dialogue: a self-healing approach for nurses and clients, Am. J. Nurs. **81**:1191-1193, June 1981.

Cook, C.B., and Mandrillo, M.: Perceived stress and situational supports, Nurs. Management **13**:31-34, September 1982.

Cousteau, V.: How to swim with sharks: a primer, Am. J. Nurs. **81**:1960, October 1981.

Curtin, L.: Enough of reality shock, burnout, and identity crisis! (editorial), Supervisor Nurse **11**:7, October 1980.

Dohrenwend, B., and Dohrenwend, B.: Stress situations, birth order, and psychological symptoms, J. Abnorm. Psychol. **71**:215-223, June 1966.

Donnelly, G.: "How do I know I'm on the right track?" RN **43**:44-46, September 1980.

Edwards, M., and Powers, R.: Turning staff frustration to satisfaction, Nurs. Management **13**:51-52, January 1982.

Engelke, M.K.: It's time to take charge, Nurs. Management **14**:71-73, February 1983.

Flaherty, M.J.: Perspectives: on being fully alive—as a person and as a nurse, Nurs. Management **14**:50-51, July 1983.

Friedman, E.: Stress and intensive-care nursing, Heart Lung **1**:753-754, November-December 1972.

Gambacorta, S.: Head nurses face reality shock, too! Nurs. Management **14**:46-48, July 1983.

Gazzaniga, M.: The split brain in man, Sci. Am. **217**:24-29, February 1967.

Gentry, W., Foster, S., and Froehling, S.: Psychologic response to situational stress in intensive and nonintensive nursing, Heart Lung **1**:793-796, November-December 1972.

Gruber, K., and Schniewind, H.: Letting anger work for you, Am. J. Nurs. **76**:1450-1452, September 1976.

Gunderson, K., et al.: How to control professional frustration, Am. J. Nurs. **77**:1180-1183, July 1977.

Hoffmann, R.: Stress and the critical care nurse, Supervisor Nurse **12**:20-23, August 1981.

Huckabay, L., and Jagla, B.: Nurses' stress factors in the intensive care unit, J. Nurs. Adm. **9**:21-26, February 1979.

Hutchinson, J., and Murphy, E.C.: Practical management course: module 12: professional survival for nurse managers, Nurs. Management **15**:51-53, June 1984.

Ivancevich, J., and Matteson, M.: Nurses and stress: time to examine the potential problem, Supervisor Nurse **11**:17-22, June 1980.

Johnson, S.: Preventing group burnout, Nurs. Management **13**:34-38, February 1982.

Knowles, R.: Managing anxiety, Am. J. Nurs. **81**:110-111, January 1981.

Knowles, R.: Control your thoughts, Am. J. Nurs. **81**:353, February 1981.

Knowles, R.: positive self-talk, Am. J. Nurs. **81**:535, March 1981.

Knowles, R.: Disputing irrational thoughts, Am. J. Nurs. **81**:735, April 1981.

Knowles, R.: Handling depression through positive reinforcement, Am. J. Nurs. **81**:1353, July 1981.

Knowles, R.: Managing guilt, Am. J. Nurs. **81**:1850, October 1981.

Knowles, R.: Handling anger: responding vs. reacting, Am. J. Nurs. **81**:2196, December 1981.

Knowles, R.: Preventing anger, Am. J. Nurs. **82**:118, January 1982.

Knowles, R.: Managing angry feelings, Am. J. Nurs. **82**:299, February 1982.

Knowles, R.: Affirmations, Am. J. Nurs. **82**:615, April 1982.

Krone, K., and Loomis, M.: Developing practice-relevant research: a model that worked, J. Nurs. Adm. **12**:38-41, April 1982.

Lavandero, R.: Nurse burnout: what can we learn? J. Nurs. Adm. **11**:17-23, November-December 1981.

Levenstein, A.: The art and science of supervision: days of stress, Supervisor Nurse **10**:69-72, September 1979.

Levenstein, A.: Art and science of management: theft—side-effect of burnout, Nurs. Management **12**:34-37, November 1981.

Levenstein, A.: Art and science of management: ready to snap? Nurs. Management **13**:47-48, January 1982.

Levenstein, A.: Evaluating the stressors in your life, Nurs. Management **17**:27-28, August 1986.

Levenstein, A.: Responding to a time of tension, Nurs. Management **17**:24-26, March 1986.

Levenstein, A.: Stress control, Nurs. Management **15**:20-21, June 1984.

Levenstein, A.: Staving off anxiety, Nurs. Management **14**:15-16, July 1983.

Levenstein, A.: Reducing the pressure, Nurs. Management **14**:53-54, March 1983.

Levine, S.: Stress and behavior, Sci. Am. **224**:26-31, January 1971.

Magill, K.: Burnin, burnout and the brightly burning, Nurs. Management **13**:17-21, July 1982.

Maslach, C.: Burned-out, Hum. Behav. **5**:16-21, September 1976.

Meisenhelder, J.B.: Networking and nursing, Image **14**:77-80, October 1982.

Mei-Tal, V., Meyerowitz, S., and Engel, G.: The role of psychological process in a somatic disorder: multiple sclerosis, Psychosom. Med. **32**:67-87, January-February 1970.

Michaels, D.: Too much in need of support to give any? Am. J. Nurs. **71**:1932-1935, October 1971.

Morris, C.: Relaxation therapy in a clinic, Am. J. Nurs. **79**:1958-1959, November 1979.

Mullins, A., and Barstow, R.: Care for the caretakers, Am. J. Nurs. **79**:1425-1427, August 1979.

Neal, M., and Cooper, P.: Diagnosing stress in your nursing world: a home-study course good for three contact hours of CE credit, Nurs. Careers **2**:15-22, September 1980.

O'Connor, A.B.: Ingredients for successful networking, J. Nurs. Adm. **12**:36-40, December 1982.

O'Flynn-Comiskey, A.: Stress: the type A individual, Am. J. Nurs. **79**:1956-1958, November 1979.

Richter, J., and Sloan, R.: Stress: a relaxation technique, Am. J. Nurs. **79**:1960-1964, November 1979.

Rodgers, J.: Women and the fear of being envied, Nurs. Outlook **30**:344-347, June 1982.

Rosenthal, T., and Rosenthal, S.: Managing risks, Nurs. Management **14**:38-40, April 1983.

Ryan, M.A.: Professional survival, Supervisor Nurse **12**:16-17, February 1981.

Schein, E.H.: How "career anchors" hold executives to their career paths, Personnel J. **52**:11-24, May-June 1975.

Schorr, T.M.: Burnout (editorial), Am. J. Nurs. **80**:1781, October 1980.

Scully, R.: Stress in the nurse, Am. J. Nurs. **80**:912-915, May 1980.

Shubin, S.: Burnout: the professional hazard you face in nursing, Nursing 78 **8**:22-27, July 1978.

Sime, A.M., and Kelly, J.W.: Lessening patient stress in the CCU, Nurs. Management **14**:24-26, October 1983.

Smith, M., and Selye, H.: Stress: reducing the negative effects of stress, Am. J. Nurs. **79**:1953-1955, November 1979.

Sperry, R.W.: The great cerebral commissure, Sci. Am. **210**:42-52, January 1964.

Spicer, J.G.: Help for the staff nurse in crises, Supervisor Nurse **9**:82-83, September 1978.

Spilken, A., and Jacobs, M.: Prediction of illness behavior from measures of life crises, manifest distress and maladaptive coping, Psychosom. Med. **33**:251-264, May-June 1971.

Storlie, F.J.: Burnout: the elaboration of a concept, Am. J. Nurs. **79**:2108-2111, December 1979.

Stress: ten sure ways to cope, Weight Watchers **2**:10+, January 1979.

Thomas, J.: Supervisors get burned-out too, Nurs. Management **13**:47-49, May 1982.

Tierney, M.J.G., and Strom, L.M.: Stress: type A behavior in the nurse, Am. J. Nurs. **80**:915-918, May 1980.

Wadsworth, N.S., Clark, N.L., and Hollefreund, B.: Managing organizational stress in nursing, J. Nurs. Adm. **16**:21-29, December 1986.

Warnath, C.F., and Shelton, J.L.: The ultimate disappointment: the burned-out counselor, Personnel Guidance J. **55**:172-175, December 1976.

Webster, S., et al.: The support group, Nurs. Management **13**:26-30, September 1982.

Weiss, J.M.: Psychological factors in stress and disease, Sci. Am. **226**:104-113, June 1972.

Wyler, A.R., Masuda, M., and Holms, T.H.: Magnitude of life events and seriousness of illness, Psychosom. Med. **33**:115-122, March-April 1971.

Yee, B.H.: The dynamics and management of burnout, Nurs. Management **12**:14-16, November 1981.

APPENDIX

Lake View Hospital is a ninety-eight-bed general hospital. It is one of two hospitals serving an industrial community with a population of about 90,000. Because a new industry has moved to the area, the population has recently increased. Consequently, a building program that will add several units is in progress.

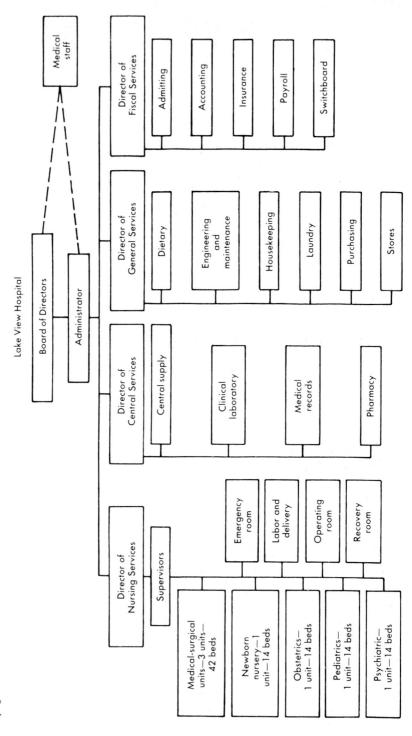

Lake View Hospital

INDEX

A

Abdominal breathing, 353
Absenteeism, 133, 157, 159, 161–163, 302–303
  dealing with, 306
  job dissatisfaction and, 239
Acceptance priority rule, 21
Acceptance rule, 20
Accommodation, 219
Accountability, 80, 100
  decentralization and, 96–97
Accounting, 44–45
Accreditation of Hospitals, Joint Commission on, 325–326, 334–335
Accrediting agencies, 325
Active listening, 248, 298
Adams, Jo Stacy, study of perceptions of equity by, 235
Adaptive model, *88*, 89
Adhocracy organizational models, 82–89
Administrators, top, function of, 35
Adult ego state, 253–254
Adult-to-adult transactions, 254
Advisory staff, 104
Affirmative action, 139–146
Age Discrimination in Employment Act (1967), 139
Agency mission, 76
Agendas, 29, 57
Aggregate management, 83–84
Aggressive behavior, 249–250, 260, 301–302; *see also* Angry employees
Aggressor, 228
Alcoholic employees, 300–301
Alcoholics Anonymous, 301, 306
Alderfer, Clayton, modified need hierarchy theory of, 232–233
All-channel network system, 242–243
Alternatives
  choosing, 6–7
  conflicting, 7
  exploring, 5–6, 221
Ambiguity in role; *see* Role ambiguity
American Arbitration Association, 322
American Hospital Association, 334
American Nurses' Association, 38, 325
  Standards of Nursing Practice, 334, 335
Anchoring, 350
Anderson, Bernice E., nursing functions identified by, 335

Anecdotal evaluation, 289
Angry employees, 301–302
Annual leave, 39
Annual review, 293–294
Appeal, right of, 311
Application forms, 134–135
Appraisal interview, 296–299
Appraisal reports, 299–300
Arbitration, 322–323
Argyris, Chris
  immaturity-maturity continuum, 188
  needs research and recommendations of, 199–200, 205
  psychological energy theory of, 234, 238
Assertive behavior, 302, 349
  barriers to, 252–253
  life positions and, 258–259
  techniques of, 259–262
  transactional analysis and, 253–258
Assessment tools, 60
Assignment systems, 146–151
Assistant staff, 103–104
Associate nurse, 150
Attendance policies, 302
Attention-getting behavior, 216
Attitudes, 22–23
Audits
  as control tool, 341–342
  internal, 342
  marketing, 59–60
  for quality assurance, 334, 337, 341
Authoritarianism, 95
Authority, 208–209
  acceptance of, 194
  ambiguous, 84–85
  in bureaucracy, 79
  of committees, 28
  delegation of, 26, 37, 95, 99–100
  line, 103
  rational legal, 193
  relationships, 108
  responsibility and, 93
  scalar chain of, 192
  staff, 103–105
Authority-obedience management, 202, *203*
Authorized penalties, 311
Autocratic behavior, 81
Autocratic manager, 22, 195, 297
Autogenic training, 355–356
Avoidance, 218–219

B

Barnard, Chester, 194
  implications of work of, for nursing adminis-
    tration, 205
BARS, 291
Basic needs theory, 233
Baths, 357
Baylor plan, 158–159
"Bear trapper" game, 257
Behavior modification; *see also* Operant condi-
  tioning
  of employee, 311–316
  for performance problems, 314–316
  techniques, 312–313
Behavioral factors, of organizational change,
  106–120
Behavioral observation scales; *see* BOS
Behavioral science, 196–204
Behaviorally anchored rating scales; *see* BARS
Behaviors, 23
Benevolent-authoritative management system,
  201
Berne, Eric, 253, 256–258
Bills, passing of, 211–213
Biofeedback, 355
Blake, Robert, managerial grid of, 202–203, 205
Blanchard, Kenneth H., model of leadership
  theory of, 187, 203–204
"Blemish" game, 257
Block scheduling, 155–156
Blocker, 229
Board of directors, function of, 35
Bookkeeping; *see* Accounting
Boredom, 302
BOS, 291–292
Boycotts, 317
Brainstorming, 5, 30, 337
Break-even calculations, 344–345
Breathing, abdominal, 353
Broken record technique, 260–261
Buck-passing, 103
Budget cycle, 43–44
Budgeting process, 50
Budgets; *see also* Cost containment; Costs
  advantages and disadvantages of, 49
  capital expenditure, 46
  cash, 46
  delegation of, 98
  operating, 45–46
  personnel, 46–47
  planning of, 43–50

Budgets—cont'd
  prerequisites to, 44–45
  review, 48
  supplementary, 48–49
Bureaucracy
  structures of, 78–81, 88
  theory of, 192–193
Burnout, 347

C

Calendar of events, 325, *326*
Capital expenditure budgets, 46
Career advancement, 146; *see also* Mentorships;
    Preceptorships
Career development programs, 110
Case method, 146
Cash budgets, 46
Catharsis, 304
Centalized scheduling, 152–153
Centering, 351–352
Centralization, 95–97
  delegation and, 97–101
  departmentalization and, 101–103
  of organization, 192
Chain communication system, 242
Change; *see also* Organizational change
  coercive, 284
  in environment, 351
  management of, 282–287
  manager's role in, 285
  process of, 283–284
  strategies for effecting, 110, 282–283
  stress and, 345–346
  types of, 284–285
Charismatic theory of leadership, 183, 193
Charitable organizations, 38
Charts
  circular, 90–91
  content analysis of, 339
  for control, 341
  decision, 226–227
  flow process, 114, *116–117*
  Gantt, 191, 205
  horizontal, 90
  organizational, 57, 82, 87, 89–91
  vertical, 89–90
Cheaper by the Dozen, 191
Checklists, 289
Child ego state, 253, 254
Childcare programs, 133

Child-to-child interactions, 254–255
Church groups, 38
Circular communication system, 242
Civil Rights Act (1964), 139
Classic organization, 192–193
Clients
  orientation of, 102–103
  profiles of, 60
Clinical systems, computerized, 16
Closed-ended questions, 137
Cluster sampling, 340
Coalition, 207–208
Codes of conduct, 311
Coercive change, 284
Coercive power, 206
Cognitive dissonance, 22–23
Collaboration, 219
Collective bargaining, 38, 324
Collective decision making, 237–238
Collegial model of management, 8, 82–83
Collegial relationships, 151
Commitment, 88
Committee chairperson, 29–30
Committee management, 192
Committee meetings, 29
Committees
  creativity in, 30–31
  in decision making, 26–31
  functioning of, 27–30
Communication
  about change, 107
  assertive, 259–262
  barriers to, 213, 246–247
  channels, 78
  diagonal, 245
  with difficult people, 249–252
  direct, 94
  downward, 243
  gaps between shifts, 157, 158
  through grapevine, 245–246
  improvement of, 247–249
  informal network of, 207
  lateral, 83, 244
  nonverbal, 298–299
  open, 82
  poor, 106
  process of, 241–242
  of regulations, 142–143
  skills, 184
  styles of, 252
  systems for, 242–243
  three-way, 202

Communication—cont'd
  time spent in, 93–94
  upward, 243–244
  vertical vs. horizontal, 83
  written, 94, 248–249
Compartmentalization, 351
Competition, 219–220
Competitors, determination of, 60
Complainers, 251
Compromise, 219
Compromiser, 228
Computers
  advantages of, 16
  applications, 16
  in scheduling, 153
  simulations, 10
  software for, 17
Conceptual thinking, 1
Conceptualization, 10
Conflict, 7
  latent, 217
  power and, 207–208
  prevention of, 231
  reactions to, 216–217
  resolution of, 218–231
  rule, 20
  sources of, 213–214
  stages of, 217–218
  theory of, 213–218
  types of, 214–216
Consensus, 83, 222; *see also* Cooperation
  difficulty in reaching, 95
  group, 87
  interdepartmental, 84
  need for, 213, 214
Consultation, 31–32
Consultative management system, 200, 201
Contingency model of leadership, 185–187, 203
Continuity of care, 157, 158, 163
Contractual model, 8
Contrast error, 288
Control, 2
  purpose of, 282
  tools for, 341–345
Control staff, 104
Control systems, 80
Conversion reaction, 217
Cook, Morris, recommendations of, 191–192
  implications of for nursing, 205
Cooperation, 194, 237
  need for, 76
Cooperative counseling, 305

Coordinator, 228
Coping behaviors, 216, 217
"Corner" game, 257
Correspondence, 5
Cost awareness, 51
Cost containment, 50–52; see also Budgets
Cost controls, 86
Costs
  break-even, 344–345
  of inventory, 342–343
  personnel, 46–47
  standard, 47–48
  variable, 344
Counseling, 304–305
  family, 306
  outplacement, 305–307
Counseling notes, 306
Counseling services, 357
Counterbalanced designs, 331–332
Country club management, 202, 203
Creative process, 5
Creative solutions, 5
Creativity, 184
  in committees, 30–31
Critic, 228
Critical incident checklist, 289
Critical-incident method, 197
Critical-path method (CPM), 14
Critical-path scheduling, 86
Criticism, dealing with, 261, 262
Cyclical scheduling, 155–156

D

Data collection, 6
Davidson, Sharon Van Sell, 336
Day
  8 hour, 5-day workweek, 156
  10 hour, 4-day workweek, 156–157
  10 hour, 7-day workweek, 157–158
  10 hour, plus 5- or 6-hour shift, 157
  12-hour shift, 7-day workweek, 158
Decentralization, 95–97, 147, 237, 238
  delegation and, 97–101
  departmentalization and, 101–103
Decentralized scheduling, 153
Deci, Edward L., study of intrinsic motivation
    by, 236
Decision(s)
  acceptance of, 20–21
  announcing, 17

Decision(s)—cont'd
  communication of, 95
  effectiveness of, 21–22
  fairness of, 20–21
  inviting discussion of, 17
  quality of, 19
  selling, 17
  tentative, 18
Decision charting, 226–227
Decision makers, 22–24
Decision making, 1
  behavioral aspects of, 17–31
  collective, 237–238
  committee aspects of, 26–31
  continuum of participation in, 17, 17–22
  diffusion of; see Centralization; Decentraliza-
      tion
  ethical aspects of, 7–9
  European-style, 83
  evaluation of, 7
  fast, 95
  by group, 18–22, 222–223
  group factors in, 24–26
  individual and, 22–24
  influence on, 240
  by middle management, 87
  process of, 4–7
  styles of, 19
  tools for, 9–17
Decision trees, 11–12
Delegation
  accountability and, 80
  of assignments, 98
  of authority, 95, 243
  in decentralized and centralized organiza-
      tions, 97–101
  factors facilitating, 97–98
  roles and, 79
  time management and, 54, 58
Delphi technique, 31
Democratic supervision, 195
Demotion, 310, 311
Departmentalization, 101–103, 108
Depression, 353
Diagnostic-related groups (DRGs), 51
Diet; see Nutrition and stress
Difficult people, communicating with, 249–252
Directing, 2; see also Leadership
  purpose of, 182
Directive counseling, 304
Disciplinary action, principles of, 308–309
Disciplinary records, 311

Discipline
  components of, 311
  need for, 307–308
  types of, 310–311
Discrimination, 140, 317; *see also* Affirmative Action; Equal Employment opportunity
Displacement, 217
Dissatisfaction, 233–234, 283
Distress, 346
Dominator, 228
DRGs; *see* Diagnostic-related groups (DRGs)
Driving forces, 285–286
Drucker, Peter, 204–205
Drug addicts, 300–301
Dual management, 78
Duty, 8

E

Education
  continuing, 5, 143–144
  in-service, 32–33, 133
Education Amendments (1972), 139
Educational institutions, policy of, 38
Educational programs, 358
Educational system, computerized, 16
Efficiency
  engineering, 191
  maximizing of, 195
  measurement of, 106
Egoism, 8
Elaborator, 228
Elite theory, 209
Emerson, Harrington, 191, 205
Empirical-rational strategies, 282
Employee policies, 36–40
Employees; *see also* Personnel; Staff; Staffing
  boredom of, 114
  counseling of, 304–305
  motivation of, 115
  termination of, 303, 305, 306, 307, 310–311
Emulative change, 284
Encourager, 228
Energizer, 228
Engineering model, 8
Environmental changes, 351
Environmental factors, 159–160
Equal Employment Act (1972), 139
Equal opportunity, 139–146
Equal Pay Act, 139
Equilibrium, 106–107

Equity theory, 235–236
Equivalent-time-samples design, 331
Esteem; *see* Self-esteem
Esteem needs, 232
Ethical considerations, 7–9
Ethical relationships, 8
European-style management, 82
Evaluation
  of decision making, 7
  of organization, 108
Exchange theory, 58–59, 209
Executive Order 11246, 139
Exercise and stress, 352–353
Exercise programs, 358
Existence-relatedness-growth theory, 232–233
Expectancy theory, 234–235
Expenses, 45–46
Experience, drawing on, 5
Experimental mortality, 328
Experimenter effect, 328–329
Expert power, 206
Exploders, 250
Exploitive-authoritative management system, 200–201
External consultant, 32
Extinction, 313

F

FAA; *see* Federal Aviation Agency
Factoral design, 330
Fair Labor Standards Act Amendments, 158
Fairness, 8
  perception of, 235–236
  rule, 20–21
Family
  counseling, 306
  as support group, 357
Fantasy, flight into, 217
Fayol, Henri, 92, 192, 193, 205
Featherbedding, 318
Federal Aviation Agency (FAA) staff rotation system, 154
Federal Mediation and Conciliation Service, 322
Feedback, 80, 221, 242, 247; *see also* Biofeedback
  change and, 107
  to and from committees, 28
  for learning, 299
  in termination process, 306
Feeling pauses, 349–350

Fiedler, Fred, leadership model introduced by, 185–187, 203, 205
Field theory, 234
Financial planning; see Budgets
Financial statements, 43
Fines, 310
First-line supervisors, 38
Fixation, 217
Flat organizational structure, 94–95
Flow diagram, 13
Flow process chart, 114, *116–117*
Fogging, 261
Follett, Mary Parker, 194, 205
Follower, 228
Forced-distribution technique, 289, 292
Force-field analysis, 285–287
Formalism, 8
Free-form organizational design, 82
Frequency distribution, 341
Frequency-rating scale, 291–292
Functional departmentalization, 101–102
Functional line organization, 87
Functional nursing, 146–147
Functional staff, 104–105
Funnel technique, 137

G

Galvanic Skin Response, 355
Game(s)
  theory, 11
  theory, of politics, 209
  transactional, 256–258
Games People Play, 256
Gantt, Henry L., 191
Gantt chart, 191, 205
Gatekeeper, 228
General staff; see Staff
Geographical location, 81
Gestalt psychology, 195
Gilbreth, Frank B., 190, 205
Gilbreth, Lillian M., 190–191, 205
Goal congruence rule, 20
Goals, 34–36, 201
  of program, 325
  reinterpretation of, 216
  setting of, 284–285, 297, 298, 348
  superordinate, 238
Graicunas, A. V., formula of, for potential relationships, 92
Grapevine, 245–246

Graphic rating scales, 290–291
Great man theory, 183
Grid of topics, 137
Grievance procedures, 308, 322, 324
Grievances, 321, 322
Group action, 83
Group cohesiveness, 26
Group conflict, resolution of, 221–230
Group creativity, 30–31
Group decision making, 18–22, 24–26, 222–223
  factors in, 24–26
Group observer, 228
Group personalities, 195
Group process, 227–228, 229
Group-task roles, 227–228
Groupthink, 25–26

H

Halo error, 288
Hamilton, General, 92
Handicapped, 140
Harassment grievances, 322
Harmonizer, 228
"Harried" game, 258
Harris, Thomas, 253
Hawthorne effect, 328
Hawthorne studies of productivity, 194–195
Head nurse, responsibilities of, 152–153
Health promotional programs, 358
Help-seeker, 229
Hersey, Paul, model of leadership theory by, 187, 203–204
Herzberg, Frederick, theory of needs motivation of, 197–198, 205, 233–234, 238–239
  comparison of with other theories, 199, *200*
Hierarchy, 78; *see also* Bureaucratic structure; Organizations
  of needs, 196–197, *199*, 205, 231–232, 239
Horizontal organizational growth, 107–108
Horns error, 288
Hostile-aggressive personalities, 249–250
Hot cargo agreements, 317
House, Robert J., leadership theory of, 187
House of Representatives, 211–212
Human relations, 193–196
  training, 87
Humor, 351
Hygiene factors, 234, 239
Hypotheses, 5

I

"I could kick myself for that" game, 258
"I feel" message, 349
Ideas, free exchange of, 30–31
Identification, 216
"If it weren't for you" game, 257
Illumination, 6
Image, 59
Imagery, mental, 356–357
Immaturity-maturity continuum, 188
Implementation, 7
Impoverished management, 202, *203*
Incidental sampling, 340
Incompetent executive, 109
Incubation, 6
Independent listing, 223
Indoctrination, 284
Inequity, perceived, 235–236
Informal power, 206–207
Information giver, 228
Information rule, 20
Information seeker, 228
Initiator-contributor, 228
Inner shouting, 350
Innovation, 6
"I'm not OK" game, 258
In-service education, 32–33, 133, 282
Instrumentation, 327–328
Integrative leadership model, 189
Intensive care nurses, 159
Interactional change, 284
Interdepartmental consensus, 84
Interdepartmental differences, 214
Intergroup conflict, 215, 229–230
Intermittent reinforcement, 313, 316
Intern programs, 133
Internal consultant, 31–32
Internship program, 143
Interpersonal conflict, 215, 220–221
Interpersonal relations, 191; *see also* Human
        relations
    power and, 207, 208
Interrole conflict, 214
Intersender conflict, 214
Interview, 135–138
    appraisal, 296–299
    corrective, 306
    to evaluate care, 338–339
    of minorities and women, 141–142
Intimacy, 258
Intragroup conflict, 215

Intrasender conflict, 214
Intrinsic motivation, 236
Intuition, 10
Inventory control, 342–343

J

James, Muriel, 253
Japanese management theory, 237–238
Jethro, 92
Job analysis, 110
Job classification analysis, 140–141
Job descriptions, 82, 98, 108, 115–120
    inadequate, 215
    samples of, 118–120
Job design, 113–115
Job enlargement, 114, 115, 237
Job enrichment, 115, 238
Job evaluation, 111–113
Job hunting assistance, 307
Job performance
    behavior modification for problems with, 314–
        316
    chronic problems with, 301
    poor, 306
Job responsibilities
    identification of, 293
Job rotation, 115, 238, 302
Job satisfaction, 157, 239–240
Job sharing, 159
Job simplification, 114
Jongeward, Dorothy, 253
Judgment errors, 288–289

K

"Kick me" game, 258
Kuder-Richardson test for reliability, 338

L

Labor law, 316–318
Labor Management Relations Act, 316–317, 320
Labor policies, 38
Labor relations, 316–324
Labor unions; *see* Unions
Labor-Management Reporting and Disclosure
        Act; *see* Landrum-Griffin Act
Landrum-Griffin Act, 316

Layoff, 310, 311
Leader-member relations, 203
Leadership
  autocratic, 22, 195, 297
  in committees, 28
  contingency model of, 203
  continuum of, 17–22
  critical dimensions of, 202–203
  effectiveness of, 185
  qualities of, 183–184
  styles of, 2, 19, 184, 187–188, 203–204
  theories of, 182–189
  of unions, 324
Learning, of role, 24
Leave without pay, 39–40
Legislative process, 211–213
Legislators, 210–211
Legitimate power, 206; see also Authority
Lesnik, M. J., nursing functions identified by, 335
"Let's you and him fight" game, 258
Lewin, Kurt
  force field analysis of, 234, 285
  group dynamics study by, 195, 205
Life and death situations, 345
Life positions, 258–259
Life-cycle theory, 187–189
Likert, Rensis, management theory of, 200–202, 205, 237
Likert Scale questionnaire, 200
Line authority, 103, 208–209
Linear programming, 15
Line-staff conflict, 105
Line-staff relationships, 103–106
Linking-pin concept, 201–202
Listening, active, 248, 298
Listening techniques, 55
Literature review, 5
Love needs, 232
"Lunch bag" game, 258

M

Majority rule, 222–223
Male-female role competition, 252
Management
  areas of, 204
  by committee, 192
  computerized information systems, 16
  European-style, 82
  functions of, 1, 4

Management—cont'd
  games, 11
  goals of, see Goals
  by objectives, 204, 205, 293–295, 297
  pool, 96
  process school, 192
  scientific, 189–192
  span of, 92–94, 108
  styles of, 17, 198–199, 202–203, 234
  team, 202–203, 297
  theories of, 189–205, 236–237
  training opportunities for, 87
  types of systems, 200–201
  unfair labor practices by, 317
Manager(s)
  as change agent, 285
  functional, 85–87
  line vs. staff, 103–106
  psychological distant, 186
  responsibilities of, 194
  termination of, 109
  underutilization of, 97
Manipulative power, 208
Manuals, 82
MAPS design technology, 287
Market, 59
  segmentation, 60–61
Marketing audit, 59–60
Marketing
  concepts of, 58–59
  implementation of, 61–62
  mix, 61
  process of, 59–62
Maslow, Abraham, hierarchy-of-needs theory of, 196–197, 199, 200, 205, 231–232, 238, 239
Massage, 353–354
Maternal Child Health programs, 333–334
Matrix organization, 84
  designs, 87–88
"Maximax" criteria, 9–10
"Maximin" criterion, 10
May, Rollo, 208
Mayo, Elton, 194, 205
MBO; see Management, by objectives
McClelland, David, basic needs theory of, 233
McGregor, Douglas, management theory of, 198–199, 200, 205, 236–238
Medicaid, 333
Medicare, 51, 333
Meditation, 356

Meetings
  length of, 56–57
  with subordinates, 99
Memoranda, 94
Memory techniques, 55
Mental imagery, 356–357
Mentorship, 145–146
Methods improvement, 113–114
Minorities, 140
  goals for, 141
  interviewing, 141–142
Model theory, 10–11
Modified need hierarchy, 232–233
Modular nursing, 149
Monistic theory, 231
Monte Carlo technique, 15
Mooney, James, 193
Morale, 37, 95, 234
Moreno, Jacob L., sociometry theory of, 195–196, 205
Moses, 92
Motion studies, 113, 205
Motivation, 231–235, 237–240
  intrinsic, 236
  process of, 197
Motivation theory, 238–239
Motivational techniques, 324
Motivation-hygiene theory, 233–234
Mouton, Jane, managerial grid of, 202–203, 205
Moving budgets, 49
Multiple time-series design, 332–333
Multiple-treatment interference, 328
Multistage sampling, 340
Music, 357

N

Narcotics Anonymous, 301
National Labor Relations Act (NLRA), 316, 317
National Labor Relations Board, 316, 319–320, 323–324
National League for Nursing, 38, 325
Natural change, 284
Need hierarchy; see Basic needs theory; Hierarchy, of needs; Modified need hierarchy
Need satisfaction, 196–200
Needs, 7–8
Negative assertion, 261, 262
Negative feelings, 349
Negative inquiry, 261, 262

Negative people, 251
Negative thinking, 350–351
Nervous tension, 353
Network analysis techniques, 14
Nominal group technique, 221–224
Nondirective counseling, 304–305
Nonequivalent control group, 331
Nonprofit Health Care Amendments, 317
Normative model, 19–22
Normative re-educative strategies, 282–283
Norms (group), 26
Not-OK feelings, 258, 259
Novelty effect, 328
"Now I've got you, you SOB" game, 257
Numerical rating scale, 289–290
Nurse administrators, politics of, 210
Nurse internship program, 143
Nurse manager(s); see also Manager(s)
  politics and, 210
  role of in collective bargaining, 324
Nurse recruiter, 132–134
Nurses
  intensive care, 159
  part-time, 163–165
  socialization of, 259
Nurses' aides, 147
Nursing
  functional, 146–147
  functions, 335
  leadership and, 182
  leveling of staff, 150–151
  management theory in, 204–205
  modular, 149
  pools, 156
  primary, 149–150
  procedures, 40–43
  qualifications, 132
  schedules, 151–159
  service goals and objectives, 32–33, 35–36
  service philosophy, 33–34
  socialization process of, 252
  team, 146, 147–149, 151
  technical, 186
Nursing care
  plan, 148
  time standards for, 161
Nursing Care Evaluation, 336
Nursing Practice and the Law, 335
Nursing services, educational, 144
Nutrition and stress, 352, 358

O

Objectives, 34–36
  management by, 293–295, 297
  policy and, 38
Observations, 341
Odiorne, George S., 204, 205
Offenses, records of, 311
OK feelings, 259
Open door policy, 98
Operant conditioning, 208, 235
Operating budgets, 45–46
Operational procedures, 109–110
Operations research, 282
Opinion giver, 228
Opinion seeker, 228
Oral reprimand, 305–306, 310
Organization(s)
  classic, 192–193
  climate of, 17
  design of, 287
  developmental stages of, 76–77
  formal, 77–78, 91
  by geographical location, 81
  goals of, 294
  informal, 77, 78, 91
  philosphy of, 17
  principles of, 78–81, 193
  as social system, 194
  by specialization, 80–81
  structure of, 77–89, 91
Organization theory, 192–193
Organizational change
  behavioral aspects of, 106–120
  to fit new needs, 76–77
  planning for, 108–110
  resistance to, 107
  strategies for, 110
  types of, 107–108
Organizational charts, 57, 82, 87, 89–91
Organizational concepts, 89–106
Organizational conflict, 230–231
Organization-man management, 202, 203
Organizing process, 1, 76
Orientation, 142–143, 308
Orientation program, 133
Orienter, 228
Outplacement counseling, 305–307
Overtime, 157

P

Paid time off, 303
Paperwork, streamlining, 54
Paraphrasing, 298–299
Parent ego state, 253, 254
Parent-to-child interactions, 255
Parent-to-parent interaction, 254
Participative management system, 200, 201–202, 297
  theory of, 237, 238–239
Passive behavior, 260, 302
Passive-aggressive behavior, 259
Pastimes, 256, 258
Path-goal theory, 187
Patient classification systems, 160–161
Peer review, 295–296
Peer support groups, 357
Perceptions, 23
Performance appraisal
  common errors in, 288–289
  methods of, 289–300
  purposes of, 287–288
Personal contacts, 94
Personality, 23; see also Type A and Type personality
Personality and interest testing, 138–139
Personnel; see also Employee(s); Staff; Staffing
  assignment of tasks, 114
  budgets, 46–47
  changes in, 108–109
  discipline of, 307–311
  evaluation of, 287–300
  files, 294
  motivation of, 110, 231–240
  policies, flexible, 133
  probationary period, 143
  problem employees, 300–305
  recruitment and hiring of, 110
  resistance of to change, 107
  retention of, 132–134
  screening of, 134–139
  skill levels of, 115
  sources of, 133
  survey of, 108
  variables affecting, 159–165
Personnel assignment(s), 87–88
  systems for, 146–151
Personnel records, 294
  cumulative evaluation, 300
  disciplinary action in, 311
Person-role conflict, 214–215

PERT, 12–14
  chart, 191
Phaneuf, Maria C., 335, 336
Philosophy of department, 33–34
Physiological needs, 232
Picket lines, 318
Planned change, 284–285
Planning, 1; *see also* Decision making; Problem
    solving
  of budget, 43–52
  for change, 108–110
  documents, 94
  long-range, 85, 88, 97
  purpose of, 4
  of time management, 52–58
Planning process
  for budget, 43–50
  goals and objectives of, 34–36
  philosophy of, 33–34
  policies and, 36–40
  procedures of, 40–43
  purpose of, 32–33
Plans, communication of, 93–94
Playboy, 229
Pluralist theory, 209
Point system of job evaluation, 111–113
Policies, 1, 5, 36–40
  communication of, 39
  statements of, 94
  written vs. oral, 37
Politics, 209–213
"Poor me" game, 258
Porter, Lyman, 234
Position power, 186, 203
Position titles, 82
Positions, 23
Positive reinforcement, 287, 312
Positive reinforcement theory, 235, 238; *see also*
    Operant conditioning
Posttest-only control group, 330
Power
  kinds of, 208
  needs for, 233
  relations, 207–208
  sources of, 206–207
  struggles, 29
Power and Innocence, 208
Power-coercive strategies, 283
Preceptorships, 144–145
Prescription, 23
Pretest sensitization, 329
Pretest-posttest control group, 329–330

Priestly model, 8
Primary nursing, 149–150
Principles of Scientific Method, The, 190
Priorities, setting, 1, 13–14
Privacy, right to, 305, 309
Probability theory, 9–10
Problem(s)
  identifying, 4–5
  symptoms vs. cause of, 4
Problem employees, 300–305
Problem-solving, 1, 4
  method, 297, 298, 306
  short-range, 86–87
  strategies for, 220
Procedural technician, 228
Procedure manuals, 40
Procedures, 40–43
  budgeting, 44
Process orientation, 101
Product orientation, 102
Productivity, 52; *see also* Time management
  decreased, 302
  lighting and, 194–195
Professional meetings, 5
Professional Standards Review Organizations
    (PSRO), 333–334
Profit center concept, 96
Program evaluation, 324–325
  invalidity sources in, 326–329
  model for, 325–326, *327*
  research designs for, 329–333
Program evaluation and review technique; *see*
    PERT
Progressive discipline policy, 303
Progressive relaxation, 354–355
Project management, 83–86
Project units, 83
Projection, 217
Promotions, 109
Psychological energy theory, 234
Psychology of Management, The, 191
Public Health Law 92–603, 333
Public Law 93–360, 317
Publics, 59
Punishment, 313
Purpose, statement of, 32–33

Q

Quality assurance, 86, 333–341
  committees, 334

Quality assurance—cont'd
  methods of data collection for, 338–339
  sampling for, 339–341
  scales for, 335–337
  validity and reliability of, 337–338
Quality circles, 237–238
Quality Patient Care Scale; *see* Qualpacs
Qualpacs, 336
Quasi-experimental designs, 330–333
Queen bee syndrome, 252–253
Questioning attitude, 5
Questionnaires, for quality assurance, 339
Queuing theory, 14–15

R

Random sampling, 328, 340
Ranking, 292–293
"Rapo" game, 257
Rating scales, 289–292
Rationalization, 216
Reaction formation, 216
Reasoning, inductive and deductive, 5
Reassurance, 304, 305
Recognition-seeker, 228
Record system, computerized, 16
Recorder, 228
Recruitment, 132–134
  of minorities and women, 141
  tool for, 144
Recurrent institutional cycle design, 333
Reference, letters of, 135
Referent power, 206
Referral services, 357
Registered nurses, 147
Regression, 217
Regression-discontinuity analysis design, 333
Rehabilitation Act (1973), 139
Reinforcement, 312
Reinforcers, 313
Relaxation techniques, 353–357
Reliability, 338
Reorganization; *see* Organizational change
Reports, 94, 341
Repression, 217
Responsibilities, 79–80, 194
  ambiguity of, 100–101
  without authority, 84–85
  delegation of, 99
  in job descriptions, 115
  of low management, 93

Restraining forces, 286
Resume service, 307
Resumes, 134–135
Retirement plans, 133
Rewards, 206
  extrinsic, 236
Rights, 8
  to privacy, 305, 309
Rituals, 256, 258
Role ambiguities, 215–216, 224
Role conflict, 24, 182, 224, 230, 240
Role contract, 226
Role enactment, 24
Role expectations, 24
Role learning, 24
Role messages, 224–225
Role models; *see* Mentorship
Role negotiations, 224–226
Role overload, 216, 224, 230
Role shock, 24
Role socialization, 24
Role stress, 24
Role structure, 23
Role theory, 23
Role-playing techniques, 196
Roles, definition of, 79
Rotating shifts, 153–155
Rothlesberger, Fritz, 194
Round-robin session, 221
Rule ethics, 8
Rules, 208
  consistent enforcement of, 309

S

Safety needs, 232
Sampling error, 341
Sampling plan, 60
Sampling technique, 339–341
Scheduling
  alternative systems of, 159
  Baylor plan, 158–159
  block or cyclical, 151–156
  centralized, 152–153
  decentralized, 153
  permanent shifts, 15
  rotating, 153–155
  shifts, 156–159
  variable, 156
Scientific management, 189–192
Screening procedure, 134–139

"See what you made me do" game, 257
Selective perception, 23, 246
Self-actualization, 196, 200, 232, 234, 238, 239
Self-appraisal, 137
Self-confessor, 229
Self-determination, 236
Self-disclosure, 262
Self-enhancing behavior, 349
Self-esteem, 231, 238–239, 258
  enhancing of, 347, 349, 357
  of nurses, 146
Self-evaluation, 295
Self-fulfilling prophecy, 23
Self-help groups, 357
Self-hypnosis, 355–356
Senate, 211–212
Separate-sample pretest-posttest control group, 332
Service loading, 14–15
Service staff, 104
Shaping, 312
Shelters for Women, 306
Shift overlap, reduction of, 51
Shifts
  permanent, 155
  rotating, 151, 153–155
Shop Management, 190
Sick leave, 39, 158
  policies, 302–303
Simulation, 10, 11
Single Parents, 306
Situation, total, 194
Situational leadership theories, 184–185
Skinner, B.F., 235, 238
Slater Scale, 335–336
Slater Stewart, Doris, scale constructed by, 335
Sleep, 353
Sniping, 250–251
Social Security Act, 333
Social services, 306
Socialization change, 284
Sociometry, 195–196
Solomon four group, 330
Solution(s), 6
Sorting, 350
Span of management, 92–94, 108
Span-of-control principle, 80–81
Spearman-Brown formula, 338
Special interest pleader, 228
Specialization, 80–81
Speed-reading, 54–55

Staff; see also Personnel
  decentralized, 153
  development of, 133, 282
  efficiency of, 57–58
  full-time, 163
  functional, 104–105
  level of, 150–151
  organization of, 151
  part-time, 163–165
  pool, 51
  purpose of, 132
  schedules, 151–159
Staff authority, 103–105, 209
Staffing, 1–2
  assignment systems, 146–151
  formulas, 161–163
  to meet fluctuating needs, 163–165
  studies, 160–163
Staff-line conflict, 105
Staff-line relationships, 103–106
Standard setter, 228
Statistical regression, 328
Statistical techniques, 60, 341
Status symbols, 247, 286
Stereotype, 23
Stratified sampling, 340
Stress, 283; see also Tension
  avoidance and regulation of, 348
  control of, 347–358
  monitoring of, 358
  response, 346
  sources of, 345–346
  symptoms of, 346–347
Stress management, 345–358; see Stress, control of
Stressors, 345–346
Strikes, 317, 320
Strokes, 256
"Stupid" game, 258
Subordinates
  delegation of responsibilities to, 100–101
  lack of confidence in, 100
  number of, 92, 93
  recognition of, 98, 99
Substance abusers, 300–301
Suggestions, soliciting, 18
Summarizing, 299
Superagreeable people, 251–252
Supervisor
  demands on, 94
  job satisfaction and, 240
Support groups, 357–358

Support services, 306
Systematic sampling, 340
Systems analysis, 282
Systems design, 88–89

T

Taft-Hartley Act, 316, 317
Tall organizational structure, 94–95
Tardiness, 306
  penalties for, 310
Task forces, 86–87
Task manager, 202
Task structure, 203
Tax Equity Fiscal Responsibility Act (1982), 51
Taylor, Frederick W.
  monistic theory of, 231
  scientific management theory of, 189-190, 193
Taylor, Paul, 205
Team building, 87, 106
Team conferences, 148
Team development, 221–224, 226
Team management, 202–203, 297
Team nursing, 146, 147–149, 151
Technocratic change, 284
Telephone, use of, 55–56
Tell-and-listen method, 296–297, 298
Tell-and-sell method, 297
Temporary help, 164
Tension, 235–236; *see also* Stress
Termination, 109, 303, 305–306
  acceptance of, 307
  as discipline, 310, 311
Theory X, 198–199, 236–238
Theory Y management, 198–200, 234, 236–238
Theory Z, 237–238
Thought stopping, 350–351
Time
  blocking, 348
  controls, 86
  estimates, 14, 57
  as factor in organization, 102
  series, 331
  standards, 160, 161
  studies, 205
Time management, 348–349
  managerial, 52–57
  organization, 57–58
Time-and-motion studies, 113
Title VI, 139
Title VII, 139

Training
  in art of interviewing, 136
  costs of, 134
  by objectives, 204
  problems of, 93
Trait theory, 183–184
Transactional analysis, 253–258
Trashing syndrome, 253
Trust, 220, 248
Tucker, Susan Martin, 336
Turnover, 134, 159, 239
Two-factor-motivation-hygiene theory, 197–198,
    199, 205, 233–234
Type A personality, 346
Type B personality, 346

U

Underdelegation, 100
Unemployment information, 307
Unfair labor practices, 317, 318
Unfavorable appraisals, 299
Union contracts, 38
Union Members' Bill of Rights, 317
Union security clause, 320
Unionization, 318–324
Unions, 308
  contract administration of, 321–323
  contract negotiations with, 320–321
  decertification of, 323–324
  organizing of; *see* Unionization
  recognition phase of, 318–320
  unfair labor practices by, 317–318
  why employees join, 316
Unresponsive people, 251
Unstructure problem rule, 20
"Uproar" game, 257
Urwick, Lyndall, 193, 205
Utilitarianism, 8

V

Valence, 234
Validity, 337–338
  measures of, 326–329
Value-laden words, 289
Values, 7, 22
Values' clarification, 347–348
Vertical organizational growth, 107
Vicarious feelings, 350

Vietnam Era Veterans Readjustment Assistance Act (1974), 139
Visualization, 356–357
Voluntary service groups, 357
Volunteers, responsibilities of, 51
Vroom, Victor, 234–235
Vroom and Yetton normative model, 19–22

W

Wagner Act; *see* National Labor Relations Act (NLRA)
Wants, 7, 8
Weber, Max, 192–193
Withdrawal, 217
Withdrawn employees, 301–302

Women
  goals for, 141
  job discrimination against, 140–141
"Wooden leg" game, 258
Workaholism, 347
Worker motions, 190
Written reprimand, 306, 310

Y

"You" messages, 349

Z

Zaibatsu, 237
Zero-base budgeting, 48